Liver Diseases: Clinical Management

Liver Diseases:
Clinical Management

Editor: Tucker Banks

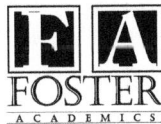

FA FOSTER
A C A D E M I C S

www.fosteracademics.com

www.fosteracademics.com

FA
FOSTER
ACADEMICS

Cataloging-in-Publication Data

Liver diseases : clinical management / edited by Tucker Banks.
   p. cm.
Includes bibliographical references and index.
ISBN 978-1-63242-683-3
1. Liver--Diseases. 2. Liver--Diseases--Prevention. 3. Liver--Diseases--Treatment.
I. Banks, Tucker.
RC845 .L58 2019
616.362--dc23

Foster Academics,
118-35 Queens Blvd., Suite 400,
Forest Hills, NY 11375, USA

ISBN 978-1-63242-683-3 (Hardback)

Contents

Permissions

List of Contributors

Index

Preface

The main aim of this book is to educate learners and enhance their research focus by presenting diverse topics covering this vast field. This is an advanced book which compiles significant studies by distinguished experts in the area of analysis. This book addresses successive solutions to the challenges arising in the area of application, along with it; the book provides scope for future developments.

Liver disease, also termed as hepatic disease, is a condition of the liver characterized by weight loss and jaundice, among many others. Some of the common liver diseases are hepatitis, fascioliasis, alcoholic liver disease, cirrhosis, fatty liver disease, liver cancer, etc. Genetic diseases such as hemochromatosis, Wilson's disease, Gilbert's syndrome, etc. can lead to liver damage. Various liver function tests that test for serum albumin, serum globulin, aspartate transaminase, etc. are used for the detection of liver diseases. Imaging techniques of ultrasound, magnetic resonance imaging and transient elastography are used for the examination of liver tissue and bile ducts. Hepatitis infections are treated using anti-viral medications. Other medications such as steroid-based drugs, ursodeoxycholic acid, etc. target specific symptoms and conditions of the liver and strive to slow down the progression of the disease. This book contains some path-breaking studies in liver diseases. The aim of this book is to present researches that have advanced the frontiers in the clinical management of liver diseases. It is a complete source of knowledge on the present status of this important field.

It was a great honour to edit this book, though there were challenges, as it involved a lot of communication and networking between me and the editorial team. However, the end result was this all-inclusive book covering diverse themes in the field.

Finally, it is important to acknowledge the efforts of the contributors for their excellent chapters, through which a wide variety of issues have been addressed. I would also like to thank my colleagues for their valuable feedback during the making of this book.

Editor

Liver Gene Therapy: Employing Surgery and Radiology for Translational Research

Luis Sendra, María José Herrero, Luis Martí-Bonmatí,
Eva M. Montalvá, Rafael López-Andújar,
Matteo Frasson, Eduardo García-Granero and
Salvador F. Aliño Pellicer

Abstract

Gene therapy is a therapeutic strategy that aims to employ nucleic acids as drugs for the transient or permanent treatment of inherited or acquired pathologies. Based on the type of vector employed for the gene transfer, gene therapy can be classified as viral gene therapy and nonviral gene therapy. Nonviral gene therapy is less efficient but safer than viral gene therapy. Hydrodynamic naked DNA transfer has shown great translational potential, achieving therapeutic levels of a human protein in the murine model. The translational process of the procedure has already been performed. Different radiologic and surgical approaches permitted pressurizing the liver in vivo by excluding its vascularization partially or totally. These approaches mediated a tissue rate of human alpha-1-antitrypsin protein translation (100–1000 copies per cell) close to those obtained with the mouse gold standard model in a safe mode that could be translated to human settings.

Keywords: gene therapy, liver, hydrodynamic, radiologic, catheterization, transplantation, surgery

1. Introduction

Gene therapy is a therapeutic strategy that uses nucleic acids, in any of their forms, as a drug for the transient or permanent treatment of inherited or acquired pathologies [1]. From a regulatory point of view, these drugs are considered in the European Regulation 1394/2007 and the Directive 2001/83/CE of the European Parliament. These, basically, establish the following:

"A gene therapy drug is a biologic drug with the following features:

a. it includes an active principle that contains a recombinant nucleic acid, or it is constituted by this, and it is employed or administered in human beings, aiming to regulate, repair, substitute, add or remove a gene sequence;

b. its therapeutic, prophylactic or diagnostic effect depends directly on the nucleic acid sequence or its expression product."

Gene therapy consists of the transfer of a gene with clinical interest to the target tissue or organ of a patient. This transfer can be mediated by a vector or vehicle or employing naked DNA. Gene therapy aims that the gene reaches the target cells with sufficient molecular bioavailability for the host cell's decoding machinery to decode the gene sequence and produce the protein encoded by it [2].

The correct production of the protein encoded by the transferred gene would permit:

a. adding a new function to the target cell

b. recovering a lost or diminished function

c. inhibiting or modulating an exacerbated function

d. editing the genome to correct the production of a defective protein

1.1. Gene therapy strategies

There are different alternatives to perform the gene transfer. Depending on the resource employed for the delivery procedure, gene therapy can be classified as viral and nonviral.

1.1.1. Viral gene therapy

Viral gene therapy employs a viral vector to carry the DNA of interest to the nucleus of the target cell [3]. This viral vector consists of the sequence of a virus, integrative or not, without the pathogenic sequences (related with its replicative ability), which are substituted by the therapeutic gene of interest. This strategy takes advantage of the viral ability to access the cells and employ their decoding machinery to translate its own genome. Viral gene therapy offers the following advantages:

a. It mediates a more efficient transfer of the gene;

b. Its administration could be systemic since the virus structure protects the gene from the circulating nucleases;

c. It permits developing permanent (employing viral vectors with the ability to integrate within the host cell genome) or transient (employing non-integrative viruses such as adenoviruses) therapies;

d. It is possible to select the target cell since some viruses present tropism.

However, they also present disadvantages to be considered:

a. Some viruses can induce intense immune responses, limiting the repeated doses (especially relevant in adenoviral vectors);

b. The exact place of the host genome where viruses integrate their genome is still unknown, hence being possible to alter the normal cell functions (insertional mutagenesis, tumor transformation);

c. Although not probable, it is possible that the viral particle without pathogenic features could recover them by genetic recombination, resulting in a potential risk for its clinical use.

1.1.2. Nonviral gene therapy

Nonviral gene therapy consists of the delivery of DNA mediated by the use of a nonviral vector [4–6] or the delivery of naked DNA [7], by physical procedures. With the aim of protecting the delivered DNA from its degradation exerted by circulating nucleases, different types of nonviral vectors have been designed. These vectors can facilitate the DNA (negative net charge) access into the cell through its plasmatic membrane, also negatively charged. Among the different models of nonviral vectors, we can find:

a. Liposomes—formed by the inclusion of DNA molecules within the lipid's concentric layers. They have the ability to protect the gene and facilitate its cell internalization by endocytosis and/or fusion with the cell membrane in order to release the DNA inside the cell [6, 8].

b. Polyplexes [6, 9]—they employ biodegradable polymers that protect the DNA from the degradation mediated by DNAses. The use of cationic lipids or polymers permits the formation of complexes with the DNA (lipoplexes and polyplexes, respectively) that facilitates its cell internalization.

Dewadvantages of nonviral vectors, they have limited utility because of their difficult formulation for clinical application. Their efficiency in 'in vitro' experiments is much higher than the efficiency observed in 'in vivo.' Furthermore, they have sometimes induced the immune response in patients.

Since viral gene therapy has offered good transfer efficiency but with the potential risk of immune reaction, or even that the recovery of virus infectivity and gene therapy mediated by nonviral vectors does not offer real advantages, physical procedures for efficient and safe naked DNA transfer have been developed. The most important alternatives of these strategies are:

a. Electroporation consists of augmenting the cell membranes' permeability by employing electric pulses [6, 10, 11]. It increases the transfer efficiency but is more targeted to muscular tissue;

b. Sonoporation consists of the application of ultrasound on a biological tissue, mediating the formation of bubbles that create a stir able to destabilize transiently the cell membrane and facilitating the access of gene [6, 12];

c. Magnetofection based on the application of a magnetic field after the transfer of a gene linked to metallic particles in order to lead the product inside the tissue. This strategy has not demonstrated important improvement [13, 14];

d. Jet injection consists of the high-speed injection of particles. It is employed specifically in muscle tissue [15–17];

e. Hydrodynamic gene transfer is mediated by changes in cell permeability induced by the intravascular injection of DNA saline solution (hydrofection). This has proved to be one of the most promising methods for naked DNA transfer and presents a great potential of clinical application in several different organs [18, 19].

1.2. Gene therapy in clinics

Since the approval of the first gene therapy clinical trial performed in patients in 1989, the number of these clinical trials, with little fluctuations, has increased constantly [20] achieving approximately 2600 in total (updated in November 2017) with a maximum rate of 169 clinical trials approved in 2015 (**Figure 1**).

The increasing use of gene therapy was possible, thanks to the development of gene constructs by employing different genes depending on the therapeutic application. Among the

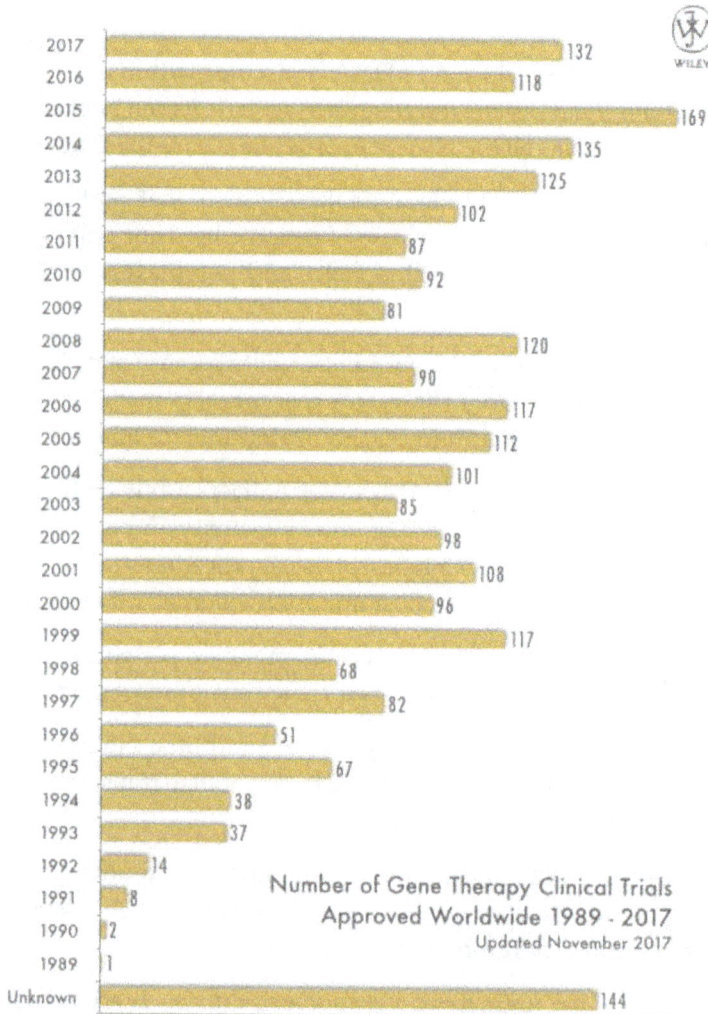

Number of Gene Therapy Clinical Trials
Approved Worldwide 1989 - 2017
Updated November 2017

The Journal of Gene Medicine, © 2017 John Wiley and Sons Ltd   www.wiley.co.uk/genmed/clinical

Figure 1. Gene therapy clinical trials approved in the world. In this figure, the number of gene therapy clinical trials approved in the world each year since 1989 until August 2016 is shown. Source: www.wiley.co.uk/genmed/clinical [21].

most employed, those modulating the immune response (by activation or repression) stand out from the others. In clinical trials, the most employed strategy for gene transfer has been viral gene transfer (around 70%). Adenoviruses (A) due to their capacity to carry large genes and express them transiently and retroviruses (R) because of their ability to integrate the gene within the host genome permitting its long-term stable expression (suitable for inherited deficiencies) are the most employed. The most employed strategies of nonviral gene therapy in clinical trials have been the lipofection and naked DNA (N), since they are the safest (**Figure 2**).

However, when clinical trials employing naked DNA for monogenic inherited diseases are searched, only six trials are found and when considering genes encoding cytokines, only one is found. Despite the different strategies to vectorize the gene and the types of treatment employed, only 0.1% of all clinical trials employing gene therapy reached phase IV (**Table 1**).

Among all the gene therapy procedures, the one that achieved the most positive benefit-risk balance has been the naked DNA hydrodynamic transfer. Given the potential interest

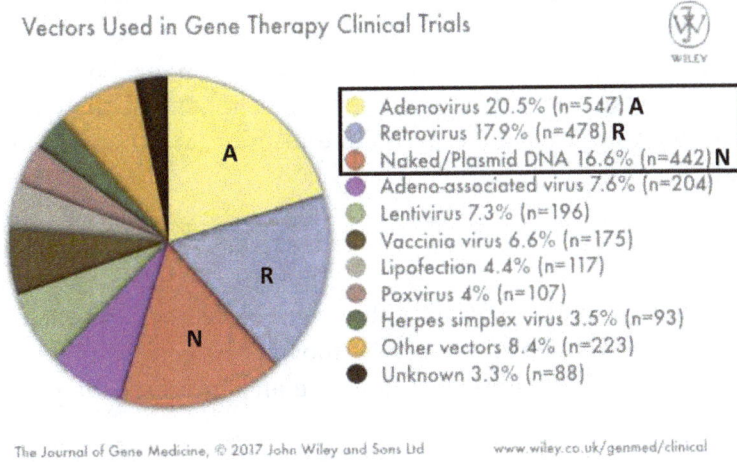

Vectors Used in Gene Therapy Clinical Trials

Adenovirus 20.5% (n=547) **A**
Retrovirus 17.9% (n=478) **R**
Naked/Plasmid DNA 16.6% (n=442) **N**
Adeno-associated virus 7.6% (n=204)
Lentivirus 7.3% (n=196)
Vaccinia virus 6.6% (n=175)
Lipofection 4.4% (n=117)
Poxvirus 4% (n=107)
Herpes simplex virus 3.5% (n=93)
Other vectors 8.4% (n=223)
Unknown 3.3% (n=88)

The Journal of Gene Medicine, © 2017 John Wiley and Sons Ltd   www.wiley.co.uk/genmed/clinical

Figure 2. Vectors used in gene therapy clinical trials. Source: www.wiley.co.uk/genmed/clinical [21].

Phase	Number of clinical trials	Ratio (%)
I	1409	57.2
I/II	500	20.3
II	429	17.4
II/III	24	1
III	91	3.8
IV	3	0.1
Single subject	5	0.2

Source: www.wiley.co.uk/genmed/clinical [21].

Table 1. Phases of gene therapy clinical trials.

of hydrodynamic gene therapy and the wide range of application in clinics (especially in the liver), the translational process of the technique has been performed from the successful murine model to human liver segments. The swine model permitted adapting the procedure for 'in vivo' liver transfer. Different radiologic and surgical approaches performed to improve the liver hydrodynamic gene transfer 'in vivo' will be discussed in this chapter.

2. Hydrodynamic naked DNA transfer

2.1. Hydrodynamic methodology

The possibility of expressing heterologous genes with high efficacy after the delivery of naked DNA was firstly described during the mid-1990s [22, 23]. In 1999, Zhang et al. [24] and Liu et al. [25] introduced the hydrodynamic gene transfer procedure. This procedure consisted of the rapid injection of a large volume (2 ml in 5–7 s) of saline solution bearing the gene of interest through the tail vein in the mouse (20 g average weight). The possibility of transferring naked DNA efficiently aroused a great interest among researchers and clinicians since the hydrodynamic procedure permitted expressing high levels of a heterologous protein, employing a safer strategy than viral gene therapy. Different research groups focused their efforts on improving the technique in order to be safer, more efficient and reproducible [26].

2.2. Hydrofection mechanism

In **Figure 3**, the sinusoid circulation within the liver before and after the retrograde injection of a saline solution containing a plasmid is shown. The gene solution injected through the tail vein reaches the liver in a retrograde sense and increases the pressure inside the

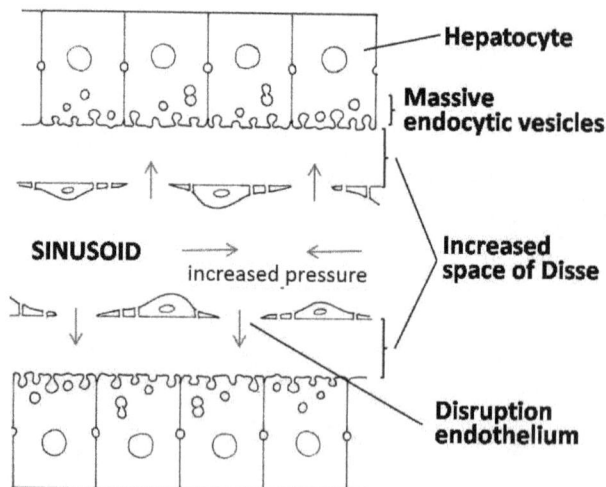

Figure 3. Schematic representation of sinusoid organization after retrograde hydrodynamic injection of gene solution. When a plasmid is injected, vessel pressure increases inducing the separation of endothelium cells. This permits the access of gene constructs to the Disse space and to the hepatocytes through the massive formation of endocytic vesicles.

vessel. This distends the wall mediating the transient separation of endothelium cells. When this occurs, the DNA leaves the blood vessels through the sinusoid pores and inter-cellular spaces and reaches the Disse space. From this space, the DNA can access the hepa-tocyte, the massive formation of endocytic vesicles playing a relevant role in this process. This DNA must reach the nucleus of the hepatocyte in order that the gene information delivered can be decoded. When this process takes place efficiently, the DNA is transcribed to RNA and this is translated to the protein, which is released into the bloodstream (in case of plasma proteins).

Employing this procedure, therapeutic plasma levels of alpha-1-protein were achieved for periods of more than 6 months in mice [27]. Nowadays, many gene therapy experiments for different pathology treatments are being studied in mice [28–30]. The possibility of achieving therapeutic levels of heterologous proteins after hydrodynamic human gene transfer in the murine model boosted the efforts of research teams to develop and adapt the procedures in larger animals aiming to translate it into the clinics, since the hemodynamic changes induced by the hydrodynamic injection are not compatible with its use in humans.

The perfusion conditions that permitted achieving the most efficient results in the mouse implied doubling the animal's volemia in a very short period of time. The procedure had to be necessarily adapted since larger animals would have not tolerated these conditions. The modifications of the procedure were directed to diminish the systemic hydrodynamic pressure. This was performed by transferring the gene of interest to the one and only target organ by image-guided catheterization procedures. Studies were performed in rats [31, 32] and rabbit [33] models but the results obtained were much less efficient than that observed in the mouse. The most recent efforts focused on developing models of liver hydrodynamic perfusion in pigs given their anatomical proximity with humans [34].

In the swine model, different strategies for minimally invasive gene transfer were designed through liver catheterization [35, 36]. Although these procedures proved to be safe, the effi-ciency achieved was not remarkable. Some authors highlighted the possibility that higher intravascular pressure within the liver could be required. For this reason, different strate-gies to block the venous backflow and employ more demanding perfusion conditions were studied. Levels of heterologous protein expression were not close to therapeutics in any case. After several works carried out by research groups around the world, no significant result was achieved [37–41]. However, given the huge interest of this procedure and its potential to be translated to human clinical practice, different groups evaluated minutely the molecular pro-cess of the transferred gene decoding in order to confirm or refuse this possibility. Evaluating at molecular level the detailed delivery, transcription and translation of a transferred gene permitted in identifying the step of the decoding process that limited the final efficacy in liver tissue and comparing this process in different animal models: mouse, pig and human. The best conditions of efficacy and safety for liver hydrodynamic gene therapy have been established in pig liver 'in vivo' (by catheterization and surgery) and the human liver 'ex vivo' (by catheterization in watertight segments). The methodology permitted comparing quantita-tively the efficiency of different procedures of liver gene transfer. These procedures included partial and complete vascular exclusion aiming to pressurize the organ without affecting the systemic hemodynamics.

2.3. Therapeutic targets

Since gene transfer can deliver a gene functionally complete to the cell, it presents a great interest for the treatment of inherited metabolic diseases [42–45], such as alpha-1-antitrypsin deficiency [46], in which the entire functional gene could be implemented.

Gene therapy can also play an important role in the treatment of different acquired pathologies. Its application for modulating the immune response in different proinflammatory conditions, such as liver transplantation, has been studied by implementing genes of anti-inflammatory cytokines such as interleukin-10 (IL10).

3. Clinical translation of hydrodynamic gene therapy

Several animal models have been employed for hydrodynamic gene transfer. The murine model has resulted in the gold standard of the procedure since therapeutic levels of the protein encoded by the transferred gene have been achieved. The translational process has been carried out in rat, rabbit, guinea pig, dog, pig and human liver segments.

The murine model consisted of the rapid injection of gene saline solution in a volume equivalent to the animal volemia. This large volume facilitates the backflow of the gene solution and provokes its retrograde access to the liver. The high heart rate of the mouse permits the injection of such volumes with animal survival. Similar conditions to those employed for mice were carried out in rats, although different adaptations for diminishing the solution volume have been proposed in order to follow up the translation process. Other researchers [47] studied different strategies to improve hydrodynamic gene delivery efficiency by targeting the right lateral liver lobe of the rat through the portal vein branch. The need for outflow blockade in the target area was reported since the portal vein pressure was too low to avoid backflow. In another attempt to improve the efficiency of the procedure, the left liver lobe was targeted in the rat and outflow occlusion was performed to compare its effect to free-flow control rats [32]. It was reported that outflow blockade is demanding to obtain efficient outcomes in transgene expression. Larger animals do not have the ability to increase the heart rate as mice and doubling their volemia would be incompatible with survival. Thus, the hydrodynamic injection had to be adapted to reduce the final volume and minimize the systemic hemodynamic impact. These adaptations focused on targeting an organ. Regarding this fact, Eastman et al. injected a gene to a single liver lobe employing a balloon catheter and to the entire organ of the rabbit with hepatic venous occlusion and achieved protein plasma expression in 2 days. The safety of the liver hydrodynamic gene transfer was also assessed in dogs to prove its feasible application in large animals [48]. They performed four successive injections in four different main liver lobes. Authors observed no significant harmful effects and rapid recovery of animals. However, the results obtained were poor.

The following step for the clinical translation of the procedure was to test its potential use in anatomically more similar animals to human beings such as pigs and primates. The techniques for gene delivery that were employed should be applicable in human settings.

Yoshino et al. [35] and Aliño et al. [36] described the first attempts performed in a pig. The total volume employed was reduced by targeting an area of liver and compared different catheter-mediated delivery strategies. These strategies included portal vein occlusion, left hepatic artery occlusion, portal vein and left hepatic artery occlusion and both vessels' occlusion with blood flow washout. Yoshino et al. injected the gene solution through the cava vein. The occlusion of portal vein and hepatic artery with the washout mediated the most efficient outcomes achieving disperse protein plasma levels for several weeks. For the first time, the procedure showed interesting results in pigs, for those proteins with low expression. In another work, hydrodynamic retrovenous gene transfer was performed in large and small areas of pigs' liver. Alino et al. [36] reported the presence of gene and protein expression in tissues, mainly within the perivenous area. Targeting smaller areas but employing same volumes of gene solution, higher plasma protein levels were achieved, much lower than those considered therapeutic. Fabre et al. [37] targeted the entire liver and isolated the hepatic segment of the inferior vena cava by clamping it suprahepatically and infrahepatically. Gene solution was transferred by a hydrodynamic procedure through two parallel syringes and, although the efficiency of gene delivery was much lower than the one observed in the mouse and rat, they confirmed the clinical feasibility of the technique as determined by systemic blood pressures, ECG, heart rate and so on.

Pressure reached within the liver during the hydrodynamic injection played an important role. For this reason, Fabre et al. [40] focused their work on pressurizing individual lobes of the liver by isolating them. Aiming to achieve localized high pressure without affecting the systemic circulation, they proposed individualizing the lobe by employing catheters with balloon and ligation. Although most of the authors suggested blood pressure to be the most important feature of hydrodynamic injection for efficient gene transfer, others have pointed other characteristics such as impulse [49] and flow rate [50, 51] to be relevant. However, nearly all authors agree to the need for isolating target areas or the entire liver to improve the procedure efficiency. This vascular isolation could be partial or complete.

Firstly, the implication of the complete vascular exclusion in the final efficacy of the procedure should be evaluated in order to determine its relevance. As previously reported, the complete liver vascularization of the pig can be occluded up to 20 min without neither hepatic injury nor systemic damage [52]. Considering this fact, Carreño et al. [50] described in pigs a surgical procedure to completely exclude liver vascularization 'in vivo' and perform hydrodynamic gene delivery, targeting the entire organ. A complete midline laparotomy was carried out, exposing all the abdominal organs. The clamping sequence was as follows: first, the hepatic artery, then the portal vein and finally the infrahepatic vena cava, to interrupt hepatic inflow. The suprahepatic vena cava was clamped last, to secure total hepatic vascular exclusion. Depending on the flow sense of gene transfer, three different models were designed. In model 1 the portal vein was clamped, and only a longitudinal incision was made on the anterior surface of the cava vein to insert the perfusion cannula. In model 2, the process was the same as in model 1 but with the clamping of the vena cava and perfusion through the portal vein. In model 3 (**Figure 4**), the gene solution was injected simultaneously through suprahepatic IVC (Inferior Vena Cava) and the portal vein employing two catheters connected by a Y connector and a high-volume pump. After solution perfusion, the liver was kept under total vascular exclusion for no more than 5 min to allow gene penetration into the cell nuclei.

In all three models, when suprahepatic IVC was occluded and liver vasculature was completely excluded, the systemic pressure decreased rapidly. However, 1 min after revascularization this parameter was entirely normalized and animals recovered in few hours. Due to the invasiveness of the surgical procedure that included a laparotomy, same authors designed a technique for liver venous sealing mediated by image-guided catheterization [53]. Two strategies with different degrees of liver vasculature closure were proposed:

a. Inject the gene solution through a balloon catheter placed in a single lobe (**Figure 5**), and only target this part of the liver and

b. Place simultaneously three catheters with balloons within suprahepatic IVC, infrahepatic IVC and portal vein around the liver entry (**Figure 6**) in order to close its vasculature. The gene solution is injected through the catheter placed in suprahepatic IVC and the entire organ is targeted.

These three procedures, surgery and open and closed catheterization, proved to be safe. After gene transfer and animal awakening, their recovery was very fast and presented normal

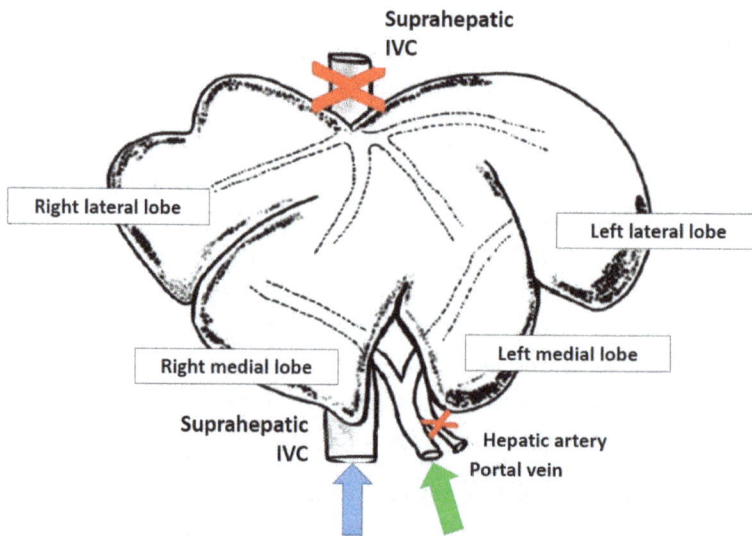

Figure 4. Schematic figure of liver simultaneous cava and porta perfusion with laparotomy surgery. Suprahepatic inferior vena cava and hepatic artery are ligated, and gene solution is transferred simultaneously by portal vein and infrahepatic inferior vena cava. Modified from [50].

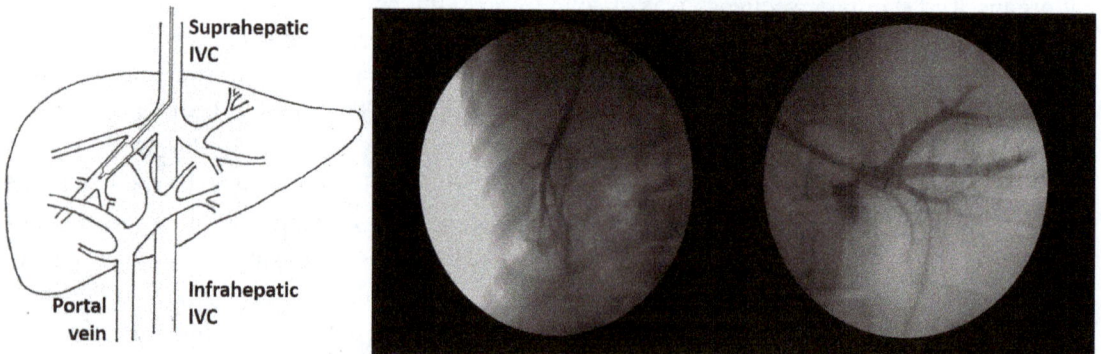

Figure 5. Single-lobe catheterization by balloon-catheter. Left panel is a schematic figure of catheter localization. Only the hepatic vein employed for gene transfer is occluded. Suprahepatic IVC, infrahepatic IVC and portal vein are not closed. Right panel shows two radiologic images of catheter position and iodinated contrast solution injection in single lobes defining the area affected by solution injected. The gene solution is injected through hepatic veins. The backflow is blocked by inflated balloon [54].

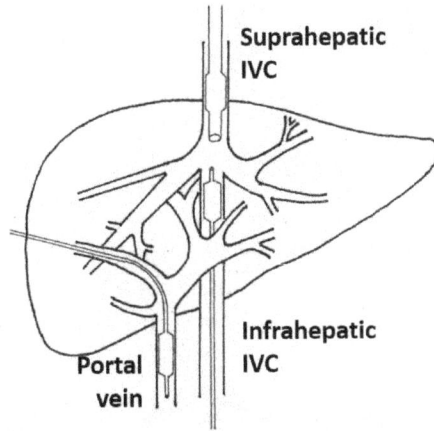

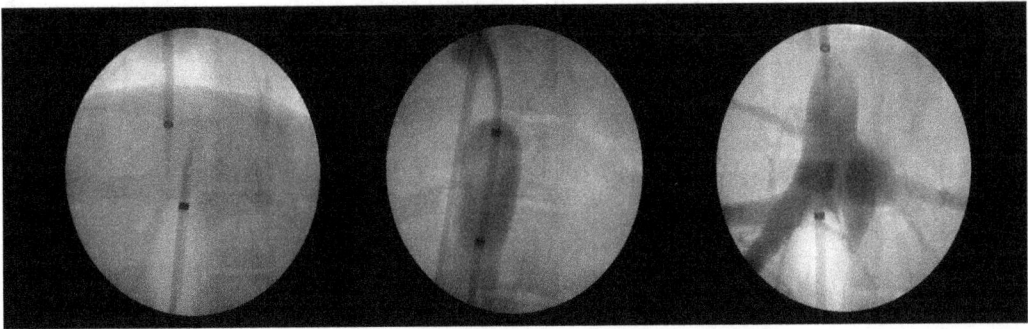

Figure 6. Whole liver catheterization by balloon-catheters. Upper panel is a schematic figure of catheters localization. Infrahepatic IVC and portal vein are closed at liver access by inflated balloon-catheters. Lower left panel shows a radiologic image of supra and infrahepatic IVC catheters position. Lower mid panel shows an inflated balloon-catheter placed at portal vein blocking its exit. Lower right panel shows the iodinated contrast solution injection in the entire liver. The gene solution is injected through suprahepatic inferior vena cava [54].

behavior few hours after the intervention. Furthermore, all of them mediated tissue expression of the protein encoded by the transferred gene. The rate of protein translation showed a direct relation with the degree of vasculature closure: surgery-mediated complete liver vasculature exclusion > catheterization-mediated venous vasculature closure > catheterization-mediated single lobe without organ vasculature closure.

Transferring the human alpha-1-antitrypsin, the single liver lobe strategy mediated 20,000 copies of protein per cell in the liver. Targeting the entire organ with the closure of suprahepatic IVC, infrahepatic IVC and portal vein mediated a higher translation rate up to 100,000 copies per cell. The complete exclusion of liver vasculature by occlusion IVC, portal vein and hepatic artery with surgical procedure increased this rate up to 400,000 copies per cell in the liver tissue. The highest rate of tissue translation achieved was only 10-fold lower than the one obtained with the successful gold standard procedure performed in the mouse. This suggests that the hydrodynamic procedure of liver gene therapy with vascular exclusion mediated by radiological and surgical strategies mediated efficient delivery with efficacious translation protein.

Once proved the efficiency of these procedures in pig and the confirmation of their safety for gene transfer 'in vivo,' the following step of translational process consisted of demonstrating the efficacy in human liver tissue.

In this sense, human liver segments proceeding from surgical resection in patients with cancer were injected with different genes to evaluate the potential transferability of this technique. Given their precedence, the vasculature of these human liver segments is entirely excluded so they are watertight and hence, pressurized. The gene is retrogradely transfected through a catheter placed in a hepatic vein (**Figure 7**) and the segment remains watertight for 5 min.

The first studies of gene transfer with human liver segments [56] used the eGFP tracer gene in order to easily determine its expression efficacy, and it was demonstrated that the gene could be efficiently delivered and the protein was produced within the liver tissue as observed by fluorescence microscopy. After confirming the feasibility of the technique in this type of tissue, genes with clinical interest were employed to define the translational potential to clinical real settings.

Sendra Gisbert et al. [55] transferred a plasmid bearing the human interleukin-10 gene (IL10). Interleukin-10 is an immunomodulatory protein with pleotropic effects with potential interest for the treatment of inflammatory diseases or for inducing tolerance in organ transplantation. The rate of tissue protein translation achieved was around 1000 copies per cell, this meaning the potential therapeutic production of protein (IC50 of IL10 for TNFa = 124 pg) if compared with other results of the same group.

Our group also transferred in similar human liver segments a plasmid with the same human alpha-1-antitrypsin employed in mice and pigs but modified. In order to permit differing endogenous and exogenous genes and proteins, a sequence of nucleotides encoding the flag peptide was added. Preliminary experiments demonstrate that the procedure is efficient and the use of a human gene in human tissue favors the production of protein. First, results prove a rate of tissue protein translation of 10^4–10^5 copies of hAAT-flag protein per cell, this accounting for up to 22% of all the hAAT proteins present in the liver tissue in 1 week.

The efficacy of gene transfer can be measured by different techniques and authors have studied many variables to present their results and evaluate how efficient a procedure is. This requires the use of a more detailed analysis that allows to identify the effectiveness of each of the stages of the process of delivery of the gene, its decoding of protein and its subsequent location.

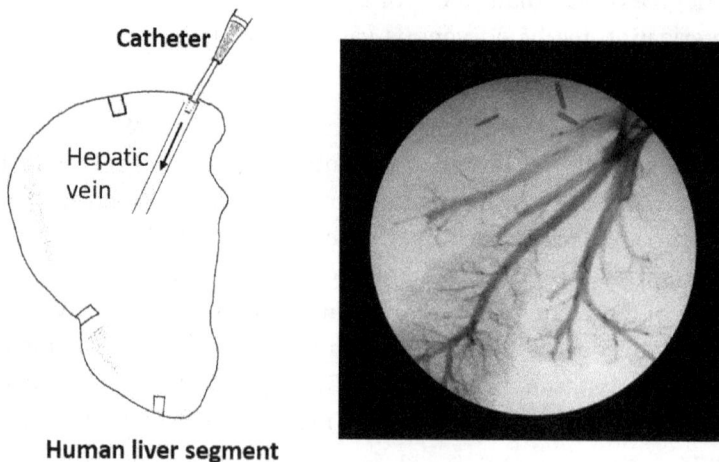

Figure 7. Catheterization of human liver segment. Left panel shows a schematic figure of a human liver segment with a catheter placed in a hepatic vein. Right panel is a radiographic image of a human liver segment injected with iodinated contrast solution through hepatic vein. Modified from [55].

The molecular quantitative evaluation of decoding is demanding for a correct interpretation of the process. Quantitative determination of the molecular process provides real data of delivery, transcription and translation indexes. It would be important that researches achieved an agreement in data quantitation and expression to be able to objectively compare results and define the better conditions for gene transfer. The units should be expressed in molecular units (as number of copies or moles) or other units of mass. It is also very important that the data are referred to a common circumstance, such as a standard or 'normalized cell.' The normalized cell is defined as 'typical mammalian hepatocyte with defined content of total DNA' (genome weight of each specific animal, for instance, human: 6.6 pg), RNA (20 pg) and protein (500 pg).

This strategy offers an objective analysis that permits expressing the data as the copy number of each molecular specie, considering the standard content of DNA, RNA and protein in a normalized cell. This offers a more comprehensive interpretation of the entire process and permits comparing the results among different works and research groups.

To sum up, the hydrodynamic procedure is an efficient strategy for gene delivery demonstrated by the levels of tissue protein that is observed. The more the vasculature is occluded, the better is the final protein expression. The surgical procedure permits, excluding liver, entire vasculature and mediates the higher expression rate. However, non-invasive image-guided catheterization permits good levels of protein production without the need of a laparotomy incision.

Acknowledgements

This work has been partially supported by Spanish Ministerio de Economía y Competitividad (SAF2011-27002, SAF2007-64492) and Grifols ALTA Award 2017.

Author details

Luis Sendra[1,2], María José Herrero[1,2]*, Luis Martí-Bonmatí[3], Eva M. Montalvá[4], Rafael López-Andújar[4], Matteo Frasson[5], Eduardo García-Granero[5] and Salvador F. Aliño Pellicer[1,2]

*Address all correspondence to: maria.jose.herrero@uv.es

1 Pharmacology Department, Medicine Faculty, University of Valencia, Valencia, Spain

2 Pharmacogenetics Unit, La Fe Health Research Institute, La Fe University and Polytechnic Hospital, Valencia, Spain

3 Radiology Department and Biomedical Imaging Research Group (GIBI230), La Fe University and Polytechnic Hospital, Valencia, Spain

4 Unit of Hepato-Biliary-Pancreatic Surgery and Transplantation, La Fe University and Polytechnic Hospital, Valencia, Spain

5 Department of General Surgery, Digestive Surgery Unit, La Fe University and Polytechnic Hospital, Valencia, Spain

References

[1] Kresina TF, Branch AD. In: Kresina TF, editor. An Introduction to Molecular Medicine and Gene Therapy. New York: Wiley-Liss; 2001. pp. 1-24

[2] Kay MA. State-of-the-art gene-based therapies: The road ahead. Nature Reviews Genetics. 2011;**12**:316-328

[3] Kay MA, Glorioso JC, Naldini L. Viral vectors for gene therapy: The art of turning infectious agents into vehicles of therapeutics. Nature Medicine. 2001;**7**(1):33-40

[4] Yin H, Kanasty RL, Eltoukhy AA, Vegas AJ, Robert Dorkin J, Anderson DG. Non-viral vectors for gene-based therapy. Nature Reviews Genetics. 2014;**15**(8):541-555

[5] Ibraheem D, Elaissari A, Fessi H. Gene therapy and DNA delivery systems. International Journal of Pharmaceutics. 2014;**459**(1-2):70-83

[6] Kamimura K, Suda T, Zhang G, Liu D. Advances in gene delivery systems. Pharmaceutical Medicine. 2011;**25**(5):293-306

[7] Taniyama Y, Azuma J, Kunugiza Y, Iekushi K, Rakugi H, Morishita R. Therapeutic option of plasmid-DNA based gene transfer. Current Topics in Medicinal Chemistry. 2012;**12**(15):1630-1637

[8] Dasí F, Benet M, Crespo J, Crespo A, Aliño SF. Asialofetuin liposome-mediated human alpha 1-antitrypsin gene transfer in vivo results in stable long-term gene expression. Journal of Molecular Medicine. 2001;**79**:205-212

[9] Chemin I, Moradpour D, Wieland S, et al. Liver-directed gene transfer: A linear polyethlenimine derivative mediates highly efficient DNA delivery to primary hepatocytes in vitro and in vivo. Journal of Viral Hepatitis. 1998;**5**:369-375

[10] Li S. Electroporation gene therapy. Preface. Methods in Molecular Biology. 2008;**423**:v-vii

[11] Heller LC, Heller R. Electroporation gene therapy preclinical and clinical trials for melanoma. Current Gene Therapy. 2010;**10**(4):312-317

[12] Tomizawa M, Shinozaki F, Motoyoshi Y, Sugiyama T, Yamamoto S, Sueishi M. Sonoporation: Gene transfer using ultrasound. World Journal of Methodology. 2013;**3**(4):39-44

[13] Plank C, Anton M, Rudolph C, et al. Enhancing and targeting nucleic acid delivery by magnetic force. Expert Opinion on Biological Therapy. 2003;**3**:745-758

[14] Dobson J. Gene therapy progress and prospects: magnetic nanoparticle-based gene delivery. Gene Therapy. 2006;**13**:283-287

[15] Yang NS, Burkholder J, Roberts B, et al. In vivo and in vitro gene transfer to mammalian somatic cells by particle bombardment. Proceedings of the National Academy of Sciences of the United States of America. 1990;**87**:9568-9572

[16] Wang S, Joshi S, Lu S. Delivery of DNA to skin by particle bombardment. Methods in Molecular Biology. 2004;**245**:185-196

[17] Langer B, Renner M, Scherer J, Schüle S, Cichutek K. Safety assessment of biolistic DNA vaccination. Methods in Molecular Biology. 2013;**940**:371-388

[18] Herweijer H, Wolff JA. Gene therapy progress and prospects: Hydrodynamic gene delivery. Gene Therapy. 2007;**14**(2):99-107

[19] Suda T, Liu D. Hydrodynamic gene delivery: Its principles and applications. Molecular Therapy. 2007;**15**:2063-2069

[20] Ginn SL, Alexander IE, Edelstein ML, Abedi MR, Wixon J. Gene therapy clinical trials worldwide to 2012—An update. The Journal of Gene Medicine. 2013;**15**:65-77

[21] Wiley database on Gene Therapy Trials Worldwide. http://www.wiley.com/legacy/ wileychi/genmed/clinical/

[22] Budker V, Zhang G, Knechtle S, Wolff JA. Naked DNA delivered intraportally expresses efficiently in hepatocytes. Gene Therapy. 1996;**3**:593-598

[23] Zhang G, Vargo D, Budker V, Armstrong N, Knechtle S, Wolff JA. Expression of naked plasmid DNA injected into the afferent and efferent vessels of rodent and dog livers. Human Gene Therapy. 1997;**8**:1763-1772

[24] Zhang G, Budker V, Wolff JA. High levels of foreign gene expression in hepatocytes after tail vein injections of naked plasmid DNA. Human Gene Therapy. 1999;**10**:1735-1737

[25] Liu F, Song Y, Liu D. Hydrodynamics-based transfection in animals by systemic administration of plasmid DNA. Gene Therapy. 1999;**6**:1258-1266

[26] Wang Z, Qiu SJ, Ye SL, Tang ZY, Xiao X. Combined IL-12 and GM-CSF gene therapy for murine hepatocellular carcinoma. Cancer Gene Therapy. 2001;**8**(10):751-758

[27] Aliño SF, Crespo A, Dasí F. Long-term therapeutic levels of human alpha-1 antitrypsin in plasma after hydrodynamic injection of nonviral DNA. Gene Therapy. 2003;**10**(19):1672-1679

[28] Gao M, Ma Y, Cui R, Liu D. Hydrodynamic delivery of FGF21 gene alleviates obesity and fatty liver in mice fed a high-fat diet. Journal of Controlled Release. 2014;**185**:1-11

[29] Ma Y, Liu D. Hydrodynamic delivery of adiponectin and adiponectin receptor 2 gene blocks high-fat diet-induced obesity and insulin resistance. Gene Therapy. 2013;**20**(8):846-852

[30] Sun H, Liu D. Hydrodynamic delivery of interleukin 15 gene promotes resistance to high fat diet-induced obesity, fatty liver and improves glucose homeostasis. Gene Therapy. 2015;**22**(4):341-347

[31] Zhang X, Collins L, Sawyer GJ, Dong X, Qiu Y, Fabre JW. In vivo gene delivery via portal vein and bile duct to individual lobes of the rat liver using a polylysine-based nonviral DNA vector in combination with chloroquine. Human Gene Therapy. 2001;**12**:2179-2190

[32] Sawyer GJ, Zhang X, Fabre JW. Technical requirements for effective regional hydrodynamic gene delivery to the left lateral lobe of the rat liver. Gene Therapy. 2010;**17**:560-564

[33] Eastman SJ, Baskin KM, Hodges BL, et al. Development of catheter-based procedures for transducing the isolated rabbit liver with plasmid DNA. Human Gene Therapy. 2002;**13**:2065-2077

[34] Herrero MJ, Dasi F, Noguera I, et al. Mouse and pig nonviral liver gene therapy: Success and trials. Gene Therapy and Molecular Biology. 2005;**9**:169-180

[35] Yoshino H, Hashizume K, Kobayashi E. Naked plasmid DNA transfer to the porcine liver using rapid injection with large volume. Gene Therapy. 2006;**13**:1696-1702

[36] Aliño SF, Herrero MJ, Noguera I, Dasí F, Sánchez M. Pig liver gene therapy by noninvasive interventionist catheterism. Gene Therapy. 2007;**14**:334-343

[37] Fabre JW, Grehan A, Whiterhorne M, et al. Hydrodynamic gene delivery to the pig liver via an isolated segment of the inferior vena cava. Gene Therapy. 2008;**15**:452-462

[38] Sawyer GJ, Rela M, Davenport M, Whitehorne M, Zhang X, Fabre JW. Hydrodynamic gene delivery to the liver: Theoretical and practical issues for clinical application. Current Gene Therapy. 2009;**9**(2):128-135

[39] Kamimura K, Suda T, Xu W, Zhang G, Liu D. Image-guided, lobe-specific hydrodynamic gene delivery to swine liver. Molecular Therapy. 2009;**17**(3):491-499

[40] Fabre JW, Whitehorne M, Grehan A, et al. Critical, physiological and surgical considerations for hydrodynamic pressurization of individual segments of the pig liver. Human Gene Therapy. 2011;**22**(7):879-887

[41] Kamimura K, Suda T, Zhang G, Aoyagi Y, Liu D. Parameters affecting image-guided, hydrodynamic gene delivery to swine liver. Molecular Therapy Nucleic Acids. 2013;**2**:e128

[42] Strauss M. Liver-directed gene therapy: Prospects and problems. Gene Therapy. 1994;**1**:156-164

[43] Davern TJ. Molecular therapeutics of liver disease. Liver Disease. 2001;**52**:381-414

[44] O'Connor TP, Crystal RG. Genetic medicines: Treatment strategies for hereditary disorders. Nature Reviews Genetics. 2006;**4**:261-282

[45] Brunetti-Pierri N, Ng P. Progress & prospects: Gene therapy for genetic diseases with helper-dependent adenoviral vectors. Gene Therapy. 2008;**15**:553-560

[46] Janciauskiene SM, Bals R, Koczulla R, Vogelmeier C, Köhnlein T, Welte T. The discovery of α1-antitrypsin and its role in health and disease. Respiratory Medicine. 2011;**105**(8):1129-1139

[47] Zhang X, Dong X, Sawyer GJ, Collins L, Fabre JW, Zhang X, et al. Regional hydrodynamic gene delivery to the rat liver with physiological volumes of DNA solution. The Journal of Gene Medicine. 2004;**6**(6):693-703

[48] Kamimura K, Kanefuji T, Yokoo T, Abe H, Suda T, Kobayashi Y, Zhang G, Aoyagi Y, Liu D. Safety assessment of liver-targeted hydrodynamic gene delivery in dogs. PLoS One. 2014;**9**(9):e107203

[49] Hackett PB Jr, Aronovich EL, Hunter D, Urness M, Bell JB, Kass SJ, Cooper LJ, McIvor S. Efficacy and safety of sleeping beauty transposon-mediated gene transfer in preclinical animal studies. Current Gene Therapy. 2011;**11**(5):341-349

[50] Carreño O, Sendra L, Montalvá E, Miguel A, Orbis F, Herrero MJ, Noguera I, Aliño SF, Lopez-Andujar R. A surgical model for isolating the pig liver in vivo for gene therapy. European Surgical Research. 2013;**51**(1-2):47-57

[51] Sendra L, Carreño O, Miguel A, Montalvá E, Herrero MJ, Orbis F, Noguera I, Barettino D, López-Andújar R, Aliño SF. Low RNA translation activity limits the efficacy of hydrodynamic gene transfer to pig liver in vivo. The Journal of Gene Medicine. 2014;**16**(7-8):179-192

[52] de Groot GH, Reuvers CB, Schalm SW, Boks AL, Terpstra OT, Jeekel H, ten Kate FW, Bruinvels J. A reproducible model of acute hepatic failure by transient ischemia in the pig. The Journal of Surgical Research. 1987;**42**(1):92-100

[53] Sendra L, Miguel A, Pérez-Enguix D, Herrero MJ, Montalvá E, García-Gimeno MA, Noguera I, Díaz A, Pérez J, Sanz P, López-Andújar R, Martí-Bonmatí L, Aliño SF. Studying closed hydrodynamic models of "In Vivo" DNA perfusion in pig liver for gene therapy translation to humans. PLoS One. 2016;**11**(10):e0163898

[54] Sendra L, Pérez D, Miguel A, Herrero MJ, Noguera I, Díaz A, Barettino D, Martí-Bonmatí L, Aliño SF, Human AAT. Gene transfer to pig liver improved by using a perfusion isolated organ endovascular procedure. European Radiology. 2016;**26**(1):95-102

[55] Sendra Gisbert L, Miguel A, Sabater L, Herrero MJ, Sabater L, Montalvá EM, Frasson M, Abargues R, López-Andújar R, García-Granero E, Aliño SF. Efficacy of hydrodynamic interleukin 10 gene transfer in human liver segments with interest in transplantation. Liver Transplantation. 2017;**23**(1):50-62

[56] Herrero MJ, Sabater L, Guenechea G, Sendra L, Montilla AI, Abargues R, Navarro V, Aliño SF. DNA delivery to 'ex vivo' human liver segments. Gene Therapy. 2012;**19**(5):504-512

2

Stereotactic Body Radiation Therapy for Hepatocellular Carcinoma in Cirrhotic Liver

Hiroshi Doi, Hiroya Shiomi and Ryoong-Jin Oh

Abstract

In the medically inoperable patients with solitary hepatocellular carcinoma (HCC), local therapies, such as radiofrequency ablation and transarterial chemoembolization, are used as alternatives. However, several factors, including anatomic and vascular variants, make procedures more challenging. Radiotherapy has historically been used as a palliative option for unresectable HCC. However, recent advances in modern radiotherapy, such as stereotactic body radiation therapy (SBRT), have dramatically increased the use of radiotherapy as a curative modality, particularly in cases ineligible for local ablation therapy or surgical resection. SBRT is a modern approach for delivering ablative high doses of irradiation in small volumes. SBRT in liver tumors, including HCC, provided local control with potential survival benefits in patients with inoperable status. However, the following issues remain to be addressed: the difference between primary and metastatic liver cancers; SBRT-related toxicity and prevention; pathological features of liver cancers; and potential SBRT strategies, including radiobiology-based SBRT and SBRT combined with immunotherapy. We summarized the effectiveness of SBRT and patient tolerance of the therapy. In addition, we present the current status and future perspective of SBRT as a treatment option for HCC.

Keywords: radiotherapy, stereotactic body radiation therapy, stereotactic ablative radiotherapy, hepatocellular carcinoma, cirrhosis, liver

1. Introduction

Hepatocellular carcinoma (HCC) is the most common primary malignancy of the liver [1]. Liver cancers have the seventh highest age-adjusted incidence rate in the world, with 0.8 million cases diagnosed a year [2]. The development of cirrhosis is associated with a high risk for developing HCC with most common risk factors including alcohol, viral hepatitis such as hepatitis C virus (HCV), and nonalcoholic fatty liver disease (NAFLD). Due to the wide prevalence of HCC, it carries a significant economic burden on society at large, especially in the East Asian countries that have hepatitis B virus (HBV). Surveillance programs halve also been implemented to screen for HCC in high-risk individuals, which is more cost-effective than the treatment of HCC. Hepatotropic viruses such as HBV and HCV have a strong association with the development of HCC; thus, the worldwide distribution of HCC mirrors the distributions of such viral infections [3]. Around 80–90% of HCC cases occur in the setting of underlying cirrhosis [4]. In addition, there is an incremental effect of the presence of more than one risk factor responsible for HCC as the presence of HBV/HCV coinfections increases the risk of HCC by two- to sixfolds. Similarly, alcohol abuse further increases this risk [5, 6]. Subsequently, we describe the role of radiotherapy in the treatment of HCC, including conventional to modern techniques, possible beneficial cases of radiotherapy, and future direction of liver stereotactic body radiation therapy (SBRT).

2. General approaches and conventional radiotherapy in the treatment of HCC

The initial approach in the management of HCC is to determine if either surgical resection or liver transplantation is feasible and best survival. The Barcelona Clinic Liver Cancer staging system is the most accepted staging system in clinical settings [7]. Orthotopic liver transplantation is the most efficient option for the treatment of HCC even though the insufficient number of donors makes challenging [8]. Therefore, local therapy is anticipated to be not only a bridging therapy but also a radical therapy in the treatment of HCC. Surgical resection is the standard local therapy for HCC [7]. Since the majority of HCC cases develop in cirrhotic patients, surgical interventions can become challenging, and the treatment has been directed toward liver transplantation. Other local therapies, such as radiofrequency ablation (RFA) and transarterial chemoembolization (TACE), are used as alternatives in patients with HCC [7–9]. However, radical treatment for liver tumors can be challenging due to poor liver function, tumor location, and anatomical barriers. Furthermore, the preservation of residual liver function is required, as liver tumors have a high recurrence potential [9].

Radiotherapy is a local treatment modality and has also been used for palliative care in liver tumors. Conventional radiotherapy has been used approximately 50 Gy in a conventional fractionated schedule which could lead to a response rate as approximately 50–70% [10–14]. High doses of radiation, which are required for HCC, would sometimes exceed the levels tolerated by the background liver [15, 16]. However, modern radiotherapies, including stereotactic body radiation therapy (SBRT), also known as stereotactic ablative radiation therapy (SABR), have recently attracted increasing attention as a therapeutic modality for various malignancies including HCC and have dramatically increased the use of radiation therapy as a curative modality [17–40]. However, certain issues regarding the current use of SBRT in HCC need to be addressed (e.g., ideal prescription doses, prevention of adverse events, and possible microscopic extension). In this chapter, we document the clinical utility and the present status of SBRT in the management of HCC, including clinical messages and pitfalls in liver cirrhosis and the probable treatment-related toxicities and their prevention, and summarize recent significant updates on biology-based SBRT strategies.

3. SBRT for HCC

The use of SBRT for extracranial tumors was developed by Blomgren et al. [17]. The major feature that distinguishes SBRT from conventional radiation treatment is the delivery of large doses of radiation in a few fractions, which results in a high biologically effective dose (BED). In addition, Zheng et al. have reported that a shortened delivery time could significantly increase the cell killing using *in vitro* experimentation [41]. The use of a high precision technique is critical to deliver a high dose of radiation to the target and keep rapid fall-off doses away from the target, thereby achieving a maximum treatment efficacy with minimal toxicity to normal tissues [42]. SBRT is now widely accepted as a treatment option for lung and liver tumors characterized by their small size and limited numbers [43].

Current advantages and challenges of SBRT in the liver are presented in **Table 1**. The clinical outcomes of SBRT for HCC in the previous reports are shown in **Table 2**. SBRT has been reported to provide 1-, 2-, and 3-year local control rates of 56–100, 53–95, and 51–92%, and 1-, 2-, and 3-year survival rates of 32–100, 55–100, and 21–82% for HCC, respectively [19–38]. **Figure 1** indicates the local control and overall survival after SBRT, $BED_{10} \geq 75$ Gy in ≤ 10 fractions (e.g., 40 Gy/4 fr), for HCC at our institute. **Figure 2** indicates a typical course of SBRT for HCC in cirrhotic liver. Recent reports indicated that SBRT was as effective as TACE and RFA, although there are only a small number of randomized trials examining the use of SBRT in HCC [34, 35, 38]. However, additional prospective studies involving large sample sizes are required to consolidate the evidences on SBRT with aim to standardize liver SBRT.

Advantages

- High possibility of local control

- Minimally invasive treatment modality, no requirements for anesthesia or injections

- High possibility to overcome anatomical limitations, including poorly defined tumors on ultrasound and tumors which are difficult to puncture

- No concern regarding the location close to major vessels, including the portal vein, inferior vein cava, and bile duct

- Possible to treat complicated forms of tumors, particularly using IMRT

- Short treatment term (usually within 2 weeks), possibility of benefit to the patient's quality of life and reduced medical cost

- Possibility to enhance the immune reaction to tumors

Current issues

- Poor outcomes and high possibility of toxicity with large tumors

- Challenges involved in the treatment of tumors close to critical organs, such as the gastrointestinal tract

- Effects of re-irradiation are unclear

- Inaccuracy due to respiration and the presence of ascites

Abbreviations: SBRT = stereotactic body radiation therapy; IMRT = intensity modulated radiation therapy.

Table 1. Features of SBRT for liver tumors.

Author [Ref]	Year	Prospective/ retrospective	Patient number	Total dose/ fraction (median, range)	BED$_{10}$ (Gy)	Median follow-up (range) (months)	Local control	Overall survival	Adverse events Acute response	Late response
Kwon et al. [19]	2010	Retrospective	42	33 (30-39) Gy/3 fr (70–85% isodose line covered the PTV)	69.2 (60-89.7)	29	1-year 72% 3-year 68%	1-year 92.9% 3-year 58.6%	35.7% G1 Constitutional symptoms; 31.0% G1-2 Elevated liver enzyme; 19.0% G1-2 Leukopenia; 2.4% G1 hyperbilirubinemia and ALP	2.4% (1 patient) G4 Liver failure
Seo et al. [20]	2010	Retrospective	38	33-57 Gy/3 fr or 40-44 Gy/4 fr (60.5% patients received 39-57 Gy/3 fr)	69.3-165.3 or 80-92.4 (89.7–165.3)	15	1-year 78.5% 2-year 66.4%	1-year 68.4% 2-year 61.4% 3-year 42.1%	(57.9% G1-2 acute toxicities); 10.5% G1-2 hyperbilirubinemia; 2.6% G1 albumin; 5.3% G1 AST/ALT; 2.6% G1 ALP; 44.7% G1–2 Nausea, vomiting; 7.9% G1 anorexia; 13.2% G1-2 abdominal pain; 2.6% G2 Paralytic ileus; 2.6% G2 radiation dermatitis	2.6% G3 soft tissue toxicity (the right upper quadrate of the abdomen)

Author [Ref]	Year	Prospective/ retrospective	Patient number	Total dose/ fraction (median, range)	BED$_{10}$ (Gy)	Median follow-up (range) (months)	Local control	Overall survival	Adverse events — Acute response	Adverse events — Late response
Andolino et al. [21]	2011	Prospective	60	Child-Pugh A (60%): 44 Gy/3 fr; Child-Pugh B (40%): 40 Gy/5 fr (80% isodose line, encompassing PTV)	Child-Pugh A: 108.5; Child-Pugh B: 85.5	27	3-year 90%	3-year 67%	n = 56 (93%) 23.2% G1-2 fatigue, nausea, and/or right upper quadrant discomfort	1.8% G2 chest wall toxicity; 16.1% G3 liver enzymes elevation and/or hyperbilirubinemia; 16.1% G3 thrombocytopenia; 3.6% PT-INR; 12.5% G3 albumin (17 patients of 21 patients with G3 hypoalbuminemia preexisting Grade 2 dysfunction); 1.8% G4 thrombocytopenia and hyperbilirubinemia; 20.0% Child-Pugh classification progression
Kang et al. [22]	2012	Prospective	47	57 (42-60) Gy/3 fr (70–80% isodose line covered at least 97% of the PTV)	165.3 (100.8–180.0)	17	2-year 94.6%	2-year 68.7%	4.3% G3 hyperbilirubinemia (pre-existing Grade 1 or 2 hyperbilirubinemia and/or thrombocytopenia); 10.6% G3 Thrombocytopenia; 4.3% G3 Ascites; 6.4% G3, 4.3% G4 Gastrointestinal ulcer (3 of 5 patients had pre-existing ulcer, 2 patients experienced Grade 4 gastric ulcer perforation at 7 months and 10 months after SBRT)	

Author [Ref]	Year	Prospective/ retrospective	Patient number	Total dose/ fraction (median, range)	BED_{10} (Gy)	Median follow-up (range) (months)	Local control	Overall survival	Adverse events Acute response	Late response
Huang et al. [23]	2012	Retrospective	36	37 (25-48) Gy/4-5 fr (70-83% isodose line, encompassing PTV)	NA(31.2-105.6)	14	1-year 87.6% 2-year 75.1%	2-year 64%	36.1% G1-2 fatigue 25.0% G1-2 anorexia 13.9% G1-2 nausea/vomiting 5.6% G1-2 abdominal pain 2.8% G2, 2.8% G3 gastric ulcer (Both of 2 patients had gastritis before SBRT) 2.8% G1 musculoskeletal	5.6% RILD (2 patients with Child-Pugh B)
Honda et al. [24]	2013	Retrospective	30	48 Gy/4 fr (86.7% of patients) or 60 Gy/8 fr (13.3% of patients) (isocenter prescription)	105.6 or 105.0	12.3	CR:96.3%	1-year 100% 2-year 100%	93.3% G1-2, 6.7% G3 leukocytopenia 96.7% G1-2, 3.3% G3 thrombocytopenia 100% G1-2 hemoglobin G1-2 hyperbilirubinemia G1 AST/ALT G1 ALP	3.3% Child-Pugh class progression

Author [Ref]	Year	Prospective/ retrospective	Patient number	Total dose/ fraction (median, range)	BED$_{10}$ (Gy)	Median follow-up (range) (months)	Local control	Overall survival	Adverse events Acute response	Late response
Bae et al. [25]	2013	Retrospective	35	45 (30-60) Gy/3-5 fr (56–83% isodose line of the maximum dose or D95 prescription of 91–100% prescription doses for PTV)	101 (58–180)	14	1-year 69% 3-year 51%	1-year 52% 3-year 21%	(23% of patients experienced grade ≥ 3 toxicity) 8.6% G3 AST (1 patient also had grade 3 hyperbilirubinemia, all patients had pre-existing grade 2 elevation of AST or hyperbilirubinemia and experienced progression of intrahepatic HCC) 2.9% G3 Hepatic failure (1 month after SBRT) 2.9% G3 colonic ulcer (1 month after SBRT)	2.9% G4 Myelitis (18 months after SBRT, spine Dmax = 31 Gy/4 fr) 2.9% G3 gastric ulcer perforation (7 months after SBRT) 2.9% G5 duodenal ulcer bleeding (5 months after SBRT) 2.9% G4 colonic ulcer (3 months after SBRT)

Author [Ref]	Year	Prospective/ retrospective	Patient number	Total dose/ fraction (median, range)	BED$_{10}$ (Gy)	Median follow-up (range) (months)	Local control	Overall survival	Adverse events Acute response	Late response
Bujold et al. [26]	2013	Prospective	102	36 (24-54) Gy/6 fr	57.6 (33.6–102.6)	31	1-year 87%	NA (median 17 months)	1.0% G3 fatigue; 10.9% AST/ALT; 3.0% G3, 2.0% G4 hyperbilirubinemia; 1.0% G3 creatinine; 2.0% G3 hemoglobin; 1.0% G3 leukocytes; 9.0% G3 platelets; 29% (3-month), 6% (12-month) Child-Pugh class progression; 46% (3-month), 17% (12-month) Child-Pugh score progression; 1.0% G3, 1.0% G4, 4.9% G5 Liver failure; 1.0% G5 cholangitis (HCC invaded the common bile duct); 1.0% G3, 1.0% G5 gastritis/gastrointestinal bleeding (G5 occurred 7.7 months after SBRT)	
Jang et al. [27]	2013	Retrospective	82 (95 HCC)	51 (33-60) Gy/3 fr (70–80% isodose line covered at least 97% of the PTV)	137.7 (69.3–180.0)	30	2-year 87% 5-year 82%	2-year 63% 3-year 39%	1.2% G3 hyperbilirubinemia (pre-existing G1) 2.4% G3 ascites; 7.3% non-classic RILD (worsening of CTP score by ≥2, ≤3 months after SBRT, 2 of 6 with disease progression); 1.2% G3 soft tissue toxicity (this patient had a large tumor near the skin); 6.1% G3–4 GI toxicity (gastroduodenal ulcer in 2 patients, clonic ulcer in 1 patient, and gastroduodenal perforation in 2 patients, gastroduodenal perforation in 2 patients)	

Author [Ref]	Year	Prospective/ retrospective	Patient number	Total dose/ fraction (median, range)	BED$_{10}$ (Gy)	Median follow-up (range) (months)	Local control	Overall survival	Adverse events	
									Acute response	Late response
Sanuki et al. [28]	2014	Retrospective	185	Child-Pugh A (74.1%): 40 Gy/5 fr; Child-Pugh B (25.9%): 35 Gy/5 fr (70–80% isodose line, encompassing PTV)	Child-Pugh A: 72.0; Child-Pugh B: 59.5	24	1-year 99% 2-year 93% 3-year 91%	1-year 95% 2-year 83% 3-year 70%	4.9% mild fatigue; 3.2% G3 laboratory abnormalities (prior to SBRT)	10.3% Child-Pugh score progression (by two points); 1.1% G5 liver failures (both 2 patients were classified as Child-Pugh B before SBRT 3, 6 months after SBRT)
Takeda et al. [29]	2014	Retrospective	63	Child-Pugh A (69.8%): 40 Gy/5 fr; Child-Pugh B (30.2%): 35 Gy/5 fr (70 or 80% isodose line, encompassing PTV)	Child-Pugh A: 72.0; Child-Pugh B: 59.5	31.1	1-year 100% 2-year 95% 3-year 92%	1-year 76% 2-year 87% 3-year 73%	*n = 63; 7.9% mild fatigue; 15.8% G3 subacute liver toxicity (6.3% before SBRT)	*n = 63; 20.6% G3 liver toxicity
Yamashita et al. [30]	2014	Retrospective	79	48 Gy/4 fr (40 Gy/4 fr-60 Gy/10 fr)	96 (75-106)	15.9	2-year 74.1%	2-year 52.9%	n = 130 (79 HCC, 51 liver metastases); 2.3% G2 gastrointestinal toxicity (gastric inflammation in 2 patients 1 month after SBRT, gastric ulcer in 1 patient; 27 months after SBRT); 3.1% G3 gastrointestinal toxicity (duodenal ulcer 17 months, intestinal tract bleeding 5, 6 months, transverse colon ulceration 5 months, respectively, after SBRT); 0.8% G4 gastro-duodenal artery rupture (5 months after SBRT); 0.8% chest wall pain (combined with TACE)	

Author [Ref]	Year	Prospective/ retrospective	Patient number	Total dose/ fraction (median, range)	BED_{10} (Gy)	Median follow-up (range) (months)	Local control	Overall survival	Adverse events Acute response	Late response
Culleton et al. [31]	2014	Prospective	29	34.4 (20.9–48.7) Gy/6 (5-15) fr (Mean dose to PTV) or 30.9 (197-46.8) Gy/6 (5-15) fr (D95 prescription for PTV)	54.1 (28.2–88.2) 46.8 (26.2–83.3) (Calculated presupposed with 6 fractions)	NA	6-month 69.7% 1-year 55.5%	1-year 32.3% (median 7.9 months)	48.3% G1-2 fatigue; 20.7% G1 nausea; 10.3% G1-2 vomiting; 10.3% G1-2 diarrhea; 10.3% G1 abdominal pain; 10.3% G1-2 abdominal distension; Child-Pugh score progression (24.1, 24.1, 10.3% by 1 point, 2 points, 3 points, respectively, at 1 month after SBRT); 17.2% G3 thrombocytopenia (3 months after SBRT); 6.9% G3, 3.4% G4 transaminase elevation (1 month after SBRT); 3.4% G4 AST (3 months after SBRT)	
Huertas et al. [32]	2015	Retrospective	77 (97 HCC)	45 Gy/3 fr (prescribed to the 80% isodose line, encompassing PTV)	112.5	12	1-year 99% 2-year 99%	1-year 81.8% 2-year 56.6%	1.3% G1, 1.3% G2 asthenia; 2.6% G1, 2.6% G2, 1.3% G3 ascites; 1.3% G1 rib pain; 1.3% G1 anorexia; 2.6% G1 nausea; 3.9% G1 epigastric pain; 1.3% Classic RILD; 3.9% Non-classic RILD; 1.3% G5 Hematemesis	1.3% G2 asthenia; 1.3% G1 radiation dermatitis; 2.6% G1 nausea; 2.6% G1, 3.9% G2, 3.9% G3 ascites; 1.3% G2 colic ulcer; 1.3% G3, 1.3% G4 gastric ulcer

Author [Ref]	Year	Prospective/ retrospective	Patient number	Total dose/ fraction (median, range)	BED$_{10}$ (Gy)	Median follow-up (range) (months)	Local control	Overall survival	Adverse events	
									Acute response	Late response
Takeda et al. [33]	2016	Prospective	90	Child-Pugh A: 40 Gy/5 fr Child-Pugh B: 35 Gy/5 fr (prescribed to the 60–80% isodose line, encompassing PTV, D95 prescription for PTV)	Child-Pugh A: 72.0 Child-Pugh B: 59.5	41.7	3-year 96.3%	3-year 66.7%	2.2% transaminase elevation 5.6% thrombocytopenia 8.9% Child-Pugh score progression (by two points)	
Wahl et al. [34]	2016	Retrospective	63	30 or 50 Gy/3 or 5 fr (D99.5 prescription for PTV, the 75 to 85% isodose line encompassing PTV	100 (NA)	13.0	1-year 97.4% 2-year 83.8%	1-year 74.1% 2-year 46.3%	1.6% G3 RILD 1.6% G3 gastrointestinal bleeding 1.6% G3 worsening ascites	8.3% G3 luminal gastrointestinal toxicity (at 2 years after SBRT) 3.3% G3 biliary toxicity (at 2 years after SBRT) *Child-Pugh score progression by average 1.2 points) (at 12 months after SBRT)
Su, et al. [35]	2017	Retrospective	82	42–48 Gy/3–5 fr (67 (57–80) % isodose line encompassing PTV)	NA (77.3–124.8) (Calculated presupposed with 42 Gy/5 fr–48 Gy/3 fr)	33.0	NA (one patient experienced local progression) (PFS; 1-year 81.4%, 3-year 50.2%, 5-year 40.7%	1-year 96.3% 3-year 81.8% 5-year 70.0%	4.9% G1, 3.7% G2, 1.2% G3 nausea 1.2% G1, 1.2% G2, 2.4% G3 weight loss 3.7%, G1, 1.2% G2 fatigue 3.7% G1 hyperbilirubinemia 3.7% G1 ALT 4.9% G1 anemia 6.1%, 3.7% Child-Pugh progression (1, 2 points, respectively)	

Author [Ref]	Year	Prospective/ retrospective	Patient number	Total dose/ fraction (median, range)	BED$_{10}$ (Gy)	Median follow-up (range) (months)	Local control	Overall survival	Adverse events	
									Acute response	**Late response**
Lo et al. [36]	2017	Retrospective	89	25–60 Gy/4-6 fr (40 Gy/5 fr (19 patients), 45 Gy/5 fr (18 patients), 50 Gy/5 fr (14 patients))	72 (40 Gy/5 fr), 85.5 (45 Gy/5 fr), 100 (50 Gy/5 fr)	NA	3-year 78.1%	1-year 45.9% 3-year 24.3%	24.7% G1, 4.5% G2 fatigue 13.5% G1, 2.2 G2 anorexia 13.5% G1, 12.4% G2, 1.1% G3 nausea/ vomiting 4.5% G1 abdominal distension 19.1 G1, 7.9% G2, 2.2% G3 abdominal pain 3.4% G2, 2.2% G3 gastritis/gastric ulcer 2.2% G1, 4.5% G2 duodenal ulcer 1.1% G1, 2.2% G2 diarrhea 1.1% G1, 2.2% G2 dermatitis 11.2% RILD (1.1% classic RILD, 9.0% non-classic RILD (including 2 patients developed fatal non-classic RILD), 1.1% fulfilled the criteria of both types)	
Uemoto, et al. [37]	2018	Retrospective	121 (146 HCCs)	45 (30–64) Gy/5 (4-20) fr	80 (48–106)	21	2-year 91.5%, 5-year 89.8%	2-year 73.7%, 5-year 57.0%	0.7≤G2, 0.7% G3 cholangiectasis 1.5% G1 pneumonitis 0.7% mucositis 0.7% G1 rib fracture 25.2% ascites 2.2 jaundice 1.5% pleural effusion (no hematological abnormality changed from the baselines)	

Abbreviations: NA = not applicable, HCC = hepatocellular carcinoma, SBRT = stereotactic body radiation therapy, NA = not applicable; BED = biologically effective dose, G = grade, PTV = planning target volume, AST = aspartate transaminase elevation, ALT = alanine transaminase elevation, ALP = alkaline phosphatase elevation, PT-INR = prothrombin time-international normalized ratio prolongation, RILD = radiation-induced liver disease, TACE = transcatheter arterial chemoembolization, PFS = progression-free survival.

Table 2. Summary of studies of hepatocellular carcinoma.

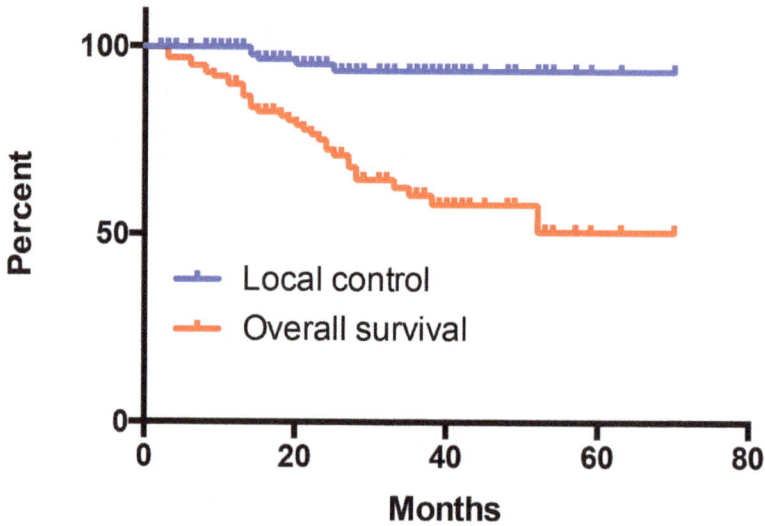

Figure 1. Local control and overall survival of HCC after SBRT. Local control (LC) and overall survival (OS) were described using the Kaplan Meier method in 100 patients with 116 HCCs underwent SBRT of BED_{10} ≥75 Gy in ≤10 fractions, between July 2007 and August 2016 at Miyakojima IGRT Clinic (Osaka, Japan, approval no. 9). The 1-, 2- and 3-year LC rate was 100.0, 95.4 and 93.5%, respectively. The 1-, 2- and 3-year OS rate was 83.7, 72.6 and 60.5%, respectively. Abbreviations: HCC, hepatocellular carcinoma; SBRT, stereotactic body radiation therapy.

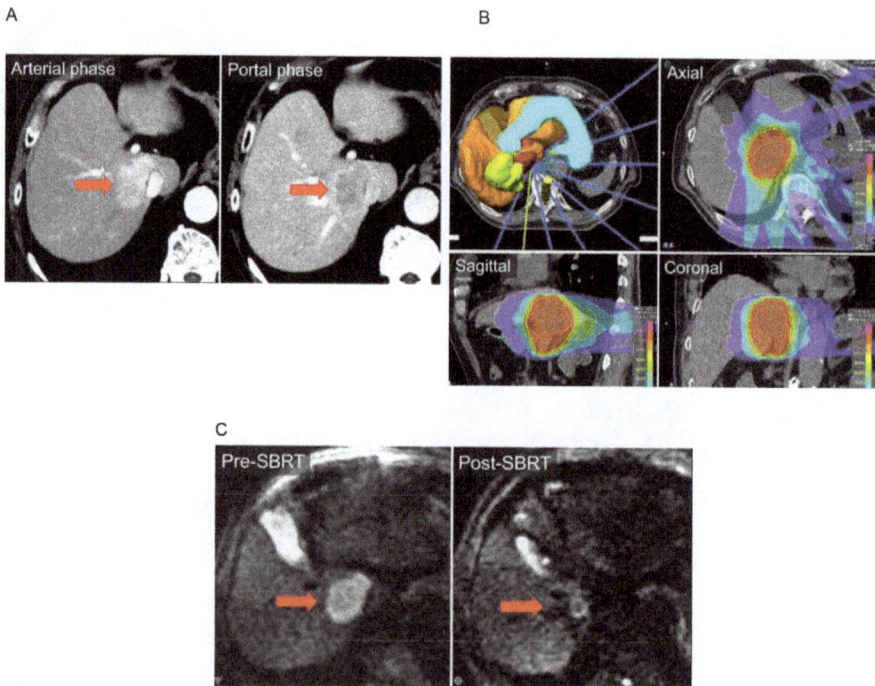

Figure 2. Typical course of SBRT for HCC in cirrhotic liver. An 86-year-old man developed HCC in S8. HCC with 50 mm in diameter existed (A, contrast-enhanced CT, arrowhead). SBRT of 40 Gy in four fractions (BED_{10} = 80.0 Gy) (B, treatment plan). The high intensity area that observed before SBRT in diffusion-weighted imaging of MRI (C, left) disappeared three months after SBRT (C, right). Abbreviations: HCC, hepatocellular carcinoma; CT, computed tomography; MRI, magnetic resonance imaging; SBRT, stereotactic body radiation therapy; BED, biologically effective dose.

4. Radiotherapy in the management of HCC with tumor thrombus in vessels

Portal vein tumor thrombosis (PVTT), the most common form of macrovascular invasion of HCC, could propagate further, obstruct the whole vein lumen, and lead to poor prognoses ranging from only 2 to 4 months after supportive care [44, 45]. One of the treatment modalities is surgical resection that could lead to median survival time of 8–64 months, 1-, 2-, and 3-year overall survival rates of 31–87, 0–76, and 0–71%, respectively [46]. In addition, there is a potential survival benefit by surgical resection [47]. However, tumor thrombectomy can be associated with high morbidity and mortality rates, up to 23.7% [48]. TACE might be contraindicated for HCC patients with PVTT because of the potential risk of hepatic ischemic damages due to TACE. In addition, PVTT is not an indication for RFA because of the potential cooling effect and challenging status of percutaneous intervention.

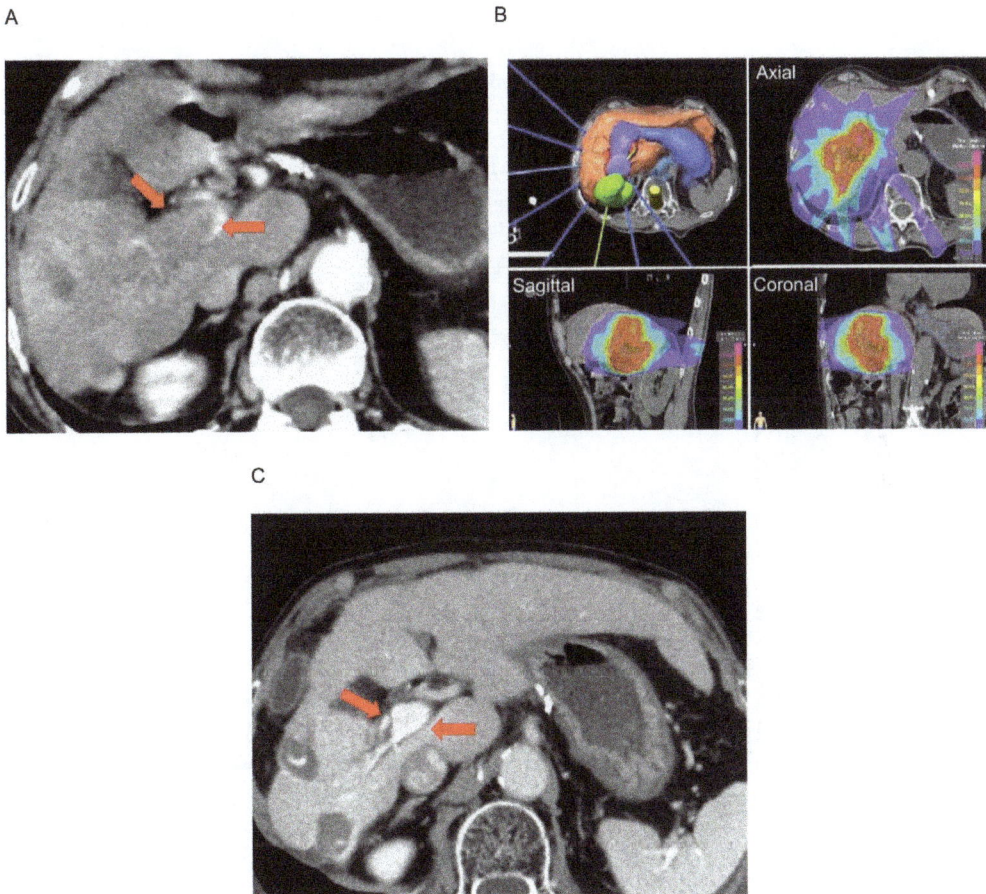

Figure 3. SBRT for PVTT. A 77-year-old man developed HCC due to hepatitis C with tumor thrombus in right portal vein (A, arrows, contrast-enhanced CT). The patient underwent SBRT of 60 Gy in 15 fractions (BED_{10} = 84.0 Gy) (B). The tumor thrombus disappeared after three months after SBRT. Contrast-enhanced CT indicates disobliteration of the right portal vein after SBRT (C, arrows). Abbreviations: SBRT, stereotactic body radiation therapy; PVTT, portal vein tumor thrombosis; HCC, hepatocellular carcinoma; CT, computed tomography; BED, biologically effective dose.

Although the efficacy of radiotherapy has been reported in patients with tumor thrombus using conventional schedule, the evidence of the survival benefit is insufficiently strong [39–41, 49–51]. In addition, Lin et al. have reported that radiotherapy can recanalize at a rate of 79% in 14 patients with PVTT [51]. However, there are only a few comparison studies among the techniques of radiotherapy [39, 51]. Matsuo et al. have reported, in a retrospective study, that the response rate of PVTT or inferior vena cava tumor thrombosis to radiotherapy was 67 and 46% in SBRT and 3D-CRT groups, respectively (P = 0.04) [39]. Moreover, SBRT has an advantage with regard to the shortened treatment term. Radiotherapy including SBRT may have the potential to be the standard technique of radiotherapy in the treatment of PVTT. **Figure 3** indicates a case of SBRT for HCC with PVTT.

Radiotherapy can overcome anatomical barriers such as major vessels and achieve a promising local control with minimal invasion. Therefore, a combined multimodal approach including radiotherapy would be needed in the treatment of the HCC with PVTT in order to maximize tumor control and to keep the normal liver damages due to treatment within a safe limit.

5. Prescription doses of SBRT for HCC

A dose-response relationship has been reported for conventional fractionated and stereotactic radiotherapy, although the best prescription dose of radiotherapy for HCC remains undecided [12, 27, 52].

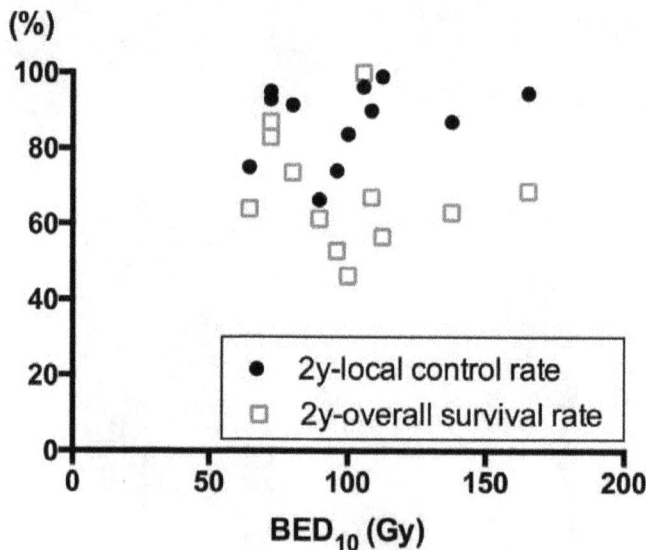

Figure 4. Dose-response relationship in SBRT for HCC. Previous reports that clearly indicates 2-year local control and overall survival were plotted in the scatter diagram [20–24, 27–30, 32, 34, 37]. X- and Y-axis indicates total doses radiotherapy in term of BED_{10} and the rates of 2-year local control and overall survival, respectively. No apparent dose-response relationship was observed in local control (r = 0.2828 and P = 0.3732) and overall survival (r = -0.1872 and P = 0.5602) at 2 years after SBRT. Abbreviations: SBRT, stereotactic body radiation therapy; HCC, hepatocellular carcinoma; BED, biologically effective dose.

Bae et al. reported 85% local control rates at 2 years after an SBRT of 50 Gy in 10 fractions, 75 Gy in terms of biologically effective dose (BED) using the linear-quadratic (LQ) model assuming an α/β = 10 Gy for tumors (BED_{10}) [53]. Lausch et al. have reported that the administration of a biologically equivalent total dose in 2-Gy fractions (EQD2) of 84 Gy (BED_{10} = 100.8 Gy) could achieve a 90% probability of a 6-month local control [54]. Jang et al. estimated that a 90% probability of a 2-year local control required 51.1 Gy in three fractions (BED_{10} = 138.1 Gy) [27]. Sanuki et al. and Takeda et al. reported a more than 90% 3-year local control rate with 40 Gy in five fractions (BED_{10} = 72 Gy) that was intended to enclose the planning target volume (PTV) by 80% isodose line of the maximum dose [28, 29]. **Figure 4** shows no dose–response relationship between a 2-year local control and overall survival rates and the total BED of SBRT with the range of prescription doses of ≥72 Gy. Notably, previous reports include various prescription definitions such as the prescription dose for the iso-center (isocentric prescription), a certain percent isodose line of the maximum dose (marginal prescription), and the dose to cover 95% of the PTV (D95 prescription). Based on these data, HCC has been treated with ≥80 Gy of BED_{10} and achieved a good local control at our institute as we hypothesized [37].

6. Adverse events of SBRT for HCC in cirrhotic liver, risk factors, and prevention

Manifestations of liver SBRT toxicity have fatigue, damage to the liver, gastrointestinal tract and biliary duct, cytopenia, dermatitis, and rib fractures (**Table 2**) [18–37]. Adverse events of radiotherapy depend on the treatment site, and the irradiated doses and volume and are categorized into either acute (typically within 3 months of radiotherapy) or late (months to years after radiotherapy), based on their time of onset [55]. The acute phase of radiation-induced injury is characterized by inflammation, in response to therapy, while the late phase is characterized by fibrosis and sclerosis of vessels leading to focal ischemia and chronic inflammation. To distinguish acute and late phases of toxicities is often difficult since liver damage with serum abnormalities can be observed weeks or months later after SBRT [16]. We summarize with focusing on the major toxicities in the liver, gastrointestinal tract, and central bile duct.

6.1. Liver toxicity

Liver toxicity, such as classic and non-classic radiation-induced liver disease (RILD), is one of the most common dose-limiting toxicities in liver radiotherapy [15, 16, 56, 57]. Clinical RILD occurs between 2 weeks and 7 months, typically within 4–8 weeks following hepatic radiotherapy. The patient presents with fatigue, weight gain, increased abdominal girth, hepatomegaly, anicteric ascites, and an elevation in alkaline phosphatase (over twice the upper limit of the normal values). Treatment options for RILD are limited, and the condition can become fatal due to liver failure [56, 58–61]. Non-classic RILD occurs in patients with underlying chronic hepatic disease, such as cirrhosis and viral hepatitis, and is characterized by jaundice and/or markedly elevated serum transaminases (over five times the upper limit of the normal values), developing between 1 week and 3 months after the completion of hepatic radiotherapy [19, 61]. The mean dose of less than 30 Gy has been considered as safe but radiation tolerance of the liver in a conventional radiotherapy [19]. However, the actual mean doses appropriate for liver irradiation in SBRT have not been adequately investigated. Furthermore, radiotherapy has the potential to reactivate hepatitis B virus and differentiating patients may be necessary [62, 63]. There are differences in radiosensitivity between patients with normal and cirrhotic livers; cirrhotic liver may yield a higher radiosensitivity than normal liver [16, 57]. In addition, Child-Pugh B, particularly scores of ≥8, was considered a significant risk factor for severe hepatic toxicity and poor prognosis [21, 31, 64]. Culleton et al. reported that 63% of 29 HCC patients with Child-Pugh B or C, receiving SBRT, declined Child-Pugh score by two points after 3 months [31].

As the liver is widely accepted as a parallel organ, a part of it can receive a high dose of irradiation as long as the functions as a whole organ are preserved [65–67]. Indeed, Schefter et al., Olsen et al., and Kang et al. used dose constraint, as the liver volume was >700 mL when the dose administered was less than 15 and 17 Gy in three fractions [22, 68, 69]. However, intrahepatic recurrence often occurs after a radical treatment for liver tumors because of chronic liver diseases, and such tumors have a chance to receive second radical treatment [9, 70]. Thus, the prediction of the volume of liver dysfunction is essential in order to spare the residual liver volume. After SBRT, focal dysfunction was noted in the irradiated background liver. Sanuki et al. have shown that the threshold dose of focal liver dysfunction was 30 and 25 Gy in five fractions in patients with Child-Pugh A and B, respectively, using magnetic resonance imaging (MRI) [71]. Similarly, Doi et al. have reported that focal liver dysfunction can occur at 40 and 70 Gy of BED_2 in the cirrhotic and normal liver, respectively, at a minimum dose [57]. **Figure 5** indicates a focal liver damage 3 months after SBRT. We have presented SBRT strategy with checkpoints to ensure safe treatment modality in SBRT for liver tumor [72]. To prevent RILD-related mortality, we evaluate the mean doses for the liver first and then analyze the potential loss of hepatic function in terms of BED (**Figure 6**).

6.2. Gastrointestinal injury

Ionizing radiation exerts an anticancer effect by reacting with molecular oxygen and water to generate reactive oxygen species that can attack deoxyribose in deoxyribonucleic acid (DNA). Sublethal doses of radiation can cause non-repairable DNA damage [73]. Intestine is a radiosensitive tissue because of the rapid turnover rate, and this can be a dose-limiting factor in SBRT. Gastrointestinal injuries including bleeding, ulcers, and perforations have been described, and the incidence of symptomatic gastrointestinal toxicities was less than 10% in majority of the previous reports (**Table 2**). However, severe toxicities, which can be lethal, have also been described in SBRT in the upper abdomen including liver [22, 30, 74–76]. Kang et al. have highlighted the possible association between severe gastrointestinal toxicity and the existence of mucosal ulceration prior to radiotherapy [22]. Barney et al. reported that the combination of SBRT and vascular endothelial growth factor inhibitor increased the risk of grade 3 or greater gastrointestinal toxicities [77]. Careful assessment is therefore required prior to the implementation of combined treatments, such as targeted therapy.

For the prevention of severe gastrointestinal injury, analyses of dose-volume responses have been reported. Kopek et al. recommended V21Gy ≤1 cc for the duodenum in abdominal SBRT in their analyses in 29 patients with cholangiocellular carcinoma (CCC) underwent SBRT (45 Gy/3 fractions) [78]. Bae et al. concluded that Dmax of 35 and 38 Gy in three fractions was associated with a probability of 5 and 10% severe gastroduodenal toxicity, respectively [79].

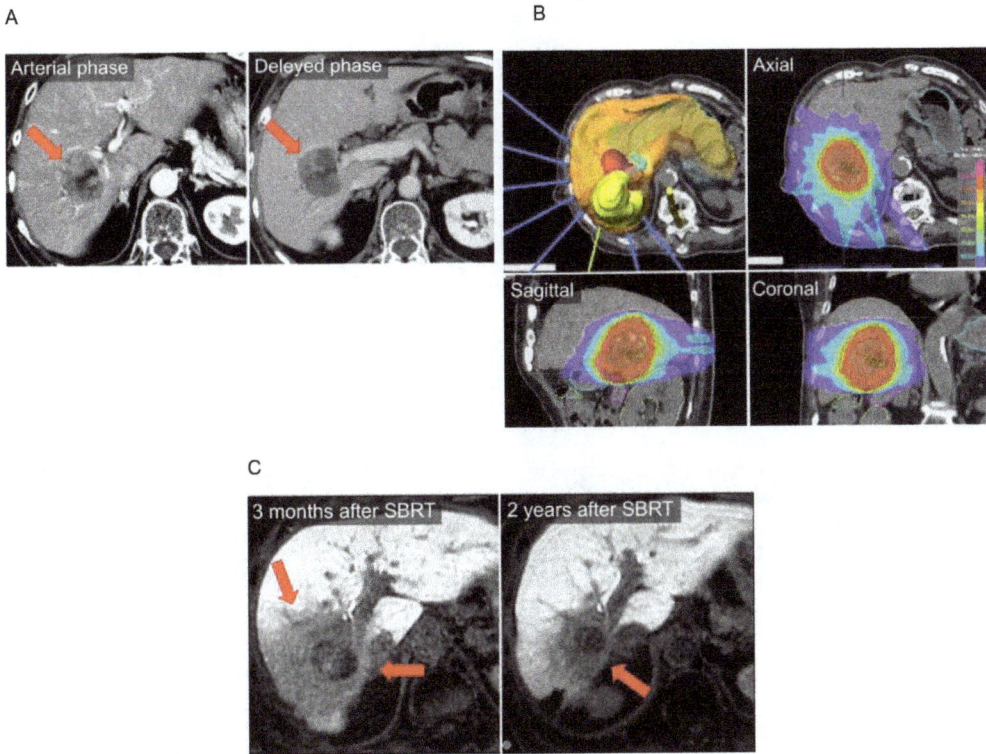

Figure 5. Focal liver dysfunction after SBRT in the follow-up MRI. A 77-year-old woman developed HCC due to hepatitis B. (A) Contrast-enhanced CT images indicate HCC in S7 area. Arterial phase showed patchy high density area (arrow, left) and contrast washed-out was observed later in delayed phase (arrow, right). (B) SBRT of 55 Gy in 10 fractions (BED_{10} = 85.3 Gy) was performed for the tumor. (C) Low intensity area was found in accordance with the irradiated area of treatment plan in Gd-EOB-DTPA enhanced-MRI three months after SBRT (left, arrows) and focal liver atrophy was observed later (right, arrow). Abbreviations: SBRT, stereotactic body radiation therapy; MRI, magnetic resonance imaging; CT, computed tomography; HCC, hepatocellular carcinoma; BED, biologically effective dose; Gd-EOB-DTPA, gadolinium ethoxybenzyl-diethylenetriamine pentaacetic acid.

Kavanagh et al. recommended that the volume of stomach receiving >22.5 Gy should be ideally minimized to <5 cc, with Dmax of <30 Gy in three fractions [80]. Sanuki et al. suggested that SBRT could be performed with the avoidance of severe toxicities when the target had a distance of >2 cm from the bowel [81]. An increased number of fractions may reduce BED for normal tissues in SBRT for liver tumors close to the gastrointestinal tract [57]. Since there are no established strategies for the prevention and treatment of radiation-induced gastrointestinal injury, efforts should be required to minimize radiation doses for gastrointestinal tracts [82].

6.3. Central hepatobiliary tract toxicity

Eriguchi et al. documented asymptomatic bile duct stenosis in 2/50 patients, receiving >20 Gy in five fractions to the central liver [83]. One of these patients received SBRT on two occasions to the central liver tumors and developed abnormalities in liver enzymes. The abnormal region visible on a computed tomography scan corresponded to the site irradiated up to a cumulative maximum dose of 88 Gy in two sessions of SBRT. The authors concluded that SBRT for liver tumors in the hepatic hilum was feasible with minimal biliary toxicity.

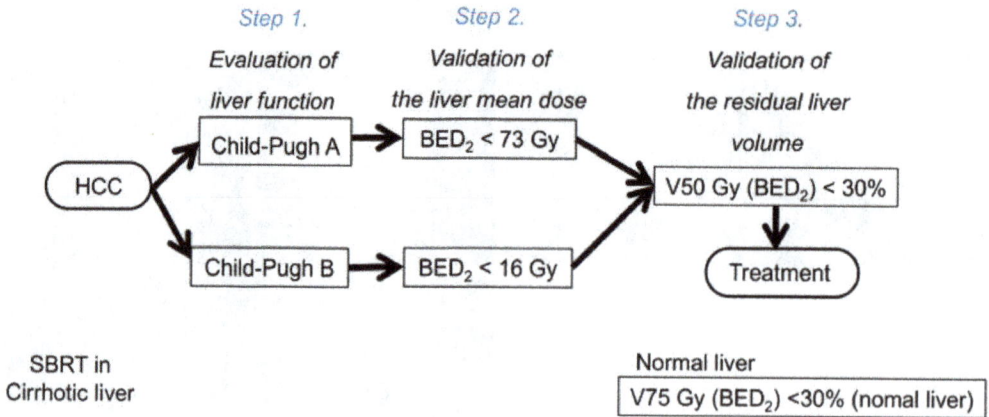

Figure 6. The current recommended treatment protocol to provide a safe SBRT for HCC in cirrhotic liver. To minimize the risk of radiation-induced liver disease and liver damage, two different checkpoints were included. Herein, we propose a safe treatment protocol for SBRT of liver tumors. First, liver function is evaluated according to the Child–Pugh classification (Step 1). Next, the liver doses are evaluated to prevent RILD. A mean BED_2 of less than 73 and 16 Gy for the whole liver should be maintained to prevent RILD in patients with Child–Pugh A and B liver function, respectively (Step 2). Finally, the volume of hepatic dysfunction is assessed to estimate the residual liver volume (Step 3). Abbreviations: SBRT, stereotactic body radiation therapy; HCC, hepatocellular carcinoma; BED, biologically effective dose.

Osmundson et al. analyzed 96 patients with liver tumors, including 20 CCCs, who received different schedules of SBRT, and reported that the incidence of hepatobiliary toxicity ≥Grade 2 and 3 was 24.0 and 18.8%, respectively [84]. Furthermore, CCC, biliary stent, $V_{BED10}72 \geq 21$ cc, $V_{BED10}66 \geq 24$ cc, and $DmeanBED_{10} \geq 14$ Gy to central hepatobiliary tract were associated with hepatobiliary toxicity [81]. The same groups reported radiation-induced pathological changes of the bile duct in resected surgical specimens 25 months after SBRT and concluded that liver toxicity should be considered while treating central liver lesions [85]. The same group has also reported a dose-volume association between ≥Grade 3 hepatobiliary toxicity and doses for central biliary tract and suggested $V_{BED10}40 < 37$ cc and $V_{BED10}30 < 45$ cc as dose-volume constraints in SBRT for primary liver tumors [86].

The anatomical structures in the hepatic hilum make radical treatment for liver tumors, such as surgery and RFA, more challenging. In such a scenario, SBRT can be a better option in comparison to other modalities, and to the best of our knowledge, there is no apparent consensus on the use of SBRT with few reports addressing this point. Further studies are required to determine the dose constraints for the bile duct, as there can be potential dose constraints due to the central hepatobiliary tract toxicity.

7. Current issues and future perspective of liver SBRT

Liver SBRT is a well-established and promising treatment for a limited number of small tumors. We have set out the difference between primary and metastatic liver cancers, considering the occurrence and prevention of toxicities. However, further questions regarding the pathological features of liver cancers, and potential SBRT strategies, including radiobiology-based SBRT and SBRT combined with immunotherapy, have not yet been fully addressed.

7.1. Potent strategies of SBRT based on radiation biology

Brown et al. reported that a greater endothelial cell damage and vascular damage, leading cancer cell apoptosis, can be caused by SBRT, and reoxygenation can increase antitumor effect in fractionated radiotherapy [87]. Shibamoto et al. concluded that reoxygenation could be promoted by a 72-h break period in SBRT [88]. No prospective clinical trials exist in terms of evaluation of the benefit of a break in SBRT. However, a longer overall treatment time (e.g., 1–2 fractions per week: 2-week schedule) may yield better local control outcomes in SBRT [89, 90]. SBRT for larger tumors has still unclear roles and is challenging because they are usually in exclusion criterion. In addition, large tumor size (≥2–4 cm) has been reported to be a predictive factor for poor outcomes after SBRT for HCC [23, 30, 32]. Further biological assessment might yield potential factors that improve treatment outcomes such as escalated doses, treatment schedule with a break, combined therapy with ideal chemotherapy, individualized treatment, and particle therapies.

7.2. Potential needs of clinical tumor volume margin in liver SBRT

Definition of clinical tumor volume (CTV) is the volume that includes both gross and microscopic disease and is created by adding several mm to 1.5 cm to gross tumor volume (GTV), in order to allow for microscopic extension. However, CTV is frequently equal to GTV in SBRT [91]. It is still poorly understood whether CTV margins are necessary, as there are limited reports of microscopic extension of liver tumors as premises for radiotherapy. HCC is characterized by direct invasion and a potential high presence of daughter nodules around the tumor that may lead to locoregional recurrence [92]. Wang et al. reported that the potential maximum margin extending beyond the gross tumor margin was 8.0 mm, although 94.7% of patients with HCC had a microscopic extension of ≤3.5 mm [93]. Wang et al. analyzed 149 resected HCCs with a mean diameter of 5.8 cm (range: 1.0–22.0 cm) and found that microinvasion was not present in 47.0% patients [94]. Microinvasion distances of ≤2 mm were found in 96.1% of patients with tumor dimensions of ≤5 cm. Uemoto et al. have first reported that a larger margin to GTV inclined to improve local control and survival outcomes in clinical data, suggesting the benefit of CTV margins [37]. Further clinical translational studies should be conducted in order to assess the optimal CTV margins.

7.3. Current knowledge of Immuno-SBRT

Regression of tumors outside the radiation field after local radiotherapy, due to systemic induction of antitumor immunity, is called the abscopal effect [95]. SBRT combined with immune checkpoint inhibitor has recently resulted in unexpected clinical complete responses from distant sites from the irradiated areas, in various malignancies [96–98]. Recently, synergistic effects of radiotherapy combined with immunotherapy have been reported in both preclinical and clinical studies, with the high possibility of the abscopal effect, which may significantly change the treatment strategies for metastatic diseases [96–105]. However, the optimal treatment schedule and doses in the combined setting of radiotherapy and immunotherapy are poorly understood at present. Young et al. reported an enhanced efficacy of immune-radiotherapy administered concurrently with radiotherapy [101]. In a meta-analysis of preclinical data, Marconi et al. reported that the probability of abscopal effects is 50% when a BED of 60 Gy is generated [102]. Moreover, SBRT may provide smaller target volumes, and in a clinical trial involving patients with pancreatic cancer, Wild et al. found that hypofractionation could minimize the toxic effects on circulating lymphocytes [106]. By expanding its application range from small tumors to metastases, SBRT might have good potential to achieve newer objectives in systematic disease, although further investigations are required.

8. Advantages of particle therapy in treatment for HCC in cirrhotic liver

The use of particle therapy, such as proton and carbon ion therapy for liver tumors, is a promising strategy to increase the dose of radiation without a concurrent increase in toxicity. Particle therapy exhibits a narrow Bragg peak at a defined depth for a defined energy [73]. Particle therapy can provide high concentrations of radiation doses to the target by positioning individual Bragg peaks to coincide with the areas of the target. In photon radiotherapy, the doses that the liver receives have a strong positive relationship with the irradiated target volume, and unacceptable higher doses might be irradiating to the background liver in the treatment of large live tumors [72]. Particle therapy can reduce the liver volume that receives low to intermediate doses, resulting in the reduction of mean liver doses with an advantage of target conformity [107, 108]. In addition, carbon ion therapy offers the added potential benefit of an increased relative biological effectiveness and a lower oxygen enhancement ratio due to the high linear energy transfer that may improve responses in hypoxic areas of tumors, which are more resistant to photon radiotherapy [73]. A relevant clinical consideration is that particle therapy can benefit relatively large tumors, such as >3 cm (particularly >5 cm) and patients with poor liver function, which are limiting for SBRT [109].

9. Conclusions

For HCC, SBRT is safe and effective, with excellent local control achieved. Tumors that are relatively small and distant from gastrointestinal tissues are strong candidate for SBRT in curative intent. Therefore, novel strategies should be developed based on new knowledge of biological responses to radiation therapy. State-of-the-art liver SBRT remains a pioneering strategy in multimodal therapy.

Acknowledgements

The authors would like to thank Messrs. Kenji Uemoto, Norihisa Masai, Koichi Yamada, and Daisaku Tatsumi from Miyakojima IGRT Clinic (Osaka, Japan).

This work was supported by Grant-in-Aid for Young Scientists (B) Grant Number 17 K16493.

Conflict of interest

None.

Author details

Hiroshi Doi[1,2]*, Hiroya Shiomi[1] and Ryoong-Jin Oh[1]

*Address all correspondence to: h-doi@med.kindai.ac.jp

1 Miyakojima IGRT Clinic, Osaka, Japan

2 Department of Radiation Oncology, Kindai University Faculty of Medicine, Osaka, Japan

References

[1] Stuver S, Trichopoulos D. Cancer of the liver and biliary tract. In: Adami HO, Hunter D, Trichopoulos D, editors. Textbook of Cancer Epidemiology. 2nd ed. New York: Oxford University Press; 2008

[2] World Health Organization, International Agency for Research on Cancer. Estimated Cancer Incidence, Mortality and Prevalence Worldwide in 2012 [Internet]. Available from: http://globocan.iarc.fr/Default.aspx. [Accessed: December 4, 2017]

[3] El-Serag HB. Hepatocellular carcinoma. The New England Journal of Medicine. 2011;**365**:1118-1127

[4] Zhang DY, Friedman SL. Fibrosis-dependent mechanisms of hepatocarcinogenesis. Hepatology. 2012;**56**:769-775

[5] Donato F, Tagger A, Gelatti U, Parrinello G, Boffetta P, Albertini A, et al. Alcohol and hepatocellular carcinoma: The effect of lifetime intake and hepatitis virus infections in men and women. American Journal of Epidemiology. 2002;**155**:323-331

[6] Fattovich G, Stroffolini T, Zagni I, Donato F. Hepatocellular carcinoma in cirrhosis: Incidence and risk factors. Gastroenterology. 2004;**127**(5, Suppl 1):S35-S50

[7] Bruix J, Reig M, Sherman M. Evidence-based diagnosis, staging, and treatment of patients with hepatocellular carcinoma. Gastroenterology. 2016;**150**:835-853

[8] Soyama A, Eguchi S, Egawa H. Liver transplantation in Japan. Liver Transplantation. 2016;**22**:1401-1407

[9] Tateishi R, Shiina S, Yoshida H, Teratani T, Obi S, Yamashiki N, Yoshida H, Akamatsu M, Kawabe T, Omata M. Prediction of recurrence of hepatocellular carcinoma after curative ablation using three tumor markers. Hepatology. 2006;**44**:1518-1527

[10] Zeng Z-C, Fan J, Tang Z-Y, Zhou J, Qin L-X, Wang J-H, et al. A comparison of treatment combinations with and without radiotherapy for hepatocellular carcinoma with portal vein and/or inferior vena cava tumor thrombus. International Journal of Radiation Oncology Biology Physics. 2005;**61**(2):432-443

[11] Park W, Lim D-H, Paik SW, Koh KC, Choi MS, Park CK, et al. Local radiotherapy for patients with unresectable hepatocellular carcinoma. International Journal of Radiation Oncology Biology Physics. 2005 Mar 15;**61**(4):1143-1150

[12] Park HC, Seong J, Han KH, Chon CY, Moon YM, Suh CO. Dose-response relationship in local radiotherapy for hepatocellular carcinoma. International Journal of Radiation Oncology Biology Physics. 2002;**54**:150-155

[13] Ben-josef E, Lawrence TS. Radiotherapy for unresectable hepatic malignancies. Seminars in Radiation Oncology. 2005 Oct;**15**(4):273-278

[14] Fuss M, Salter BJ, Herman TS, Thomas CR. External beam radiation therapy for hepato-cellular carcinoma: Potential of intensity-modulated and image-guided radiation ther-apy. Gastroenterology. 2004 Nov;**127**(5 Suppl 1):S206-S217

[15] Emami B, Lyman J, Brown A, Coia L, Goitein M, Munzenrider JE, Shank B, Solin LJ, Wesson M. Tolerance of normal tissue to therapeutic irradiation. International Journal of Radiation Oncology, Biology, Physics. 1991;**21**:109-122

[16] Pan CC, Kavanagh BD, Dawson LA, Li XA, Das SK, Miften M, Ten Haken RK. Radiation-associated liver injury. International Journal of Radiation Oncology, Biology, Physics 2010;**76**:S94-100

[17] Blomgren H, Lax I, Näslund I, et al. Stereotactic high dose fraction radiation therapy of extracranial tumors using an accelerator: Clinical experience of the first thirty-one patients. Acta Oncologica. 1995;**34**:861-870

[18] Wulf J, Guckenberger M, Haedinger U, et al. Stereotactic radiotherapy of primary liver cancer and hepatic metastases. Acta Oncologica. 2006;**45**:838-847

[19] Kwon JH, Bae SH, Kim JY, et al. Long-term effect of stereotactic body radiation therapy for primary hepatocellular carcinoma ineligible for local ablation therapy or surgical resection. Stereotactic radiotherapy for liver cancer. BMC Cancer. 2010;**10**:S27-S10

[20] Seo YS, Kim MS, Yoo SY, et al. Preliminary result of stereotactic body radiotherapy as a local salvage treatment for inoperable hepatocellular carcinoma. Journal of Surgical Oncology. 2010;**102**:209-214

[21] Andolino DL, Johnson CS, Maluccio M, Kwo P, Tector AJ, Zook J, Johnstone PA, Cardenes HR. Stereotactic body radiotherapy for primary hepatocellular carcinoma. International Journal of Radiation Oncology, Biology, Physics. 2011;**81**:e447-e453

[22] Kang JK, Kim MS, Cho CK, Yang KM, Yoo HJ, Kim JH, Bae SH, Jung DH, Kim KB, Lee DH, Han CJ, Kim J, Park SC, Kim YH. Stereotactic body radiation therapy for inoper-able hepatocellular carcinoma as a local salvage treatment after incomplete transarterial chemoembolization. Cancer. 2012;**118**:5424-5431

[23] Huang WY, Jen YM, Lee MS, et al. Stereotactic body radiation therapy in recurrent hepa-tocellular carcinoma. International Journal of Radiation Oncology, Biology, Physics. 2012;**84**:355-361

[24] Honda Y, Kimura T, Aikata H, et al. Stereotactic body radiation therapy combined with transcatheter arterial chemoembolization for small hepatocellular carcinoma. Journal of Gastroenterology and Hepatology. 2013;**28**:530-536

[25] Bae SH, Kim MS, Cho CK, Kim KB, Lee DH, Han CJ, Park SC, Kim YH. Feasibility and efficacy of stereotactic ablative radiotherapy for barcelona clinic liver cancer-C stage hepatocellular carcinoma. Journal of Korean Medical Science. 2013;**28**:213-217

[26] Bujold A, Massey CA, Kim JJ, et al. Sequential phase I and II trials of stereotactic body radiotherapy for locally advanced hepatocellular carcinoma. Journal of Clinical Oncology. 2013;31:1631-1639

[27] Jang WI, Kim MS, Bae SH, et al. High-dose stereotactic body radiotherapy correlates increased local control and overall survival in patients with inoperable hepatocellular carcinoma. Radiation Oncology. 2013;8:250

[28] Sanuki N, Takeda A, Oku Y, Mizuno T, Aoki Y, Eriguchi T, Iwabuchi S, Kunieda E. Stereotactic body radiotherapy for small hepatocellular carcinoma: A retrospective outcome analysis in 185 patients. Acta Oncologica. 2014;53:399-404

[29] Takeda A, Sanuki N, Eriguchi T, Kobayashi T, Iwabutchi S, Matsunaga K, Mizuno T, Yashiro K, Nisimura S, Kunieda E. Stereotactic ablative body radiotherapy for previously untreated solitary hepatocellular carcinoma. Journal of Gastroenterology and Hepatology. 2014;29:372-379

[30] Yamashita H, Onishi H, Matsumoto Y, Murakami N, Matsuo Y, Nomiya T, Nakagawa K. Local effect of stereotactic body radiotherapy for primary and metastatic liver tumors in 130 Japanese patients. Radiation Oncology. 2014;9:112

[31] Culleton S, Jiang H, Haddad CR, Kim J, Brierley J, Brade A, Ringash J, Dawson LA. Outcomes following definitive stereotactic body radiotherapy for patients with Child-Pugh B or C hepatocellular carcinoma. Radiotherapy and Oncology. 2014;111:412-417

[32] Huertas A, Baumann AS, Saunier-Kubs F, et al. Stereotactic body radiation therapy as an ablative treatment for inoperable hepatocellular carcinoma. Radiotherapy and Oncology. 2015;115:211-216

[33] Takeda A, Sanuki N, Tsurugai Y, et al. Phase 2 study of stereotactic body radiotherapy and optional transarterial chemoembolization for solitary hepatocellular carcinoma not amenable to resection and radiofrequency ablation. Cancer. 2016;122:2041-2049

[34] Wahl DR, Stenmark MH, Tao Y, Pollom EL, Caoili EM, Lawrence TS, Schipper MJ, Feng M. Outcomes after stereotactic body radiotherapy or radiofrequency ablation for hepatocellular carcinoma. Journal of Clinical Oncology. 2016;34:452-459

[35] Su TS, Liang P, Liang J, et al. Long-term survival analysis of stereotactic ablative radiotherapy versus liver resection for small hepatocellular carcinoma. International Journal of Radiation Oncology, Biology, Physics. 2017;98:639-646

[36] Lo CH, Yang JF, Liu MY, et al. Survival and prognostic factors for patients with advanced hepatocellular carcinoma after stereotactic ablative radiotherapy. PLoS One. 2017;12:e0177793

[37] Uemoto K, Doi H, Shiomi H, Yamada K, Tatsumi D, Yasumoto T, Takashina M, Koizumi M, Oh RJ. Clinical assessment of micro-residual tumors during stereotactic body radiation therapy for hepatocellular carcinoma. Anticancer Research. 2018;38:945-954

[38] Nugent FW, Qamar A, Stuart KE, Galuski K, Flacke S, Molgaard C, Gordon F, Iqbal S, Hunter KU, Hartnett E, Gunturu K. A randomized phase II study of individualized stereotactic body radiation therapy (SBRT) versus transarterial chemoembolization (TACE)

with DEBDOX beads as a bridge to transplant in hepatocellular carcinoma (HCC). In: 2017 Gastrointestinal Cancer Symposium; Jan 19-21; San Fransisco, CA, USA; 2017. 223

[39] Matsuo Y, Yoshida K, Nishimura H, Ejima Y, Miyawaki D, Uezono H, Ishihara T, Mayahara H, Fukumoto T, Ku Y, Yamaguchi M, Sugimoto K, Sasaki R. Efficacy of stereotactic body radiotherapy for hepatocellular carcinoma with portal vein tumor thrombosis/inferior vena cava tumor thrombosis: Evaluation by comparison with conventional three-dimensional conformal radiotherapy. Journal of Radiation Research. 2016;57:512-523

[40] Xi M, Zhang L, Zhao L, Li QQ, Guo SP, Feng ZZ, Deng XW, Huang XY, Liu MZ. Effectiveness of stereotactic body radiotherapy for hepatocellular carcinoma with portal vein and/or inferior vena cava tumor thrombosis. PLoS One. 2013;8:e63864

[41] Zheng X-K, Chen L-H, Yan X, Wang H-M. Impact of prolonged fraction dose-delivery time modeling intensity-modulated radiation therapy on hepatocellular carcinoma cell killing. WJG. 2005 Mar 14;11(10):1452-1456

[42] Benedict SH, Yenice KM, Followill D, et al. Stereotactic body radiation therapy: The report of AAPM task group 101. Medical Physics. 2010;37:4078-4101

[43] Timmerman RD, Herman J, Chinsoo Cho L. Emergence of stereotactic body radiation therapy and its impact on current and future clinical practice. Journal of Clinical Oncology. 2014;32:2847-2854

[44] Yin J, Bo W-T, Sun J, Xiang X, Lang J-Y, Zhong J-H, et al. New evidence and perspectives on the management of hepatocellular carcinoma with portal vein tumor thrombus. Journal of Clinical and Translational Hepatology. 2017 Jun 28;5(2):169-176

[45] Schöniger-Hekele M, Müller C, Kutilek M, Oesterreicher C, Ferenci P, Gangl A. Hepatocellular carcinoma in Central Europe: Prognostic features and survival. Gut. 2001;48: 103-109

[46] Jiang J-F, Lao Y-C, Yuan B-H, Yin J, Liu X, Chen L, et al. Treatment of hepatocellular carcinoma with portal vein tumor thrombus: Advances and challenges. Oncotarget. 2017 May 16;8(20):33911-33921

[47] Kokudo T, Hasegawa K, Matsuyama Y, Takayama T, Izumi N, Kadoya M, et al. Survival benefit of liver resection for hepatocellular carcinoma associated with portal vein invasion. Journal of Hepatology. 2016 Nov;65(5):938-943

[48] Tang Q-H, Li A-J, Yang G-M, Lai ECH, Zhou W-P, Jiang Z-H, et al. Surgical resection versus conformal radiotherapy combined with TACE for resectable hepatocellular carcinoma with portal vein tumor thrombus: A comparative study. World Journal of Surgery. 2013 Jun;37(6):1362-1370 Oncotarget; 2017

[49] Chan SL, Chong CCN, Chan AWH, Poon DMC, Chok KSH. Management of hepatocellular carcinoma with portal vein tumor thrombosis: Review and update at 2016. WJG. 2016 Aug 28;22(32):7289-7300

[50] Choi BO, Choi IB, Jang HS, et al. Stereotactic body radiation therapy with or without transarterial chemoembolization for patients with primary hepatocellular carcinoma: Preliminary analysis. BMC Cancer. 2008;8:351

[51] Lin CS, Jen YM, Chiu SY, et al. Treatment of portal vein tumor thrombosis of hepatoma patients with either stereotactic radiotherapy or three-dimensional conformal radiotherapy. Japanese Journal of Clinical Oncology. 2006;**36**:212-217

[52] Goodman KA, Wiegner EA, Maturen KE, et al. Dose-escalation study of single-fraction stereotactic body radiotherapy for liver malignancies. International Journal of Radiation Oncology, Biology, Physics. 2010;**78**:486-493

[53] Bae SH, Park HC, Lim DH, et al. Salvage treatment with hypofractionated radiotherapy in patients with recurrent small hepatocellular carcinoma. International Journal of Radiation Oncology, Biology, Physics. 2012;**82**:e603-e607

[54] Lausch A, Sinclair K, Lock M, et al. Determination and comparison of radiotherapy dose responses for hepatocellular carcinoma and metastatic colorectal liver tumours. The British Journal of Radiology. 2013;**86**:20130147

[55] Cox JD, Stetz J, Pajak TF. Toxicity criteria of the radiation therapy oncology group (RTOG) and the European Organization for Research and Treatment of cancer (EORTC). International Journal of Radiation Oncology, Biology, Physics. 1995;**31**:1341-1346

[56] Jackson A, Haken Ten RK, Robertson JM, et al. Analysis of clinical complication data for radiation hepatitis using a parallel architecture model. International Journal of Radiation Oncology, Biology, Physics. 1995;**31**:883-891

[57] Doi H, Shiomi H, Masai N, Tatsumi D, Igura T, Imai Y, Oh RJ. Threshold doses and prediction of visually apparent liver dysfunction after stereotactic body radiation therapy in cirrhotic and normal livers using magnetic resonance imaging. Journal of Radiation Research. 2016;**57**:294-300

[58] Dawson LA, Ten Haken RK, Lawrence TS. Partial irradiation of the liver. Seminars in Radiation Oncology 2001;**11**:240-246

[59] Ohara K, Okumura T, Tsuji H, et al. Radiation tolerance of cirrhotic livers in relation to the preserved functional capacity: Analysis of patients with hepatocellular carcinoma treated by focused proton beam radiotherapy. International Journal of Radiation Oncology, Biology, Physics. 1997;**38**:367-372

[60] Cheng JCH, Wu JK, Huang CM, et al. Radiation-induced liver disease after three-dimensional conformal radiotherapy for patients with hepatocellular carcinoma: Dosimetric analysis and implication. International Journal of Radiation Oncology, Biology, Physics. 2002;**54**:156-162

[61] Xu ZY, Liang SX, Zhu J, Zhu XD, Zhao JD, Lu HJ, Yang YL, Chen L, Wang AY, Fu XL, Jiang GL. Prediction of radiation-induced liver disease by Lyman normal-tissue complication probability model in three-dimensional conformal radiation therapy for primary liver carcinoma. International Journal of Radiation Oncology, Biology, Physics. 2006;**65**:189-195

[62] Chou CH, Chen PJ, Lee PH, et al. Radiation-induced hepatitis B virus reactivation in liver mediated by the bystander effect from irradiated endothelial cells. Clinical Cancer Research. 2007;**13**:851-857

[63] Kim JH, Park JW, Kim TH, et al. Hepatitis B virus reactivation after three-dimensional conformal radiotherapy in patients with hepatitis B virus-related hepatocellular carcinoma. International Journal of Radiation Oncology, Biology, Physics. 2007;**69**:813-819

[64] Cardenes HR, Price TR, Perkins SM, et al. Phase I feasibility trial of stereotactic body radiation therapy for primary hepatocellular carcinoma. Clinical & Translational Oncology. 2010;**12**:218-225

[65] Ingold JA, Reed GB, Kaplan HS, Bagshaw MA. Radiation hepatitis. The American Journal of Roentgenology, Radium Therapy, and Nuclear Medicine. 1965;**93**:200-208

[66] Lawrence TS, Haken Ten RK, et al. The use of 3-D dose volume analysis to predict radiation hepatitis. International Journal of Radiation Oncology, Biology, Physics. 1992;**23**:781-788

[67] Withers HR, Taylor JM, Maciejewski B. Treatment volume and tissue tolerance. International Journal of Radiation Oncology, Biology, Physics. 1988;**14**:751-759

[68] Schefter TE, Kavanagh BD, Timmerman RD, Cardenes HR, Baron A, Gaspar LE. A phase I trial of stereotactic body radiation therapy (SBRT) for liver metastases. International Journal of Radiation Oncology, Biology, Physics. 2005;**62**:1371-1378

[69] Olsen CC, Welsh J, Kavanagh BD, Franklin W, McCarter M, Cardenes HR, Gaspar LE, Schefter TE. Microscopic and macroscopic tumor and parenchymal effects of liver stereotactic body radiotherapy. International Journal of Radiation Oncology, Biology, Physics. 2009;**73**:1414-1424

[70] Yoshida H, Shiratori Y, Moriyama M, et al. Interferon therapy reduces the risk for hepatocellular carcinoma: National surveillance program of cirrhotic and non-cirrhotic patients with chronic hepatitis C in Japan. IHIT study group. Inhibition of Hepatocarcinogenesis by interferon therapy. Annals of Internal Medicine. 1999;**131**:174-181

[71] Sanuki N, Takeda A, Oku Y, Eriguchi T, Nishimura S, Aoki Y, Mizuno T, Iwabuchi S, Kunieda E. Threshold doses for focal liver reaction after stereotactic ablative body radiation therapy for small hepatocellular carcinoma depend on liver function: Evaluation on magnetic resonance imaging with Gd-EOB-DTPA. International Journal of Radiation Oncology, Biology, Physics. 2014;**88**:306-311

[72] Doi H, Masai N, Uemoto K, Suzuki O, Shiomi H, Tatsumi D, Oh RJ. Validation of the liver mean dose in terms of the biological effective dose for the prevention of radiation-induced liver damage. Reports of Practical Oncology and Radiotherapy. 2017;**22**:303-309

[73] Hall EJ, Giaccia AJ. Radiobiology for the Radiologist. 7th ed. Philadelphia: Lippincott Williams & Wilkins; 2011

[74] Høyer M, Roed H, Traberg Hansen A, Ohlhuis L, Petersen J, Nellemann H, Kiil Berthelsen A, Grau C, Aage Engelholm S, Von der Maase H. Phase II study on stereotactic body radiotherapy of colorectal metastases. Acta Oncologica. 2006;**45**:823-830

[75] Høyer M, Roed H, Sengelov L, et al. Phase-II study on stereotactic radiotherapy of locally advanced pancreatic carcinoma. Radiotherapy and Oncology. 2005;**76**:48-53

[76] Onishi H, Ozaki M, Kuriyama K, et al. Serious gastric ulcer event after stereotactic body radiotherapy (SBRT) delivered with concomitant vinorelbine in a patient with left adrenal metastasis of lung cancer. Acta Oncologica. 2012;**51**:624-628

[77] Barney BM, Markovic SN, Laack NN, et al. Increased bowel toxicity in patients treated with a vascular endothelial growth factor inhibitor (VEGFI) after stereotactic body radiation therapy (SBRT). International Journal of Radiation Oncology, Biology, Physics. 2013;**87**:73-80

[78] Kopek N, Holt MI, Hansen AT, et al. Stereotactic body radiotherapy for unresectable cholangiocarcinoma. Radiotherapy and Oncology. 2010;**94**:47-52

[79] Bae SH, Kim MS, Cho CK, Kang JK, Lee SY, Lee KN, Lee DH, Han CJ, Yang KY, Kim SB. Predictor of severe gastroduodenal toxicity after stereotactic body radiotherapy for abdominopelvic malignancies. International Journal of Radiation Oncology, Biology, Physics. 2012;**84**:e469-e474

[80] Kavanagh BD, Pan CC, Dawson LA, Das SK, Li XA, Ten Haken RK, Miften M. Radiation dose-volume effects in the stomach and small bowel. International Journal of Radiation Oncology, Biology, Physics. 2010;**76**:S101-S107

[81] Sanuki N, Takeda A, Kunieda E. Role of stereotactic body radiation therapy for hepatocellular carcinoma. World Journal of Gastroenterology. 2014;**20**:3100-3111

[82] Lalla RV, Bowen J, Barasch A, et al. MASCC/ISOO clinical practice guidelines for the management of mucositis secondary to cancer therapy. Cancer. 2014;**120**:1453-1461

[83] Eriguchi T, Takeda A, Sanuki N, Oku Y, Aoki Y, Shigematsu N, Kunieda E. Acceptable toxicity after stereotactic body radiation therapy for liver tumors adjacent to the central biliary system. International Journal of Radiation Oncology, Biology, Physics. 2013;**85**:1006-1011

[84] Osmundson EC, Wu Y, Luxton G, Bazan JG, Koong AC, Chang DT. Predictors of toxicity associated with stereotactic body radiation therapy to the central hepatobiliary tract. International Journal of Radiation Oncology, Biology, Physics. 2015;**91**:986-994

[85] Shaffer JL, Osmundson EC, Visser BC, Longacre TA, Koong AC, Chang DT. Stereotactic body radiation therapy and central liver toxicity: A case report. Practical Radiation Oncology. 2015;**5**:282-285

[86] Toesca DAS, Osmundson EC, Eyben RV, Shaffer JL, Lu P, Koong AC, Chang DT. Central liver toxicity after SBRT: An expanded analysis and predictive nomogram. Radiotherapy and Oncology. 2017;**122**:130-136

[87] Brown JM, Carlson DJ, Brenner DJ. The tumor radiobiology of SRS and SBRT: Are more than the 5 Rs involved? International Journal of Radiation Oncology, Biology, Physics. 2014;**88**:254-262

[88] Shibamoto Y, Miyakawa A, Otsuka S, Iwata H. Radiobiology of hypofractionated stereotactic radiotherapy: What are the optimal fractionation schedules? Journal of Radiation Research. 2016;**57**:i76-i82

[89] Shibamoto Y, Hashizume C, Baba F, et al. Stereotactic body radiotherapy using a radio-biology-based regimen for stage I non-small-cell lung cancer: Five-year mature results. Journal of Thoracic Oncology. 2015;**10**:960-964

[90] Matsuo Y, Shibuya K, Nagata Y, et al. Prognostic factors in stereotactic body radio-therapy for non-small-cell lung cancer. International Journal of Radiation Oncology, Biology, Physics. 2011;**79**:1104-1111

[91] Nagata Y, editor. Stereotactic Body Radiation Therapy: Principles and Practices. 1st ed. Tokyo: Springer; 2015

[92] Jwo SC, Chiu JH, Chau GY, et al. Risk factors linked to tumor recurrence of human hepatocellular carcinoma after hepatic resection. Hepatology. 1992;**16**:1367-1371

[93] Wang W, Feng X, Zhang T, Jin J, Wang S, Liu Y, et al. Prospective evaluation of micro-scopic extension using whole-mount preparation in patients with hepatocellular car-cinoma: Definition of clinical target volume for radiotherapy. Radiation Oncology. 2010;**5**:73

[94] Wang MH, Ji Y, Zeng ZC, et al. Impact factors for microinvasion in patients with hepa-tocellular carcinoma: Possible application to the definition of clinical tumor volume. International Journal of Radiation Oncology, Biology, Physics. 2010;**76**:467-476

[95] Le QT, Shirato H, Giaccia AJ, et al. Emerging treatment paradigms in radiation oncol-ogy. Clinical Cancer Research. 2015;**21**:3393-3401

[96] Postow MA, Callahan MK, Barker CA, et al. Immunologic correlates of the abscopal effect in a patient with melanoma. The New England Journal of Medicine. 2012;**366**:925-931

[97] Hiniker SM, Chen DS, Reddy S, et al. A systemic complete response of metastatic mela-noma to local radiation and immunotherapy. Translational Oncology. 2012;**5**:404-407

[98] Golden EB, Demaria S, Schiff PB, et al. An abscopal response to radiation and ipili-mumab in a patient with metastatic non-small cell lung cancer. Cancer Immunology Research. 2013;**1**:365-372

[99] Hiniker SM, Reddy SA, Maecker HT, et al. A prospective clinical trial combining radia-tion therapy with systemic immunotherapy in metastatic melanoma. International Journal of Radiation Oncology, Biology, Physics. 2016;**96**:578-588

[100] Seung SK, Curti BD, Crittenden M, et al. Phase 1 study of stereotactic body radio-therapy and interleukin-2–tumor and immunological responses. Science Translational Medicine. 2012;**4**:137ra74

[101] Young KH, Baird JR, Savage T, et al. Optimizing timing of immunotherapy improves control of tumors by hypofractionated radiation therapy. PLoS One. 2016;**11**:e0157164

[102] Marconi R, Strolin S. Bossi et al. a meta-analysis of the abscopal effect in preclini-cal models: Is the biologically effective dose a relevant physical trigger? PLoS One. 2017;**12**:e0171559

[103] Shehade H, Kariolis MS, Stehr H, et al. Reprogramming the immunological microenvi-ronment through radiation and targeting Axl. Nature Communications. 2016;**7**:13898

[104] Twyman-Saint Victor C, Rech AJ, et al. Radiation and dual checkpoint blockade activate non-redundant immune mechanisms in cancer. Nature. 2015;**520**:373-377

[105] Deng L, Liang H, Burnette B, et al. Irradiation and anti-PD-L1 treatment synergistically promote antitumor immunity in mice. The Journal of Clinical Investigation. 2014;**124**:687-695

[106] Wild AT, Herman JM, Dholakia AS, et al. Lymphocyte-sparing effect of stereotactic body radiation therapy in patients with Unresectable pancreatic cancer. International Journal of Radiation Oncology, Biology, Physics. 2016;**94**:571-579

[107] Abe T, Saitoh JI, Kobayashi D, et al. Dosimetric comparison of carbon ion radiotherapy and stereotactic body radiotherapy with photon beams for the treatment of hepatocellular carcinoma. Radiation Oncology. 2015;**10**:187

[108] Toramatsu C, Katoh N, Shimizu S, Nihongi H, Matsuura T, Takao S, Miyamoto N, Suzuki R, Sutherland K, Kinoshita R, Onimaru R, Ishikawa M, Umegaki K, Shirato H. What is the appropriate size criterion for proton radiotherapy for hepatocellular carcinoma? A dosimetric comparison of spot-scanning proton therapy versus intensity-modulated radiation therapy. Radiation Oncology. 2013;**8**:48

[109] Mizumoto M, Oshiro Y, Okumura T. Proton beam therapy for hepatocellular carcinoma: A review of the University of Tsukuba experience. International Journal of Particle Therapy. 2016;**2**:570-578

3

Nonalcoholic Fatty Liver Disease: The Future Frontier of Hepatology for South Asia

Shahinul Alam, Thupten Kelsang Lama,
Golam Mustafa, Mahabubul Alam and
Nooruddin Ahmad

Abstract

This review is to know the magnitude of nonalcoholic fatty liver disease (NAFLD) among general population and risk group populations of the South Asian countries. A thorough search of evidence-based literature was conducted using the PubMed database with key words. Databases searched from inception to February 2017. Systematic search of the literature was conducted for studies pertaining. Prevalence of NAFLD in South Asia varies from 13 to 34%. The Highest rate is in Bangladesh (34.34%) and lowest in Pakistan (13.5%). Prevalence of NAFLD is 15–80% among obese people, 25–60% with dyslipidemia and 33–55% in pre diabetics and diabetics. Nonalcoholic steatohepatitis (NASH) is present in about 50% of the NAFLD cases that can lead to fibrosis, cirrhosis or even hepatocellular carcinoma (HCC). NAFLD is not the disease for only obese people, but it is also common in nonobese in this region. About 11.11% hepatocellular carcinoma developed from NASH. Incidence rate of diabetes and coronary artery disease is high among NAFLD patients. NAFLD is becoming a future challenge for South Asia region. Prevalence and severity has been remarkably increasing for last few years. The health system should get ready to confront burden of NAFLD in future for South Asia.

Keywords: nonalcoholic fatty liver disease, nonalcoholic steatohepatitis, South Asia

1. Introduction

Nonalcoholic fatty liver disease (NAFLD) is a characterized by excessive accumulation of fat (defined as the presence of lipid in >5% of hepatocytes or a lipid content >5% of liver weight) [1] in the liver, who consume little (<20 g of alcohol/d) or no alcohol [1, 2]. It is the most common cause of chronic liver injury [3]. Worldwide millions of people are affected by the NAFLD and it is prophesied to be the following universal epidemic [4]. Universally its prevalence rate is 25.24 with highest in the Middle East and South America and lowest in Africa [5]. The NAFLD with necroinflammation, defined as nonalcoholic steatohepatitis (NASH) [2]. According to Younossi ZM, universally overall mortality for NAFLD is 1.05; and incidence of hepatocellular carcinoma (HCC) and liver-specific mortality among NAFLD is 0.44 and 0.77 per 1000 person-years respectively. About 30% NAFLD progress to NASH, it can be lead to fibrosis, cirrhosis or even hepatocellular carcinoma [6]. HCC is one of the most common cancers worldwide and its burden is highest in the South-East Asia [7]. Countries with higher economic status tend to present a higher prevalence of NAFLD [8]. But it is not uncommon in low economic countries like countries of South Asia. The prevalence of NAFLD has increased remarkably over the years in South Asia and South-East Asia affecting 5–34% of general population [9, 10]. Metabolic syndrome common in people from South Asia is an important risk factor for NAFLD and Bangladeshi ethnicity is an important independent risk factor for NAFLD [3]. It is commonly described as hepatic manifestation of metabolic syndrome and insulin resistance. Though prevalence of NAFLD markedly increased in obese population, presence of NAFLD is further more challenging to diagnose and manage in lean population. In this study we aimed to know the prevalence NAFLD among general population and risk group populations of the South Asian countries. We also explored the prevalence of NASH and its associated conditions.

2. Materials and methods

We performed a systematic PubMed/MEDLINE literature search with the following key words: "Non-alcoholic Fatty Liver Disease/epidemiology"[Mesh], "Non-alcoholic steatohepatitis" [Text word] AND "Liver Transplantation/etiology"[Mesh], "Obesity"[Mesh], "Diabetes Mellitus"[Mesh], "Global," "Afghanistan," "Pakistan," "India," "Sri Lanka," "Maldives," "Nepal," "Bangladesh," and "Bhutan." Databases searched from inception to February 2017. Exclusions included data on alcohol consumption or other liver diseases. Relevant full article, abstract, review, mini review, editorial and conference proceeding are included in this review.

3. Global epidemiology

Nonalcoholic fatty liver disease (NAFLD) is the commonest liver disease with global prevalence of approximately 25.24% of the general population [5]. Nonalcoholic steatohepatitis (NASH) and NAFLD are not only a Western disease. NAFLD and NASH have increasingly been diagnosed in all regions of Asia [11]. A study using the National Health and Nutrition Examination Survey (NHANES) found a 30% prevalence of NAFLD in the United States between 2011 and 2012 [12]. NAFLD is the most common cause of chronic liver disease in Western countries. It affects about 1 billion individuals worldwide [13]. Increasing prevalence of NASH is closely associated with prevalence diabetes and obesity, which may defined as epidemic worldwide. At least 1.46 billion obese adult is persisting in the world. Approximately 6 million individuals in the USA are in the risk of developing NASH and about 0.6 million

Region	Population studied	Prevalence of NAFLD in these populations (%)
USA	Pediatric population	13–14
	General population	27–34
Europe	Pediatric population	2.6–10
	General population	20–30
Middle East	General population	20–30
Far East	General population	15
South Asia	General population	5–30

Table 1. Estimated prevalence of NAFLD and NASH among different areas of the word.

to develop NASH-related cirrhosis [14]. **Table 1** shows estimated prevalence of NAFLD and NASH. Reports on the prevalence of NAFLD and NASH vary substantially due to varying definitions, differences in the populations studied, and the diagnostic methods used [14].

4. Delineation of South Asia and its population diversity

According to the United Nations geographic region ordering, South Asia comprised with Afghanistan, Bangladesh, Bhutan, India, Maldives, Nepal, Pakistan, and Sri Lanka (**Figure 1**). Topographically, it is dominated by the Indian Plate; the terms "Indian subcontinent" and "South Asia" are sometimes used interchangeably [15]. South Asia is the most populated region in the world [16]. Socially it is very mixed, consisting of many language groups and religions, and social practices in one region that are vastly different from those in another [17].

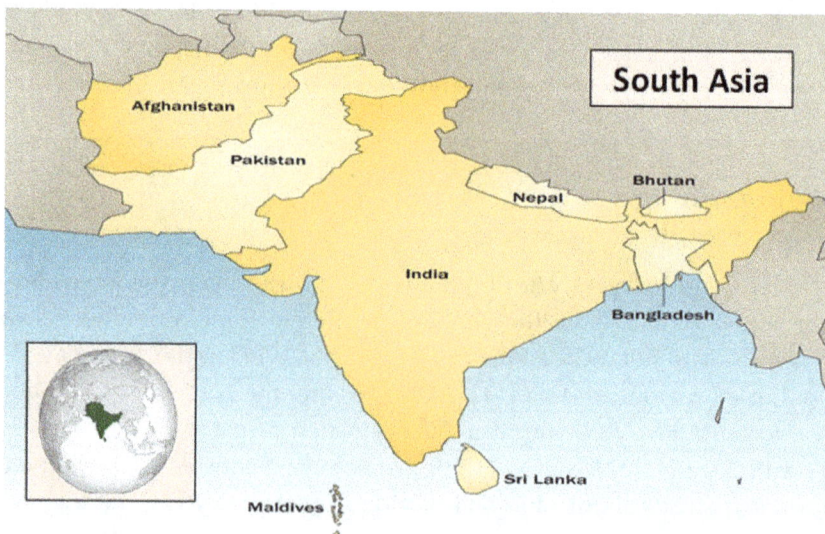

Figure 1. Geographical position and area of South Asia [16].

5. Prevalence of NAFLD among South Asian people

Recent socioeconomic changes have resulted in an emerging epidemic of non-communicable diseases such as type 2 diabetes and nonalcoholic fatty liver disease. The prevalence of nonalcoholic fatty liver disease in Asian Pacific countries now approximates and even overrides levels encountered in Western countries in some studies [18]. NAFLD is the emerging challenge for public health issue in Asia [19]. This has a potential burden not only on liver disease but also on metabolic syndrome related morbidity: obesity, diabetes, and atherosclerotic cardiovascular disease [19]. Largest population of the world inhabiting in Asia are passing through an economic growth and shift of focus from a dominant physical activity to knowledge, capital and physical inactivity. An increasing GDP is paralleled by a rising body mass index (BMI) in an almost linear fashion [19]. Countries with higher economic status tend to present a higher prevalence of NAFLD [8]. It is believed to provide a distinctive epidemiologic perspective to global situation of NAFLD. Especially for South Asia, according to increasing with their economy the prevalence of NAFLD is increasing day by day.

Most of the available epidemiological studies in NAFLD from Asia are ultrasound based and hence detect prevalence of hepatic steatosis alone initially, correlating it with anthropometric, biochemical, and demographic features of the population (**Table 2**). The community prevalence of NAFLD in South Asia and South-East Asia ranges from 5 to 30% [9, 10]. Recently a hospital based study in Pakistan had shown a frequency of approximately 14%. In India, it varies from 5 to 28% in general population, especially those who are undergoing health check-ups. Indians have increased propensity for visceral fat accumulation which may present from birth [9]. Prevalence of NAFLD in general population of Bangladesh has been estimated to vary from 4 to 34.34% [20, 21], which exceeds previous reports and it jumps up to 49.8% in diabetic patients [22, 23]. And in Sri Lanka the prevalence rate was found 32.6 in an urban based study [24]. So it is seen that, among South Asian countries the highest magnitude of NAFLD is in Bangladesh and lowest is in Pakistan (**Figure 2**).

Country	Population and place	Sample size (n)	Prevalence of NAFL
India	Selected population Mumbai	1168	16.6%
	General population West Bengal (rural)	1911	167 (8.7%)
	General population Chennai (urban)	541	173 (32%)
Bangladesh	General population Nation wide	2621	900 (34.34%)
	Selected Population Camilla (rural)	665	219 (33%)
Sri Lanka	General population (urban)	2985	974 (32.6%)
Pakistan	Tertiary care hospital, Karachi	952	129 (13.5%)

Table 2. Prevalence of NAFLD among the Indian, Sri Lanka and Pakistani people.

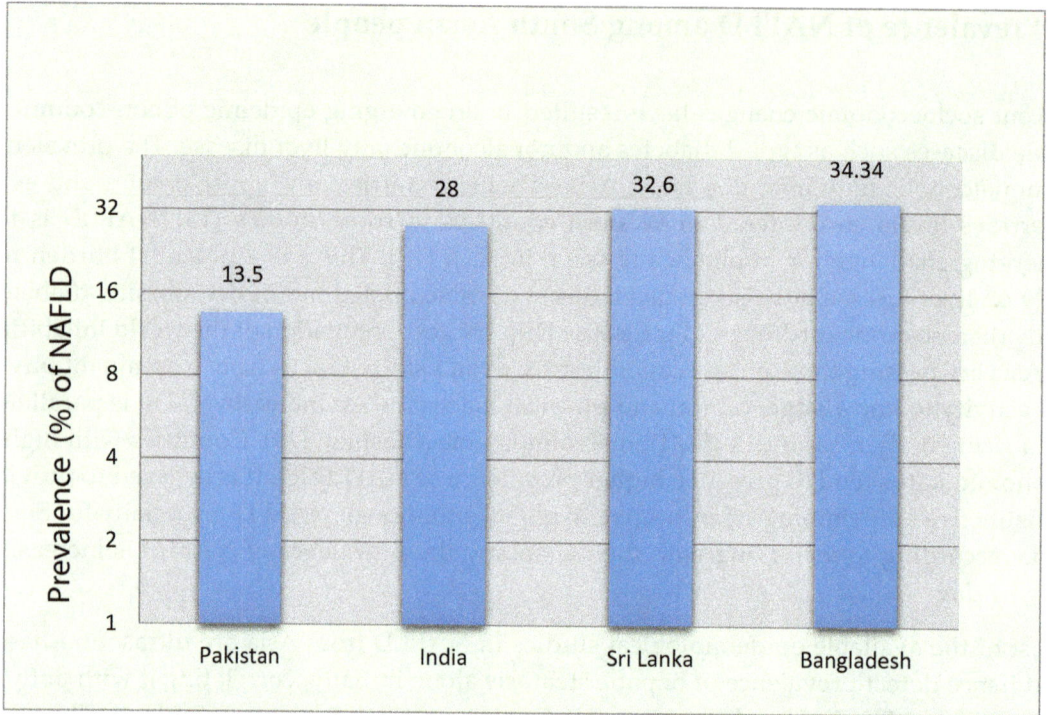

Figure 2. Prevalence of NAFLD in different countries of South Asia.

From the study of Alazawi et al. the prevalence of recorded NAFLD varied considerably by ethnic group. This study identified that Bangladeshi ethnicity as an independent risk factor for NAFLD. Diagnosed NAFLD was significantly more prevalent among people of Bangladesh ethnicity (1.8% of the adult population) than other ethnic group, including other South Asian groups. Among Bangladeshis, there are higher rates of type 2 diabetes and cardiovascular disease that may have a genetic basis. Transaminase were measured on 218,032 patients, of whom 31,627 had elevated serum transaminases. In a multivariate analysis, independent risk factors for NAFLD included Bangladeshi ethnicity, diabetes, raised BMI, hypertension, and hypercholesterolaemia. As expected, the prevalence of NAFLD was significantly lower in the African and Caribbean ethnic groups [19]. Female are predominant sufferers of NAFLD in Bangladesh [25]. So the prevalence of NAFLD in South Asia has been increased from previous reports and now it ranges from 14 to 34.34% in general population. In systematic searching in PubMed/MEDLINE database, we found research articles on epidemiology of NAFLD of India, Bangladesh, Sri Lanka and Pakistan. But we did not get any article relevant to the epidemiology of NAFLD of Afghanistan, Maldives, Nepal and Bhutan.

6. Prevalence of NASH and its progression

The active form of NAFLD is non-alcoholic steatohepatitis (NASH), which is characterized by hepatocyte injury with liver inflammation, and progression of fibrosis [26]. And it has emerged as one of the most important causes of liver failure and hepatocellular carcinoma. Up to 20% of cases NASH may progress to cirrhosis [27]. According to Alam et al. "Patients with NASH are at risk for progressive liver disease (which can progress to cirrhosis, hepatocellular carcinoma, and death from chronic liver disease), as well as cardiovascular mortality and type-2 diabetes" [25].

NASH is present in 42.4–53.1% cases of Bangladeshi NAFLD patients [25]. Diabetic is the principle cause to develop NASH. A study in Indian Diabetic Mellitus (DM) patient; it reported that severe NASH is present among 9.35% Indian DM patients [28]. Ultrasound based Indian study showed the prevalence of NAFLD to be 16.6%, while a study based on liver biopsy showed the presence of NASH was 53% [29, 30]. And in Sri Lanka a liver biopsy based study were performed on 296 patients and 100 (35.1%) were diagnosed as having NASH [31]. In another Asian study proven NASH at presentation was found in 32.6% patients of NAFLD [32].

Study from the West found that disease progression from NAFLD to NASH is 44% patients [33]. Multiple factors like obesity, insulin resistance, genetic factor, immune response and lipotoxicity are involved in the progression of NAFLD to NASH [34]. In patients with cirrhotic NASH, HCC and liver failure are the main causes of morbidity and mortality. A prospective Japanese study elucidated the progression from NASH to HCC is 11.3% [35]. The prevalence of NASH (9.35–59%) among NAFLD patients is much higher in South Asian countries than that of Western countries. Severity of NAFLD in the form of NASH is also highest in Bangladesh among the South Asian countries as evidenced by recent studies from tertiary level hospitals of the country.

7. Depiction of the magnitude among different risk group

According to Alam, one fourth of the Bangladeshi NAFLD patients are nonobese; among them 53.1% cases present NASH. Male are largely dominating in nonobese group, where female are in obese group [36]. High BMI, central obesity, triglyceridemia and age are important risk factors for Bangladeshi people, and risk factors contributed about 29% risk for the occurrence of NASH [37]. After adjusting the risk factors (BMI and TG) female gender is the independent risk for Bangladeshi [38]. Although insulin resistance (IR) is strongly associated with NAFLD, But IR is not the sole predictor in the pathogenesis of NAFLD [38–40].

In India the prevalence of NAFLD is 15–80% among obese people, 25–60% in patients with dyslipidemia and 33–55% in pre-diabetics and diabetics' Indian people [41]. Most of the non-diabetic NAFLD patients are overweight/obese with higher insulin resistance, dyslipidemia, and subclinical inflammation [42]. Among 65.7% Morbidly Obese South Indian Patients has NAFLD. Among them 33.6% were of NASH, 31.3% shows fibrosis and 14.1% shows advanced fibrosis [43]. The polymorphism T-455C in APOC3 gene and elevated serum triglycerides are associated with Indian NAFLD patients [44]. In another series, 56.5% T2DM patients have NAFLD, and the prevalence is higher in females (60%) than males T2DM patients [45]. NAFLD is the commonest liver disease in Indian psoriatic patients also [46]. Coronary artery disease (CAD) is more prevalent in the NAFLD compared to non-NAFLD; It is a surrogate and fairly reliable marker of risk for CAD among type 2 diabetic patients [47]. According to Duseja NAFLD is the commonest cause of unexplained elevation of SGPT and cryptogenic cirrhosis and hepatocellular carcinoma in Indian patients. Insulin resistance and full blown metabolic syndrome are highly prevalent in Indian patients with NAFLD [48]; 51.4% of patients of NAFLD have metabolic syndrome [49]. And it is really threatening news that 3% of 5–12 years Indian children have NAFLD [50].

In Sri Lanka Incidence rate of diabetes are 64.2 per 1000 person-years among NAFLD persons [51]. NAFLD is an independent predictor of developing diabetes mellitus [51]. Increased age and presence of NAFLD conferred a higher mortality risk from ACS as predicted by GRACE score [52].

As like developed countries obesity, insulin resistance, diabetes, dyslipidemia are the major risk factors for development of NAFLD. But the paradox is that it could develop in nonobese population also and one fourth of NAFLD of South Asia is from nonobese people.

8. Global and South Asian publication trend on NAFLD

According to Zhang et al. study, with the globally increasing prevalence, nonalcoholic fatty liver disease (NAFLD) becomes the predominant cause of chronic liver disease. The global scientific research articles relevant to NAFLD revealed 6356 articles were published in 994 different journals during 1986–2013. Starting from the late 1980s, the publication on NAFLD grew slowly and entered into a highly developing period in the 21st century, especially in the last decade (**Figure 3**). Bibliometric results suggest that the obviously rapid growth of the

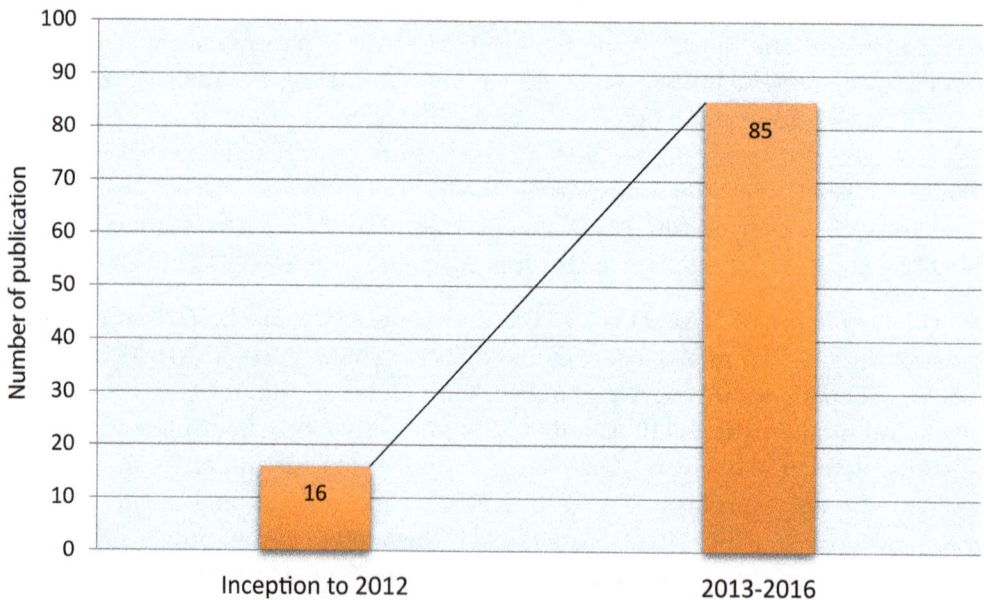

Figure 3. Trend of number of publication on NAFLD of South Asia (published in PubMed).

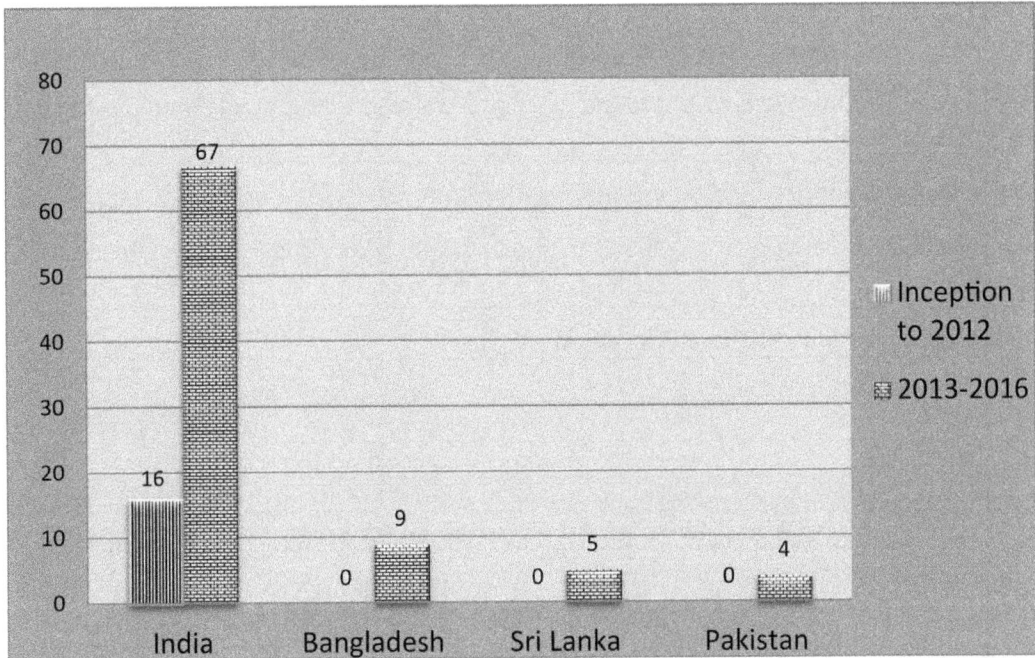

Figure 4. Article on NAFLD publication in South Asia Trend in PubMed from inception-2016.

articles in recent years appears to be associated with the accelerating incidence of NAFLD and its cofactors such as metabolic syndrome. In this study we found that, from inception to 2012 only 16 Indian research articles have been published in PubMed. Where from 2013 to 2016 total 85 research articles of India, Bangladesh, Sri Lanka and Pakistan has been published in PubMed (**Figure 4**). This phenomenon indicate that, how NAFLD is growing in South Asia.

9. Conclusion

The increase in NAFLD will continue to burden the health care system, especially because of its association with obesity, IR and metabolic syndrome. Along with globalization the prevalence of NAFLD is increasing alarmingly. The prevalence of NAFLD has been increasing remarkably for the last 12 years. Currently it is not only a disease of the Western countries but also becoming a major challenge for South Asia region. NAFLD is not the disease for only obese people, but it is also common in nonobese. And if the condition remains untreated it can turn into cirrhosis and hepatocellular carcinoma. It is really a great threat for us that, NAFLD is being seeing among our subcontinent's children also. The burden of NAFLD and its severity projects that obviously it will be the biggest frontier of Hepatology in South Asia in near future.

Author details

Shahinul Alam[1*], Thupten Kelsang Lama[2], Golam Mustafa[1], Mahabubul Alam[1] and Nooruddin Ahmad[1]

Address all correspondence to: shahinul67@yahoo.com

1 Department of Hepatology, Bangabandhu Sheikh Mujib Medical University, Dhaka, Bangladesh

2 Civil Service Hospital, Kathmandu, Nepal

References

[1] Arab JP, Candia R, Zapata R, Munoz C, Arancibia JP, Poniachik J, Soza A, Fuster F, Brahm J, Sanhueza E, Contreras J, Cuellar MC, Arrese M, Riquelme A. Management of nonalcoholic fatty liver disease: An evidence-based clinical practice review. World Journal of Gastroenterology. 2014;20:12182-12201 [PMID: 25232252]. DOI: 10.3748/wjg.v20.i34.12182

[2] Zhang TS, Qin HL, Wang T, Li HT, Li H, Xia SH, Xiang XH. Global publication trends and research hotspots of nonalcoholic fatty liver disease: A bibliometric analysis and systematic review. SpringerPlus. 2015;4:776 [PMID: 26697286]. DOI: 10.1186/s40064-015-1542-1

[3] Alazawi W, Mathur R, Abeysekera K, Hull S, Boomla K, Robson J, Foster GR. Ethnicity and the diagnosis gap in liver disease: A population-based study. The British Journal of General Practice. 2014;64:e694-e702 [PMID: 25348993]. DOI: 10.3399/bjgp14X682273

[4] Sherif ZA, Saeed A, Ghavimi S, Nouraie SM, Laiyemo AO, Brim H, Ashktorab H. Global epidemiology of nonalcoholic fatty liver disease and perspectives on US Minority populations. Digestive Diseases and Sciences. 2016;61:1214-1225 [PMID: 27038448]. DOI: 10.1007/s10620-016-4143-0

[5] Younossi ZM, Koenig AB, Abdelatif D, Fazel Y, Henry L, Wymer M. Global epidemiology of nonalcoholic fatty liver disease-meta-analytic assessment of prevalence, incidence, and outcomes. Hepatology. 2016;64:73-84. [PMID: 26707365]. DOI: 10.1002/hep.28431

[6] Chalasani N, Younossi Z, Lavine JE, Diehl AM, Brunt EM, Cusi K, Charlton M, Sanyal AJ. The diagnosis and management of non-alcoholic fatty liver disease: Practice Guideline by the American Association for the Study of Liver Diseases, American College of Gastroenterology, and the American Gastroenterological Association. Hepatology. 2012;55:2005-2023 [PMID: 22488764]. DOI: 10.1002/hep.25762

[7] Ashtari S, Pourhoseingholi MA, Zali MR. Non-alcohol fatty liver disease in Asia: Prevention and planning. World Journal of Hepatology. 2015;7:1788-1796 [PMID: 26167252]. DOI: 10.4254/wjh.v7.i13.1788

[8] Zhu JZ, Dai YN, Wang YM, Zhou QY, CH Y, Li YM. Prevalence of nonalcoholic fatty liver disease and economy. Digestive Diseases and Sciences. 2015;60:3194-3202. [PMID: 26017679]. DOI: 10.1007/s10620-015-3728-3

[9] Parkash O, Hamid S. Are we ready for a new epidemic of under recognized liver disease in South Asia especially in Pakistan? Nonalcoholic fatty liver disease. The Journal of the Pakistan Medical Association. 2013;63:95-99 [PMID: 23865141]

[10] Chan WK, Tan AT, Vethakkan SR, Tah PC, Vijayananthan A, Goh KL. Low physical activity and energy dense Malaysian foods are associated with non-alcoholic fatty liver disease in centrally obese but not in non-centrally obese patients with diabetes mellitus. Asia Pacific Journal of Clinical Nutrition. 2015;24:289-298 [PMID: 26078246]. DOI: 10.6133/apjcn.2015.24.2.15

[11] Rahman MM, Abedin T, Amin R, Rahman MR, Faiz MA. Nonalcoholic fatty liver disease—Is it always benign? Journal of Bangladesh College of Physicians and Surgeons. 2007;25(3):144-152. DOI: 10.3329/jbcps.v25i3.411

[12] Ruhl CE, Everhart JE. Fatty liver indices in the multiethnic United States National Health and Nutrition Examination Survey. Alimentary Pharmacology & Therapeutics. 2015;41:65-76 [PMID: 25376360]. DOI: 10.1111/apt.13012

[13] Munteanu MA, Nagy GA, Mircea PA. Current management of NAFLD. Clujul Medical. 2016;89:19-23. [PMID: 27004021]. DOI: 10.15386/cjmed-539

[14] LaBrecque DR, Abbas Z, Anania F, Ferenci P, Khan AG, Goh KL, Hamid SS, Isakov V, LizarzabalM, PenarandaMM, RamosJF, SarinS, StimacD, ThomsonAB, UmarM, Krabshuis J, LeMair A. World Gastroenterology Organisation global guidelines: Nonalcoholic fatty liver disease and nonalcoholic steatohepatitis. Journal of Clinical Gastroenterology. 2014;48:467-473. [PMID: 24921212]. DOI: 10.1097/mcg.0000000000000116

[15] Pandit K, Goswami S, Ghosh S, Mukhopadhyay P, Chowdhury S. Metabolic syndrome in South Asians. Indian Journal of Endocrinology and Metabolism. 2012;16:44-55. [PMID: 22276252]. DOI: 10.4103/2230-8210.91187

[16] United Nations, Department of Economic and Social Affairs, Population Division. World Urbanization Prospects: The 2014 Revision. The United Nations, New York; 2014

[17] Baten J. A History of the Global Economy. Cambridge, UK: Cambridge University Press; 2016

[18] Mahady SE, George J. The future liver of the Asia pacific: Fatter and firmer from more fructose and fortune? Journal of Clinical and Experimental Hepatology. 2013;3:106-113 [PMID: 25755484]. DOI: 10.1016/j.jceh.2012.10.011

[19] Chowdhury A, Younossi ZM. Global epidemiology and risk factors for nonalcoholic fatty liver disease. Alcoholic and Non-Alcoholic Fatty Liver Disease: Springer. 2016:21-40

[20] Alam S, Chowdhury MAB, Azam G, Ahsan M, Mustafa G, Hossain M, Khan M, Ahmed N. Prevalence of fatty liver in Bangladesh: A nation wide population based study. Hepatology International. 2017;11:S553. DOI: 10.1007/s12072-016-9783-9

[21] Hoque MK, AMM, Islam MB. Prevalence of non-alcoholic fatty liver disease in rural population of Bangladesh. Hepatology International. 2017;**11**:S961. DOI: 10.1007/s12072-016-9783-9

[22] Hoque MI. NAFLD in Bangladesh. Abstract Book 1st Conference of SASL2013. p. 69

[23] Rahman MMKM, Begum H, Haque M, Sultana N, Akhter M. Prevalence and risk factors of nonalcoholic fatty liver disease in a rural Community of South Asia. Gastroenterology Research and Practice. 2015;**148**:S1045-S1046

[24] Dassanayake AS, Kasturiratne A, Rajindrajith S, Kalubowila U, Chakrawarthi S, De Silva AP, Makaya M, Mizoue T, Kato N, Wickremasinghe AR, de Silva HJ. Prevalence and risk factors for non-alcoholic fatty liver disease among adults in an urban Sri Lankan population. Journal of Gastroenterology and Hepatology. 2009;**24**:1284-1288 [PMID: 19476560. DOI: 10.1111/j.1440-1746.2009.05831.x

[25] Alam S, Noor EASM, Chowdhury ZR, Alam M, Kabir J. Nonalcoholic steatohepatitis in nonalcoholic fatty liver disease patients of Bangladesh. World Journal of Hepatology. 2013;**5**:281-287 [PMID: 23717739]. DOI: 10.4254/wjh.v5.i5.281

[26] Wong VW-S, Chitturi S, Wong GL-H, Yu J, Chan HL-Y, Farrell GC. Pathogenesis and novel treatment options for non-alcoholic steatohepatitis. The Lancet Gastroenterology & Hepatology. 2016;**1**:56-67

[27] Matteoni CA, Younossi ZM, Gramlich T, Boparai N, Liu YC, McCullough AJ. Nonalcoholic fatty liver disease: A spectrum of clinical and pathological severity. Gastroenterology. 1999;**116**(6):1413-1419 [PMID: 10348825]

[28] Gupte P, Amarapurkar D, Agal S, Baijal R, Kulshrestha P, Pramanik S, Patel N, Madan A, Amarapurkar A. Non-alcoholic steatohepatitis in type 2 diabetes mellitus. Journal of Gastroenterology and Hepatology. 2004;**19**:854-858

[29] Yilmaz Y, Eren F. A Bayesian approach to an integrated multimodal noninvasive diagnosis of definitive nonalcoholic steatohepatitis in the spectrum of nonalcoholic fatty liver disease. European Journal of Gastroenterology & Hepatology. 2014;**26**:1292-1295 [PMID: 25171027]. DOI: 10.1097/meg.0000000000000184

[30] Duseja A, Das A, Das R, Dhiman RK, Chawla Y, Bhansali A, Kalra N. The clinicopathological profile of Indian patients with nonalcoholic fatty liver disease (NAFLD) is different from that in the West. Digestive Diseases and Sciences. 2007;**52**:2368-2374 [PMID: 17420951]. DOI: 10.1007/s10620-006-9136-y

[31] De Hewavisenthi SJ, Dassanayaka AS, De Silva HJ. Clinical, biochemical and histological characteristics of a Sri Lankan population of non-alcoholic steatohepatitis (NASH) patients. The Ceylon Medical Journal. 2005;**50**:113-116 [PMID: 16252575]

[32] Wong VW, Wong GL, Choi PC, Chan AW, Li MK, Chan HY, Chim AM, Yu J, Sung JJ, Chan HL. Disease progression of non-alcoholic fatty liver disease: A prospective study with paired liver biopsies at 3 years. Gut. 2010;**59**:969-974. [PMID: 20581244]. DOI: 10.1136/gut.2009.205088

[33] McPherson S, Hardy T, Henderson E, Burt AD, Day CP, Anstee QM. Evidence of NAFLD progression from steatosis to fibrosing-steatohepatitis using paired biopsies: Implications for prognosis and clinical management. Journal of Hepatology. 2015;62:1148-1155 [PMID: 25477264]. DOI: 10.1016/j.jhep.2014.11.034

[34] Sharma M, Mitnala S, Vishnubhotla RK, Mukherjee R, Reddy DN, Rao PN. The riddle of nonalcoholic fatty liver disease: Progression from nonalcoholic fatty liver to nonalcoholic steatohepatitis. Journal of Clinical and Experimental Hepatology. 2015;5:147-158 [PMID: 26155043]. DOI: 10.1016/j.jceh.2015.02.002

[35] Hashimoto E, Tokushige K. Prevalence, gender, ethnic variations, and prognosis of NASH. Journal of Gastroenterology. 2011;46:S63-S69 [PMID: 20844903]. DOI: 10.1007/s00535-010-0311-8

[36] Alam S, Gupta UD, Alam M, Kabir J, Chowdhury ZR, Alam AK. Clinical, anthropometric, biochemical, and histological characteristics of nonobese nonalcoholic fatty liver disease patients of Bangladesh. Indian Journal of Gastroenterology. 2014;33:452-457 [PMID: 25023045]. DOI: 10.1007/s12664-014-0488-5

[37] Majid N, Ali Z, Rahman MR, Akhter A, Rajib RC, Ahmad F, Sharmin S, Akond AK, Huq N. Histological scoring and associated risk factors of non-alcoholic fatty liver disease. Mymensingh Medical Journal. 2013;22:767-772 [PMID: 24292310]

[38] Hossain IA, Akter S, Rahman MK, Ali L. Gender specific association of serum leptin and insulinemic indices with nonalcoholic fatty liver disease in prediabetic subjects. PLoS One. 2015;10:e0142165 [PMID: 26569494]. DOI: 10.1371/journal.pone.0142165

[39] Alam S, Mustafa G, Alam M, Ahmad N. Insulin resistance in development and progression of nonalcoholic fatty liver disease. World Journal of Gastrointestinal Pathophysiology. 2016;7:211-217 [PMID: 27190693]. DOI: 10.4291/wjgp.v7.i2.211

[40] Hossain IA, Rahman Shah MM, Rahman MK, Ali L. Gamma glutamyl transferase is an independent determinant for the association of insulin resistance with nonalcoholic fatty liver disease in Bangladeshi adults: Association of GGT and HOMA-IR with NAFLD. Diabetes and Metabolic Syndrome: Clinical Research and Reviews. 2016;10:S25-S29. [PMID: 26482965]. DOI: 10.1016/j.dsx.2015.09.005

[41] Tandon RK. Emergence of non-alcoholic fatty liver disease (NAFLD). Journal of the Association of Physicians of India. 2013;61:445-446 [PMID: 24772745]

[42] Bhatt SP, Misra A, Nigam P, Guleria R, Pasha MA. Phenotype, body composition, and prediction equations (Indian fatty liver index) for non-alcoholic fatty liver disease in non-diabetic Asian Indians: A case-control study. PLoS One. 2015;10:e0142260 [PMID: 26599361]. DOI: 10.1371/journal.pone.0142260

[43] Praveenraj P, Gomes RM, Kumar S, Karthikeyan P, Shankar A, Parthasarathi R, Senthilnathan P, Rajapandian S, Palanivelu C. Prevalence and predictors of non-alcoholic fatty liver disease in morbidly obese south indian patients undergoing bariatric surgery. Obesity Surgery. 2015;25:2078-2087 [PMID: 25835982]. DOI: 10.1007/s11695-015-1655-1

[44] Puppala J, Bhrugumalla S, Kumar A, Siddapuram SP, Viswa PD, Kondawar M, Akka J, Munshi A. Apolipoprotein C3 gene polymorphisms in Southern Indian patients with nonalcoholic fatty liver disease. Indian Journal of Gastroenterology. 2014;**33**:524-529 [PMID: 25319715]. DOI: 10.1007/s12664-014-0504-9

[45] Kalra S, Vithalani M, Gulati G, Kulkarni CM, Kadam Y, Pallivathukkal J, Das B, Sahay R, Modi KD. Study of prevalence of nonalcoholic fatty liver disease (NAFLD) in type 2 diabetes patients in India (SPRINT). The Journal of the Association of Physicians of India. 2013;**61**:448-453 [PMID: 24772746]

[46] Madanagobalane S, Anandan S. The increased prevalence of non-alcoholic fatty liver disease in psoriatic patients: A study from South India. Australian Journal of Dermatology. 2012;**53**:190-197 [PMID: 22672067]. DOI: 10.1111/j.1440-0960.2012.00905.x

[47] Agarwal AK, Jain V, Singla S, Baruah BP, Arya V, Yadav R, Singh VP. Prevalence of non-alcoholic fatty liver disease and its correlation with coronary risk factors in patients with type 2 diabetes. The Journal of the Association of Physicians of India. 2011;**59**:351-354 [PMID: 21751587]

[48] Duseja A. Nonalcoholic fatty liver disease in India—A lot done, yet more required! Indian Journal of Gastroenterology. 2010;**29**:217-225 [PMID: 21191681]. DOI: 10.1007/s12664-010-0069-1

[49] Gaharwar R, Trikha S, Margekar SL, Jatav OP, Ganga PD. Study of clinical profile of patients of nonalcoholic fatty liver disease and its association with metabolic syndrome. The Journal of the Association of Physicians of India. 2015;**63**:12-16 [PMID: 26591121]

[50] Chaturvedi K, Vohra P. Non-alcoholic fatty liver disease in children. Indian Pediatrics. 2012;**49**:757-758 [PMID: 23024085]

[51] Kasturiratne A, Weerasinghe S, Dassanayake AS, Rajindrajith S, de Silva AP, Kato N, Wickremasinghe AR, de Silva HJ. Influence of non-alcoholic fatty liver disease on the development of diabetes mellitus. Journal of Gastroenterology and Hepatology. 2013;**28**:142-147 [PMID: 22989165]. DOI: 10.1111/j.1440-1746.2012.07264.x

[52] Perera N, Indrakumar J, Abeysinghe WV, Fernando V, Samaraweera W, Lawrence JS. Nonalcoholic fatty liver disease increases the mortality from acute coronary syndrome: An observational study from Sri Lanka. BMC Cardiovascular Disorders. 2016;**16**:1

4

Diagnosis and Characterization of Non-Alcoholic Fatty Liver Disease

Paula Iruzubieta, Marta González, Joaquín Cabezas,
María Teresa Arias-Loste and Javier Crespo

Abstract

Non-alcoholic fatty liver disease (NAFLD) can develop cirrhosis and even hepatocellular carcinoma, resulting in a high liver-related morbidity and mortality, being important to know those risk factors for disease progression, among which the presence of diabetes stands out. In addition, it is a disease with multisystemic behavior, becoming an independent risk factor for cardiovascular disease and extrahepatic tumors. Hence, early diagnosis and multidisciplinary management of NAFLD are really important. In this chapter, we will expose the different diagnostic and follow-up tools available for this disease, and with them we will make an algorithm according to the recommendations and the current evidence.

Keywords: NAFLD, biomarkers, transient elastography, multisystemic disease

1. Introduction

Non-alcoholic fatty liver disease (NAFLD) includes a wide spectrum of liver damage whose distinctive feature is the accumulation of intrahepatic fat, especially triglycerides, which cannot be attributed to secondary causes such as alcohol and certain drugs. NAFLD is nowadays considered to be the most common cause of chronic liver disease in western countries, showing a prevalence of around 30% in the general population [1]. Within NAFLD, two histological subtypes can be distinguished: (a) non-alcoholic fatty liver (NAFL), which includes patients with simple steatosis with or without mild inflammation and (b) non-alcoholic steatohepatitis (NASH), characterized by the presence of hepatic inflammation and hepatocyte injury (ballooning) with or without fibrosis [2, 3]. NAFL is a generally benign condition, and NASH is the progressive subtype that can lead to cirrhosis and hepatocellular carcinoma

(HCC) [4]. However, several studies with paired liver biopsies have demonstrated that both patients with NASH and those with NAFL have the potential to develop a progressive hepatic disease, and in this risk of progression there are some key factors such as diabetes mellitus [5, 6]. In general, patients with NAFLD have a higher long-term mortality than the general population, cardiovascular disease (CVD) being the principal cause of death, followed by different types of cancer [7–9] and liver-related complications, as well as the cardiovascular risk caused by the different factors of the metabolic syndrome, very frequent in this type of subjects; NAFLD is itself an independent risk factor for CVD [10]. Liver-related mortality is increased up to 10-fold in patients with NAFLD. In this sense, it should be emphasized that cirrhosis and HCC are the fifth most prevalent cause of mortality in the world. Therefore, given the hepatic and cardiovascular morbi-mortality generated by NAFLD, the early iden-tification of these patients is important to provide suitable management that can lower the mortality for all causes.

2. Screening and diagnostic criteria

The mechanisms leading to the development and progression of NAFLD are not completely known, but it is widely accepted that the initial events are dependent on the development of obesity and insulin resistance (IR) [11]. For this reason, NAFLD has a strong association with the factors constituting the metabolic syndrome, the prevalence in this group of patients being considerably heightened. This relation is especially close in morbid obesity, where NAFLD is present in more than 90% of the cases, this condition taking the form of steatohepatitis in a third of the cases, while in up to 5–10% of the subjects, the liver disease has progressed to cirrhosis [12, 13]. The association between NAFLD and IR or diabetes mellitus type 2 (DM2) has also been clearly established [14]. It has been demonstrated that DM2 is associated with a greater hepatic content of triglycerides independently of the body mass index (BMI) [15, 16]. Thus, the prevalence of NAFLD in DM2 patients can reach up to 70% [11, 17, 18]. Moreover, both prediabetes (glucose intolerance and altered glucose when fasting) and DM2 are related to the severity of liver damage, the presence of steatohepatitis, fibrosis and even HCC [1, 19, 20]. Overall, 80% of the NAFLD cases present with some of the cardiovascular risk factors that constitute the metabolic syndrome (IR, obesity, dyslipidemia and arterial hypertension), and its prevalence directly increases the number of these factors that are present [21].

As a consequence of its high prevalence, especially in subjects with the abovementioned risk factors, its prognostic implications, and given that NAFLD is generally an asymptomatic dis-ease, some authors recommend the implantation of an NAFLD-screening programme within the risk population [22, 23]. However, this topic is at present controversial given the great load on the national health systems that could be caused by these screening programmes and the lack of efficacious treatments currently available. In fact, the principal associations for the study of liver diseases (American Association for the Study of Liver Diseases (AASLD) and European Association for the Study of the Liver (EASL)) in their guidelines for clinical practice do not recommend this screening in any population [24] or they recommend it, with an A2 level of evidence, only for patients with DM2 independently of the levels of hepatic enzymes [25]. To attempt to answer this question, valid cost-utility studies are necessary in screening programmes. There is no discussion, however, about the need to act when faced with a patient suspected of having NAFLD and not to underestimate its discovery due to the limited clinical and analytical repercussion manifested at first. In our opinion, patients with NAFLD and suspected to have advanced disease must be evaluated in specialist units for their correct characterization in case of a prompt availability of specific treatment.

2.1. Clinical and analytical manifestations

A diagnosis of NAFLD is very often reached through a casual analytical discovery during a health examination after an alteration in tests of liver function, or an alteration in hepatic morphology detected through an image study done with another objective, given that it is generally an asymptomatic disease. In the cases in which the patient reports symptoms, they are usually mild and unspecific, asthenia and abdominal problems being frequent, especially in the right hypochondria. The physical exploration may be normal or detect a soft, painless hepatomegaly, although occasionally it is difficult to evaluate as these patients very often present with central-type obesity, and in the patients with advanced fibrosis and cirrhosis, we may find signs of portal hypertension such as ascites, splenomegaly or jaundice [26].

Analytically, most of the patients present tests with normal or discretely altered liver function, with a predominance of ALT (alanine aminotransferase) compared to AST (aspartate aminotransferase). On specific occasions, a discrete elevation can be appreciated in the markers of cholestasis, especially GGT (gamma-glutamyl transpeptidase), which has been related to obesity and IR [27]. Another frequent analytical discovery is the elevation of the levels of ferritin in blood and of the transferrin saturation index without having demonstrated a corresponding increase in the deposits of hepatic iron [28]. Something similar occurs with the presence of elevated autoantibodies, which appear quite frequently in NAFLD and are considered an epiphenomenon [29].

2.2. Diagnosis of steatosis

Hepatic steatosis is defined histologically as the deposit of fat ≥5% of the hepatocytes and is classified in four grades depending on the percentage of hepatocytes with steatotic vacuoles. The normal liver (S0) contains fat in less than 5% of the hepatocytes while grade 1 steatosis (S1) corresponds to less than 33% of the steatotic hepatocytes. In grade 2 and 3 steatosis, fat is present in at least 33 or 66% of the hepatocytes, respectively.

The presence of risk factors such as DM2, metabolic syndrome and obesity with the elevation of the hepatic enzymes, especially ALT, increases the possibility of fatty liver presenting. Nevertheless, although the ALT is a useful test, it is not valid for predicting the presence of this disease, or even the risk of progression, given that it can occur with normal hepatic enzymes [30]. In fact, in patients with DM2 and normal levels of ALT, a high prevalence of NAFL and NASH has been reported [31].

In clinical practice, ultrasound scan is a first-rate image technique if NAFLD is suspected due to its wide availability, low cost and safety [32]. The sensitivity of this technique is 93%

when the steatosis is greater than 33%; however, this sensitivity decreases considerably when the steatosis affects less than 30% of the hepatocytes [33, 34]. Steatosis can also be diagnosed through computerized tomography (CT), but its cost and the patient's exposure to radiation make its systematic use in long-term follow-up unadvisable in this pathology; moreover, its sensitivity does not improve substantially if the steatosis is mild [32]. Magnetic resonance imaging (MRI), including spectroscopy, can diagnose content levels of hepatic fat >5% and it is reliable to determine changes (≥0.5%) in the grade of steatosis after weight loss. Although its use has widened in many studies, its use in clinical practice is limited by its cost and duration [35, 36].

The recently developed CAP (controlled attenuation parameter), an application of transient elastography (TE), which will be discussed later, available in the latest generation devices, enables the immediate and easy quantification of steatosis. CAP measures the degree of attenuation of the ultrasound wave transmitted through the liver, which is proportional to the amount of hepatic fat, and is less influenced by the sampling error than the liver biopsy, since it explores a liver volume approximately 100 times greater. Its values oscillate between 100 and 400 dB/m and it is possible to measure the liver stiffness used for the evaluation of fibrosis simultaneously. The studies published to date indicate that CAP is capable of diagnosing steatosis in chronic liver diseases of diverse causes even in mild stages (>10%) and has a good correlation with the degree of steatosis [37–44]. These studies show different cut-offs of CAP for the different grades of steatosis, but all of them demonstrate that the cut-offs do not differ among the different causes of liver diseases, in contrast with what happens with transient elastography [40]. In this sense, a recent meta-analysis including 2735 patients has established a series of cut-offs for the different grades of steatosis: 248 dB/m for S1, 268 dB/m for S2 and 280 dB/m for S3, with a sensitivity of 69, 77 and 88%, respectively, and a specificity of 82, 81 and 78%, respectively. In this meta-analysis, etiology, BMI and diabetes showed a significant influence on the value of the CAP, so the authors suggested the cut-offs established but subtracting 10 dB/m from the value of the CAP for the patients with NAFLD, 10 dB/m for diabetics, and subtracting/adding 4.4 dB/m for each unit of BMI above/below 25 kg/m^2 in the interval of 20–30 kg/m^2 [45].

Another image technique is magnetic resonance imaging-estimated proton density fat fraction (MRI-PDFF), which is based on chemical shift-based water fat separation methods. MRI-PDFF has shown good correlation with histology-determined steatosis grade in NAFLD patients, so it could be used for follow-up and treatment-response evaluation [46].

Lastly, within the non-invasive diagnosis of steatosis, various serological tests of biomarkers have been developed to predict the existence of hepatic fat (**Table 1**) [47–51]. However, all these biomarkers may be influenced by inflammation and fibrosis, and given that they do not provide great advantages compared to image techniques and routine analysis, their use in clinical practice is not widespread; even so, the Fatty Liver Index (FLI) that uses easily available parameters could be considered, although CAP has demonstrated better performance than this test for the diagnosis of grade 2–3 steatosis [44]. Nevertheless, FLI has been associated independently to liver-related mortality, as well as to the mortality rates due to

Indices	Formula	Cut-offs	Sensitivity (%)	Specificity (%)
Hepatic Steatosis Index (HSI)	8 × ALT/AST ratio + BMI (+2, if DM; +2, if female)	30 (low cut-off) 36 (high cut-off)	93 45	40 93
Fatty liver Index (FLI)	exp(n)/1 + exp (n) × 100 (n) = 0.953 × ln(TG) + 0.139 × BMI + 0.718 × ln(GGT) + 0.053 × waist circumference − 15.745	10 (low cut-off) 60 (high cut-off)	95 44	29 91
SteatoTest	Proprietary formula (a2-macroglobulin, haptoglobin, apolipoprotein A1, GGT, bilirubin, ALT, cholesterol, triglycerides, glucose, BMI, age, gender)	0.3 (low cut-off) 0.7 (high cut-off)	90 46	54 88
NAFLD liver Fat score	−2.89 + 1.18 × metabolic Syndrome (yes: 1, no: 0) + 0.45 × Type 2 diabetes (yes: 2, no: 0) + 0.15 × insulin + 0.04 × AST − 0.94 × AST/ALT	−0.640	86	71
Lipid accumulation product (LAP)	LAP (men) = Waist circumference − 65 LAP (women) = Waist circumference − 58	20 (low cut-off) 80 (high cut-off)	99 43	16 94

Table 1. Indices for diagnosis of steatosis.

cardiovascular disease and cancer, but it seems that these associations are interfered by the risk conferred by the state of insulin resistance [52].

When steatosis is suspected in the aforementioned non-invasive methods, the liver biopsy is still the gold-standard method to conclusively diagnose NAFLD and the only one capable of distinguishing between NAFL and NASH, thus enabling the classification of the disease according to the grade of activity (inflammation and hepatocyte injury) and the stage of fibro-sis, the best predictors of the disease progression [53, 54]. The advantages and, especially, the drawbacks of the liver biopsy are dealt with later.

2.3. Initial diagnosis of NAFLD

From what has been mentioned so far, we can specify a series of characteristics that indicate a patient with NAFLD: (1) radiological evidence of steatosis or CAP >248 dB/m ± Abnormal liver blood test, (2) the presence of insulin resistance or another component of the metabolic syndrome, (3) consumption of alcohol of <30 g/d in men and <20 g/d in women and (4) exclu-sion from other causes of chronic liver disease (viral hepatitis, cholestatic diseases, autoim-mune hepatitis, hemochromatosis, α1 antitrypsin deficiency, Wilson's disease, drug-induced liver injury and celiac disease) [24, 25]. Once the initial diagnosis of NAFLD has been made, our next step is to evaluate the stage of disease and the necessity of carrying out a liver biopsy.

3. Diagnosis of steatohepatitis

A key element in the diagnosis of NAFLD is the differentiation of NASH from NAFL and the staging of the liver fibrosis, given that patients with NASH and advanced fibrosis are those at the greatest risk of developing hepatic complications and cardiovascular disease [54–56].

3.1. Liver biopsy

As it was mentioned earlier, the chosen method to evaluate the grade of histological lesion is still the liver biopsy. However, liver biopsy has well-known limitations and cannot be proposed for all patients, given the high prevalence of NAFLD worldwide. Liver biopsy is invasive and is not without complications. Besides, there are other drawbacks: (1) sampling error, since a typical liver biopsy samples only 1/50,000 of all liver tissues, and histolog-ical lesions of NASH are unevenly distributed throughout the liver parenchyma [57]; (2) inter- and intra-observer variability, as observed by Gawrieh et al. although there was a high agreement ratio in the assessment of steatosis grading and fibrosis staging between patholo-gists, the agreement was suboptimal for lobular inflammation and hepatocellular ballooning [58]; and (3) the existence of different criteria for the definition of NASH. The Non-alcoholic Steatohepatitis Clinical Research Network (NASH-CRN) proposed the system termed the NAS scoring system in order to classify NAFLD according to severities of fatty change, inflammation and hepatocellular ballooning [3]. NAS is markedly reproducible and is useful for assessing therapeutic effects in Clinical trials, but it is incapable of diagnosing NASH in patients with burned-out NASH, in whom fatty changes and inflammatory cell infiltration resolving in fibrosis have progressed [59].

Given these limitations, non-invasive methods have been developed for the diagnosis of NASH and fibrosis as a first option to examine NAFLD patients and to help determine which require a liver biopsy. The ideal test should be economical, reproducible and capable of diagnosing the whole spectrum of lesions, including within NAFLD, and even reflecting the changes produced on initiating specific treatment. Nowadays, we do not have a test available that has these characteristics, so these non-invasive methods are based on diverse complementary approaches: clinical factors, genetics, serological markers, image tests and transient elastography [60, 61].

3.2. Risk factors associated with non-alcoholic steatohepatitis and progressive disease

The best predictor of the evolution of NAFLD is the presence of necroinflammation and fibrosis in liver biopsy; however, there are more and more studies reporting no insignificant rates of progression of simple steatosis [5, 6, 62]. A first study that analyzed patients with NAFLD and paired biopsies demonstrated that even patients with simple steatosis can progress to NASH and advanced fibrosis, especially in the presence of metabolic risk factors [6]. Therefore, there is a series of non-modifiable and modifiable factors in patients associated with a greater risk of development of NASH and more progressive disease.

Various transversal studies have demonstrated that the disease is more severe in older patients, although this phenomenon could be due to the sum of pathogenic factors and a greater duration of the liver disease itself and the associated diseases [8, 63, 64]. In fact, the longitudinal studies have not managed to demonstrate that age is a factor that aggravates the disease per se [65]. The association between sex and fibrosis progression is controversial; two transversal studies show that men and post-menopause women have a greater risk of fibrosis in comparison with pre-menopause women; moreover, precocious menopause is associated with a greater risk of fibrosis [66–69]. Other non-modifiable factors are genetic; dozens of genes with multiple polymorphisms associated with NAFLD have been discovered thanks to genome-wide association studies (*GWAS*), but the number of strongly validated genes in large independent cohorts is limited to two, *patatin-like phospholipase domain containing 3* (PNPLA3) and *transmembrane 6 superfamily member 2* (TM6SF2) [70]. The presence of the single nucleotide polymorphisms (SNPs) rs738409 and rs58542926 of the genes PNPLA3 and TM6SF2, respectively, has been associated with a greater risk of NAFLD, as well as a more severe disease [71–76]. Recently, an SNP of IL28b (also implicated in the response to interferon in chronic hepatitis C patients (VHC)) has been associated with an increment in fibrosis in NAFLD patients [77]. Moreover, in a control-case study carried out by our working group, we have observed that the presence of the variants rs1421085 and rs1558902 of the fat mass and obesity-associated (FTO) gene confer a high risk of liver inflammation particularly in patients of normal weight with NAFLD (unpublished).

On the other hand, NAFLD tends to be more severe in patients with various factors of the metabolic syndrome, particularly DM2 and obesity. In fact, the reduction in weight and good glycemic control are associated with an improvement in inflammation and liver fibrosis [11, 78, 79]. However, it is known that NASH can also be present in slim subjects although it is unknown whether the natural history of the disease in these slim subjects is similar to that present in obese subjects. As for arterial hypertension, it is arguable whether its treatment improves the histology of NASH [5, 80]. Another factor of the metabolic syndrome, frequent in NAFLD patients, is dyslipidemia, fundamentally in the form of hypertriglyceridemia and atherogenic dyslipidemia [64, 81]; but moreover, a recent study has related the very low-density lipoprotein (VLDL) profile with the NAFLD severity, observing that a decrease in small VLDL particle concentration is associated with more advanced fibrosis [82]. Vitamin D deficiency is also frequent among NAFLD patients, and its levels have been correlated negatively with the severity of steatosis, inflammation and fibrosis [83, 84].

Another possible factor associated with NAFLD progression is the alcohol consumption, a controversial aspect as despite there being a limit above which the consumption of alcohol would define alcoholic steatohepatitis (≥ 60 g/d in women and ≥80 g/d in men), it is not clear that we are confronting a pathology different to NASH given that the pathogeny of these entities presents a great similarity. Moreover, the quantification of alcohol consumption is quite subjective, imprecise, habitually underestimated and not contrasted with objective determinations through biomarkers. At present, there is no agreement on the impact of light-moderate consumption of alcohol on NAFLD given that the literature available about this topic shows contradictory results relate to NAFLD progression [85, 86]. Nevertheless, it seems that all the relevant studies are in favor of a possible benefit from the moderate alcohol consumption, defined as the consumption of up to one drink a day for women and two drinks a day for men [87]. While the consumption of large doses of alcohol leads to the development of insulin resistance and to the infiltration of macrophages into the adipose tissue [88], moderate consumption has been associated with an improvement in the sensitivity to insulin and high concentrations of adiponectin [89–91]. Various studies suggest a significant association between the moderate consumption of alcohol and the less histological severity of NAFLD [92, 93]. As for the development of HCC, only one prospective study exists that evaluates the consumption of alcohol with the risk of HCC in NAFLD, finding a greater risk of this tumor with moderate use of alcohol; however, this study is carried out in patients with cirrhosis due to established NASH, without evaluating the impact of alcohol on patients with a less severe disease [94].

3.3. Non-invasive diagnosis of non-alcoholic steatohepatitis

There is still no available image test in clinical practice capable of differentiating NAFL from NASH, so various biomarkers have been evaluated to predict the existence of NASH, which are related to pathogenesis pathways of the disease (apoptosis/cellular death, inflammation and oxidative stress).

The most studied serum biomarker associated with the presence of NASH is cytokeratin 18 fragments (CK18-F), a product of the degradation resulting from the apoptosis of hepatocytes mediated by caspase 3 [95], which is measured using enzyme-linked immunosorbent assay (ELISA). Various studies have demonstrated a significant increase in CK18-F in NASH patients in comparison with NAFL patients, and a positive correlation with fibrosis and the histological components of NASH [96, 97]. However, the sensitivity and specificity of this test are quite low, around 60% [98]. Oxidized low-density lipoprotein (LDL), thiobarbituric acid reactive substances (TBARS) and malonaldehyde have been used as markers of oxidative stress, but the results are contradictory [99, 100]. Among the markers of inflammation studied include leptin, protein C reactive, interleukin 6, hyaluronic acid, adiponectin and tumor necrosis factor α (TNFα). All of them have been evaluated in short series or pilot studies in heterogeneous groups of patients with contradictory results [101].

With the aim of improving the diagnostic value of the biomarkers, predictive models have been developed that combine some of these serum biomarkers with analytical parameters and clinical variables, but they have not been adequately validated, so up to now, they are not recommendable in clinical practice [102–107] (**Table 2**).

3.3.1. Emerging fields

Emerging fields in the search for non-invasive biomarkers of NAFLD are proteomics, metabolomics and epigenetics.

Proteomics provides essential information about the biologically active entity named protein. Thanks to proteomic analysis, key changes in serum protein expression levels have been demonstrated between control subjects and patients with different stages of fatty liver [108].

In the last years, studies about the use of metabolomic to discover biomarkers of progression of NAFLD have received great interest, and not only in this liver disease [109–111]. In fact, a Spanish group has developed the so-called OWL Liver Test that consists in the determination

Model	Variables	Sensitivity (%)	Specificity (%)
HAIR score	Hypertension, ALT, insulin resistance	80	89
NASHTest	Age, gender, weight, height, cholesterol, triglycerides, α2-macroglobulin, apolipoprotein A1, haptoglobin, GGT, ALT, AST, bilirubin	88	50
NASH score	PNPLA3 genotype, insulin, AST	75	74
Nice model	Ck18, ALT, metabolic syndrome	84	86
NAFLD diagnostic panel	Diabetes, gender, BMI, triglycerides, M30, M65-M30	91	47
OxNASH	Age, BMI, AST, 13-Hydroxyoctadecadienoic acid, linoleic acid	81	–

Table 2. Predictive models for non-alcoholic steatohepatitis.

of more than 500 serum metabolites through liquid chromatography coupled with mass spectrometry (LC–MS) in NAFLD patients obtaining a metabolomic profile that enables the differentiation between NAFL and NASH with good specificity and sensitivity [112]. Moreover, the same group thanks to the study of metabolomic profiles at the serum level observed two different subtypes of NAFLD according to the involvement of the methionine metabolism, subtype M and subtype no M, distinguishing those patients that could benefit from therapy with SAMe (S-adenosyl methionine) [113].

Recently, studies in rodents suggest that epigenetic events, inheritable events not caused by changes in DNA sequence, may influence susceptibility to NASH. The three most commonly described epigenetic mechanisms are DNA (CpG) methylation, post-translational histone modifications and microRNAs (miRNAs). Several miRNAs have been identified in serum/ plasma of NAFLD patients that show diagnostic potential for distinguishing NAFL from NASH and advanced fibrosis [114].

4. Diagnosis of hepatic fibrosis

The stage of fibrosis ranges from absent (F0) to cirrhosis (F4), with stages F2–F4 considered to be clinically significant and stages F3–F4 considered to be advanced fibrosis. Apart from liver biopsy, there are two broad categories of non-invasive markers used to determine the stage of liver fibrosis: serum and radiological markers. This stratification based on markers of fibrosis is more tractable than those used for NASH and so it is currently used to identify patients who are at risk of disease progression.

4.1. Serum biomarkers

There are two large groups of predictive models of advanced fibrosis: 'simple bedside models', which use a combination of routine blood tests and clinical variables, and 'complex models', which use serum markers of fibrosis (measures of extracellular matrix deposition and turnover).

Although several of these predictive models of advanced fibrosis have been evaluated (**Table 3**) [61, 66, 115], two of the tests have been more widely studied and have easily available parameters, *Fibrosis-4 index* (FIB-4) and *NAFLD Fibrosis Score* (NFS). FIB-4 is based on age, levels of AST, ALT and platelet count. Values of this index below −1.30 enable the exclusion of the presence of advanced fibrosis with a sensitivity of 74% and a specificity of 71%, while values above 2.67 indicate advanced fibrosis with a sensitivity and specificity of 33 and 98%, respectively [115]. NFS is another formula developed and validated for the detection of advanced fibrosis that includes age, BMI, presence of diabetes or hyperglycemia, platelet count, albumin and AST/ALT ratio (http://nafldscore.com/). In a meta-analysis of 13 studies with more than 3000 patients, a value of NFS < −1.455 had a sensitivity of 90% and a specificity of 60% to exclude advanced fibrosis, while a value of >0.676 identified the presence of it with a sensitivity of 67% and a specificity of 97% [116].

Model	Variables	Cut-offs	Sensitivity (%)	Specificity (%)
FIB-4	Age, AST and ALT levels, platelets	1.30 (low cut-off)	74	71
		2.67 (high cut-off)	33	98
NAFLD fibrosis score	Age, hyperglycemia, BMV, AST/ALT ratio, albumin, platelet	−1.455 (low cut-off)	90	60
		0.675 (high cut-off)	67	97
AST to platelet ratio index (APRI)	AST, platelet	1	27	89
AST/ALT ratio	AST, ALT	0.8 (low cut-off)	90	60
		1 (high cut-off)	67	97
BAAT score	BMI, age, ALT, serum triglycerides	2	71	80
BARD score	BMI, AST/ALT ratio, diabetes	2	89	44
Enhanced liver fibrosis (ELF) test	Age, hyaluronic acid, TIMP-1, PIIINP	8.5 (low cut-off)	80	90
		11.3 (high cut-off)		
FibroTest	α2-macroglobulin, haptoglobin, GGT, bilirubin, apolipoprotein	0.3 (low cut-off)	77	77
		0.7 (high cut-off)	15	90
Hepascore	Age, gender, bilirubin, hyaluronic acid, α2-macroglobulin	0.44	75	84

AST, aspartate aminotransferase; ALT, alanine aminotransferase; BMI, body mass index; TIMP-1, tissue inhibitor of metalloproteinase 1; PIIINP, procollagen III amino-terminal peptide; GGT, gamma glutamyl transferase.

Table 3. Predictive models for significant and advanced fibrosis in NAFLD patients.

The principal drawback of all these biomarkers is that none of them is specific of the liver and their results can be influenced by co-morbidities of patients, so a critical interpretation of the result is necessary.

4.2. Imaging methods to measure fibrosis

With respect to image techniques, transient elastography (FibroScan®) is the most widely used technique in the diagnosis of liver fibrosis, not only in NAFLD but also in different chronic liver diseases [117]. TE measures the propagation velocity of low-frequency waves (50 Hz) through the hepatic parenchyma using ultrasounds and is expressed in kilo Pascal (kPa); the higher the propagation velocity, the greater the stiffness of the tissue. The advantages provided by this technique are its speed, the immediacy of the results and the ease of handling. However, proper results require careful interpretation of data, based on at least 10 successful measurements, a success rate above 60% and an interquartile range (IQR) of <30% of the median value. A limitation of TE in NAFLD is the high rate of technical failure due to the attenuation of the elastic wave by interposition of adipose tissue secondary to the central obesity, very frequent in these patients. Although an XL probe has been developed, which enables greater penetration of the wave, this difficulty is often insurmountable [118, 119]. Moreover, this technique has been initially validated in patients with chronic infection by VHC [120], while the studies focusing on evaluating its use in NAFLD are smaller and have often used different cut-offs [42, 118, 121–129] (Table 4). According to the results of several studies, the cut-offs with M probe accepted for NAFLD patients are 7.0 kPa for significant fibrosis (≥F2), 8.7 kPa for advanced fibrosis (≥F3) and 10.3 kPa for cirrhosis (F4) [124, 126, 128]. When using the XL probe, these cut-offs differ as the measure of liver stiffness with this probe is less than that with the M probe in the same patient; in this case, 6.2, 7.2 and 7.9 kPa are the cut-offs for significant fibrosis, advanced fibrosis and cirrhosis, respectively [119, 130, 131].

Another liver elasticity-based imaging technique is ARFI (*acoustic radiation force impulse imaging*). Although for the time being there are few studies that have evaluated its utility in NAFLD patients, its great advantage is that it can be easily connected to traditional ultrasound scan enabling the positioning of the zone of interest under visual control [132, 133]. Another method suitable for studying the elastic properties of the hepatic parenchyma is magnetic resonance elastography (MRE). MRE can be more reliable than TE to diagnose advanced fibrosis; moreover, it has the advantage of being able to evaluate the whole hepatic parenchyma even in obese patients, but the technique is expensive and not widely available [134, 135]. Magnetic resonance imaging is more widely available and is the basis of new software called DEMILI (*Detection of Metabolic-Induced Liver Injury*), which through computerized optical analysis of its images determines a series of optical biomarkers enabling the detection of the presence of NASH (NASHMRI) and predicting significant fibrosis (FibroMRI) in NAFLD patients. For the detection of NASH, a cut-off has been established with NASHMRI of >0.5, presenting a sensitivity and specificity of 87 and 60%, respectively. In the case of FibroMRI, the cut-off is also >0.5 for the prediction of significant fibrosis with a sensitivity of 77% and a specificity of 80% [136]. Given that this technique enables the analysis of the total volume of the liver, as well as its use in the diagnosis of NASH and significant fibrosis, it enables the potential effects of a therapy to be monitored.

A recently developed technique is multiparametric magnetic resonance (MR) that includes T_1 mapping for fibrosis/inflammation imaging, T_2* mapping for liver iron quantification and proton magnetic resonance spectroscopy (^{1}H-MRS) for liver fat quantification. In a recent study, it has demonstrated good correlation with disease severity in NAFLD patients, showing excellent accuracy in quantifying both the inflammatory and fibrotic components of NAFLD [137].

A summary of the approach to the management and characterization of NAFLD patients is shown in **Figure 1**.

Study	Patients, n	Probe	Fibrosis Stage	Cut-off (kPa)	Sensitivity (%)	Specificity (%)
Yoneda et al. [122]	67	M	$F \geq 2$	6.65	82	91
			$F \geq 3$	8.0	87	84
			$F = 4$	17.0	100	98
Yoneda et al. [125]	97	M	$F \geq 2$	6.65	74	97
			$F \geq 3$	9.8	85	81
			$F = 4$	17.5	100	97
Nobili et al. [129]	52	M	$F \geq 2$	7.4	100	92
			$F \geq 3$	10.2	100	100
			$F = 4$	–		
Wong et al. [128]	246	M	$F \geq 2$	7.0	79	76
			$F \geq 3$	8.7	84	83
			$F = 4$	10.3	92	88
Lupsor et al. [124]	72	M	$F \geq 2$	6.8	67	84
			$F \geq 3$	10.4	100	97
			$F = 4$	–		
Petta et al. [118]	169	M	$F \geq 2$	7.25	69	70
			$F \geq 3$	8.75	76	78
			$F = 4$	–		
Kumar et al. [126]	205	M	$F \geq 2$	7.0	78	79
			$F \geq 3$	9.0	85	88
			$F = 4$	11.8	90	88
Pathik et al. [121]	110	M	$F \geq 2$	9.1	–	–
			$F \geq 3$	12.0	90	80
			$F = 4$	20.0	90	80
Cassinotto et al. [123]	291	M	$F \geq 2$	6.2	90	–
			$F \geq 3$	8.2	90	–
			$F = 4$	9.5	90	–
Imajo et al. [42]	142	M	$F \geq 2$	11.0	62	100
			$F \geq 3$	11.4	86	84
			$F = 4$	14.0	100	76

Table 4. Comparative studies of FibroScan with liver biopsy in the detection of fibrosis in NAFLD.

NAFLD approach

Identify metabolic risk factors	Disease activity			Identify contributing factors	Evaluation of cardiovascular risk	Nutritional assessment	Assessment of potential therapies
	Diagnose steatosis	Diagnose liver inflammation	Diagnose liver fibrosis				
Insulin resistance/Type 2 diabetes Hypertension Dyslipidemia Central obesity	**Serum biomarkers:** Fatty Liver Index Hepatic Steatosis Index **Imaging techniques:** Ultrasound scan CAP	**Serum biomarkers:** OWL Liver Test **Imaging techniques:** NASHMRI Liver biopsy	**Serum biomarkers:** NAFLD Fibrosis Score FIB-4 **Imaging techniques:** Transient elastography FibroMRI Liver biopsy	Drugs Alcohol Vitamin D déficit OSAS/ Psoriasis / POS/ Hypothyroidism PNPLA3 (I148M) / TMGSF2 (E167K)	Electrocardiogram Ankle-brachial index Carotid ultrasound	Lifestyle Dietary habits Physical activity	Weight-los agents Insulin sensitizers Anti-diabetic drugs Hepatoprotectans Antifibrotic drugs

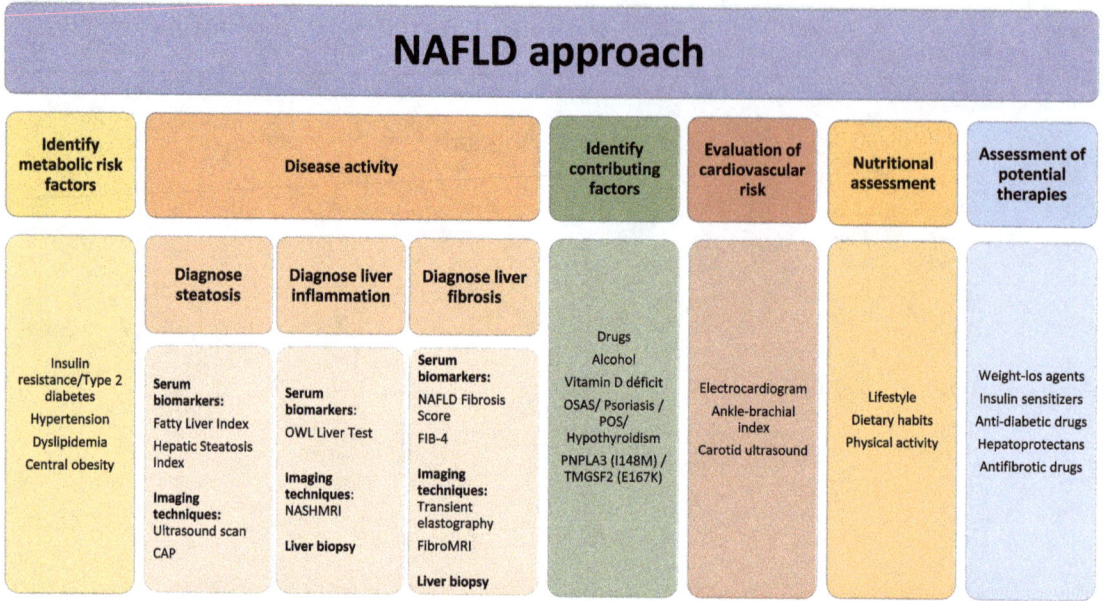

Figure 1. Practical approach to the management of patient with NAFLD.

5. Monitoring disease progression

A recent meta-analysis of 11 studies that evaluated the progression of NAFLD through the use of paired liver biopsies revealed that patients with NAFL and NASH presented a progression of fibrosis of 33.6% and an improvement of it of 22.3%, the rate of fibrosis progression being greater in patients with NASH than with NAFL (progression in a stage of 7.1 years compared to 14.3 years, respectively) [5]. However, there is a lack of homogenization in the speed of fibrosis progression in all these studies with paired biopsy, which is mostly due to the presence of characteristics of the metabolic syndrome in the patients [5–7, 62, 65, 138–144]. For this reason, due to the lack of studies that provide complete data about the differential progression of the disease in patients with different stages of NAFLD, there is no guide on the frequency of follow-up of these patients or on the means available to monitor the progression. Nevertheless, once the diagnosis of NAFLD is made, the follow-up will depend on the presence of metabolic risk factors and the severity of the hepatic disease, which will be determined by the presence of NASH and, especially, the stage of fibrosis.

The principal metabolic factor of the risk of NAFLD progression is DM2 [1, 19, 145]. Patients with DM2 have a more severe grade of NAFLD than the patients without DM2, with rates of NASH up to 80% and of advanced fibrosis of 30–40% [146, 147]. These data confirm the need for closer monitoring in these patients. Bazick et al. [147] developed a clinical model to detect NASH and advanced fibrosis in patients with NAFLD and DM2 with a sensitivity and specificity of 57 and 90%, respectively. This model includes easily accessible parameters such as BMI, circumference at the waist, HbA1c, insulin resistance, ALT, AST, albumin and ferritin, for NASH; and age, BMI, waist/hip ratio, arterial hypertension, ALT/AST ratio, alkaline phosphatase, bilirubin, globulin, albumin, serum insulin, hematocrit, INR and platelets, to predict advanced fibrosis. However, further studies are still necessary to externally validate this model. Other metabolic factors described with more evidence for the disease progression are central obesity, arterial hypertension and high levels of LDL cholesterol [7, 148–150]. No study shows cost-efficacy in the monitoring of the progression in these at-risk patients, but we recommend carrying out NFS and/or FIB-4 every 2 or 3 years in these patients with non-significant fibrosis, and if NASH and/or significant fibrosis is presented in the initial diagnosis, the follow-up will not differ from the rest of the patients.

The other factor having the greatest effect on the disease progression is liver fibrosis [151]. In general, in a period of 15 years, 13% of the patients with stage F2 and 25% of those presenting with F3 will develop cirrhosis [6, 7, 62]. These patients with significant fibrosis should be considered for pharmacological treatment, besides lifestyle modifications (diet and exercise). Moreover, NAFLD patients may develop HCC even in the absence of cirrhosis [152], given that it is the continuous hepatocyte injury that leads to a compensatory proliferation, key driver of the development of HCC [153]. Therefore, patients with NASH and significant fibrosis, which is indicative of important cellular damage, are also at risk of developing this liver tumor.

With all this information, we recommend recalculating NFS and/or FIB-4 every 4–5 years for patients with NAFL without risk factors or if the patient develops DM2; in patients with NASH without significant fibrosis, we recommend an annual follow-up with a calculation of NFS and/or FIB-4 and carrying out TE and ultrasound, and in patients with significant fibrosis, a 6-monthly follow-up is recommended with special interest in screening for HCC. The management and follow-up of the patients with advanced fibrosis/cirrhosis due to NASH does not differ from the rest of etiologies [25].

Another important question is the evaluation of the response to the therapy provided. The non-invasive methods available currently have not been reliable or have not been validated to document efficacy of the treatments, so liver biopsy is still necessary to determine this efficacy, especially in a clinical trial setting.

6. Screening of associated diseases

In recent years, several studies have confirmed that the morbimortality associated with NAFLD is not limited only to hepatic injury, yet it is a disease with multisystemic behavior with affectation of different organs.

6.1. Insulin resistance and metabolic syndrome

As was previously mentioned, the concurrent characteristics of metabolic syndrome increase the risk of developing NAFLD, and a recent study of the HepaMet group relates the severity of NAFLD with the number of factors of the metabolic syndrome present (publication pending). However, the presence of NAFLD in itself also increases the risk of developing complications such as dyslipidemia and insulin resistance [154–156]. In this sense, the diagnosis and quantification of hepatic fat can be useful in the prediction of future development of diabetes and other cardiovascular risk factors [56].

Insulin resistance is a key in the physiopathology of NAFLD, associated with the increase in the deposit of fat and fibrosis, and it substantially increases the risk of developing DM2, which indicates that NAFLD can precede the development of diabetes. Moreover, and as it was mentioned earlier, several studies have demonstrated that, especially in patients with insulin resistance and/or diabetes, liver fibrosis can progress even when a baseline hepatic histology described only simple steatosis without hepatocellular damage [62, 141]. All in all, in daily clinical practice the use of screening tools is necessary to detect the presence of diabetes (fasting blood glucose levels, HbA1c or, if available, the oral glucose tolerance test) or insulin resistance. The reference technique for the diagnosis of IR in non-diabetic patients is the hyperinsulinemic-euglycemic clamp test, although this procedure is expensive and complicated, so it is not routinely used in daily clinical practice [157]. In these cases, the calculation of HOMA-IR (*homeostatic model assessment*) is an acceptable alternative to evaluate the IR, although there is no agreement on the threshold that defines insulin resistance using this formula [158]. Nevertheless, HOMA-IR can help us during the follow-up to identify patients at risk of fibrosis progression [6, 62]. The next question once the patients with IR are identified is whether it is necessary to treat them pharmacologically or not; and, whether in diabetic patients is necessary to intensify the anti-diabetic treatment to avoid liver disease progression or not. As expected, several insulin-sensitizing agents have demonstrated an improvement in the hepatic histology [159–161], even in patients without DM2 [162, 163], given that both entities share multiple physiopathological mechanisms, so this treatment can be considered in patients with NASH and/or multiple factors of progression in which a decrease of IR cannot be achieved with diet and exercise, although the EASL and AASLD guidelines do not contemplate it. Given that IR plays an essential role in NAFLD progression but not the only one, we do not believe that it is necessary to treat DM2 differently/intensely in patients with NAFLD, independently of the grade, provided that the IR is controlled.

6.2. Cardiovascular disease

Cardiovascular disease is quantitatively the main cause of death in NAFLD patients. Besides the risk itself of the characteristics of the metabolic syndrome, multiple pathogenic conditions of NAFLD contribute to the development of cardiovascular disease. In fact, patients with NAFLD often present elevation in the markers implicated in the development of atherosclerosis, such as CD36 in its soluble form (sCD36), a membrane receptor responsible for, among other things, the transport of fatty acids [164]. The spectrum of CVD in NAFLD includes atherosclerotic coronary heart disease, heart failure and cardiac arrhythmias. This necessitates the study of probable CVD, especially subclinical atherosclerosis, in all these patients [10]. There are little data to define the optimal means of screening NAFLD patients with CVD, but it is important to be aware that there are different techniques for the detection of subclinical atherosclerosis that are bloodless and some of which are very easily performed. Among these, the measurement of ankle-brachial index and carotid ultrasound are assessments especially useful for patients with intermediate cardiovascular risk, situation affecting a very important part of the population with NAFLD [165].

6.3. Extrahepatic cancer

The second most prevalent cause of death among patients with NAFLD is cancer, both gastrointestinal (colon, esophagus, stomach and pancreas) and extraintestinal (kidney and breast), which leads to the suspicion that this liver disease might promote the development of neoplasms.

The association of insulin resistance/diabetes, obesity and metabolic syndrome with an increase in the risk of a large number of cancers is well established [166–171]. These three characteristics are closely related to NAFLD and contribute significantly to the risk of developing HCC; nevertheless, various recent studies indicate that NAFLD can be an additional and independent risk factor for extrahepatic cancers [172, 173], especially colorectal cancer (CRC) [127, 174]. In several studies, colorectal lesions, particularly tubular adenomas and carcinomas, were significantly more prevalent in NAFLD patients, regardless of age, sex and manifestations of metabolic syndrome; even the presence of NASH has been related to a greater risk in comparison with those with NAFL [174, 175]. This rise in the risk of CRC in NAFLD can be explained by the increase in insulin and pro-inflammatory cytokines and the alteration of the adipokines metabolism predominantly leptin versus adiponectin that exists in these patients and which promotes cellular proliferation, inhibition of apoptosis and angiogenesis [176, 177].

Although these data clearly suggest more rigorous screening programmes for CRC in NAFLD patients, there are no well-designed prospective studies enabling the verification of a causal relation between NAFLD and CRC or studies that evaluate the usefulness of earlier screening in this liver disease, so no guidelines make a distinction with respect to CRC screening in these patients.

6.4. Other associated diseases

There is increasing interest in the possible contribution of NAFLD to the development and progression of chronic kidney disease (CKD) [178–181]. A recent meta-analysis has revealed that the presence and severity of NAFLD are associated with an increase in the risk and severity of CKD [181]. However, it is difficult to establish NAFLD as an independent risk factor of CKD given the close relation between NAFLD and other known risk factors of CKD such as obesity and IR. Obstructive sleep apnea syndrome (OSAS) is strongly associated with NAFLD independently of other traditional factors; it is a consequence of the decrease in the lipid metabolism provoked by intermittent hypoxia [182–185]. Other described diseases associated with NAFLD include osteoporosis [186], psoriasis [187], polycystic syndrome [188] and other endocrinopathies such as hypothyroidism [189], hypopituitarism [190] and hypogonadism [191]. Until now, there is no evidence for screening of all these pathologies for the mere fact that the subject presents NAFLD, so all that needs to be studied is the presence of them if the patient has clinical manifestations related to them. Moreover, a recent study by our group has demonstrated that psychotic patients with specific pharmacological treatment have a high risk of developing NAFLD in the first years, so its early detection will enable better prevention of cardiovascular events, which are so increased in this population [192].

7. Diagnostic algorithm and follow-up

While working on the different sections of this chapter, we have detailed the fundamental elements for the development of a diagnostic algorithm and a follow-up procedure for NAFLD (**Figure 2**). This algorithm is based on clinical evidence available in the current literature with respect to the topic and on different guidelines issued by the principal international associations for the study of the liver (EASL and AASLD). In the case of monitoring and follow-up of these patients where the existing evidence is not relevant in certain aspects, our recommendations are based on the experience of our clinical group in different high-quality studies in this field.

Once the initial diagnosis of NAFLD is made, our posterior attitude will depend on the result of the non-invasive liver fibrosis methods. In general, current image techniques are quite reliable to distinguish between advanced fibrosis (≥F3) and mild fibrosis or null (F0–F1), but they are insufficient to identify those patients with significant fibrosis (≥F2). Therefore, in clinical practice, we recommend the combination of elastographic techniques with serum markers, more specifically TE and NFS due to their wide accessibility and ease of application. When these two parameters generate doubt about the grade of fibrosis or indicate possible significant fibrosis, liver biopsy is necessary. Depending on the result, we determine the posterior follow-up as can be seen in the algorithm (**Figure 2**). The presence of metabolic risk factors influences not only the therapeutic management but also the follow-up. If liver biopsy is

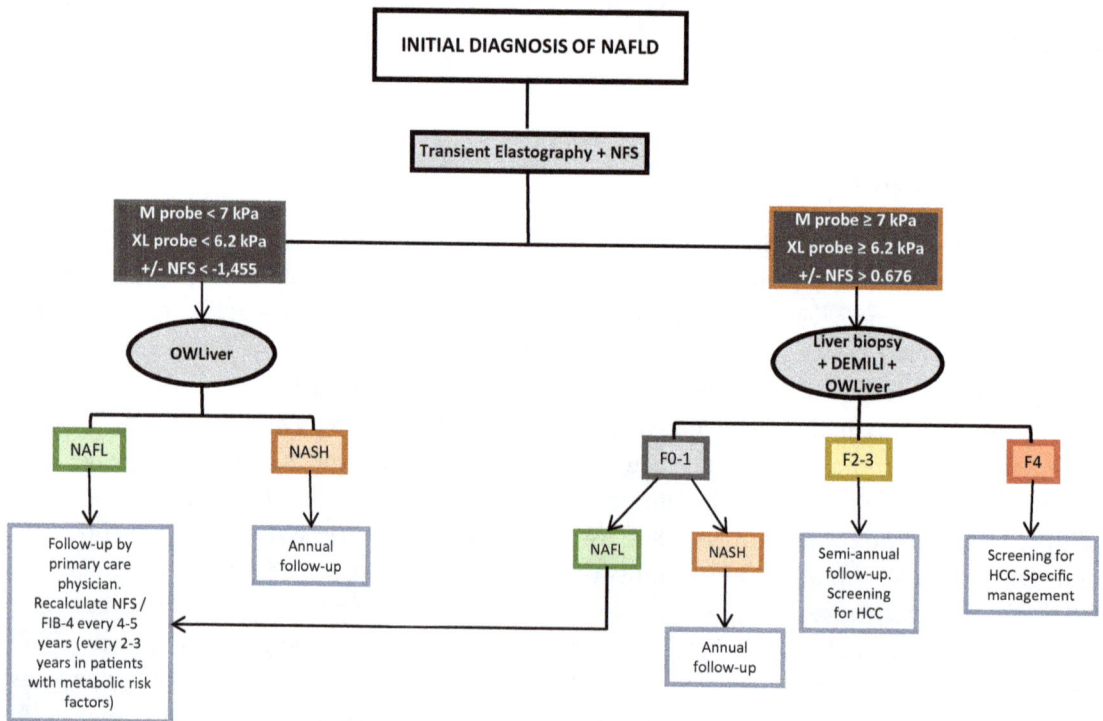

Figure 2. Clinical algorithm for the diagnosis of NAFLD and monitoring disease progression.

not to be performed on the patient with NAFLD, due to advanced age, to the absence of significant fibrosis in the non-invasive methods or to contraindication, we could evaluate the performance of the OWL Liver Test to help identify those patients with NASH who require a closer follow-up. If the patient does not present improvement in laboratory parameters even in imaging tests, we should evaluate to repeat liver biopsy 5 years after the last one, or even before if progression of the disease is suspected.

8. Conclusions

NAFLD is currently the primary cause of chronic liver disease in the western world and its growth is a consequence of its close relation to obesity and metabolic syndrome. One of the great challenges in this disease is to diagnose and classify it correctly, given that the characteristics defining NAFLD are the common denominator of many liver diseases. Its correct characterization is important as in spite of presenting a generally benign and slowly developing evolution from the hepatic viewpoint; the fatty liver can progress towards more severe forms with the development of inflammation, fibrosis, cirrhosis and HCC, thus conferring morbimortality. However, its potential morbimortality is not limited to this organ, but goes beyond; NAFLD is being considered a mediator of systemic diseases. Therefore, the early identification of these patients would help to improve its prognosis through an individualized intervention depending on the stage of liver disease, on the metabolic risk factors present and on the cardiovascular risk, which translates into the need for a systemic approach to the disease with multidisciplinary management including primary care physician, endocrinologists, nutritionists, psychologists and hepatologists.

Conflict of interest

The authors declared that they do not have anything to disclose regarding funding or conflict of interest with respect to this chapter.

Author details

Paula Iruzubieta, Marta González, Joaquín Cabezas, María Teresa Arias-Loste and Javier Crespo*

*Address all correspondence to: javiercrespo1991@gmail.com

Department of Gastroenterology and Hepatology, Marqués de Valdecilla University Hospital, Centro de Investigación Biomédica en Red de Enfermedades Hepáticas y Digestivas (CIBERehd), Infection, Immunity and Digestive Pathology Group, Research Institute Marqués de Valdecilla (IDIVAL), Santander, Spain

References

[1] Vernon G, Baranova A, Younossi ZM. Systematic review: The epidemiology and natural history of non-alcoholic fatty liver disease and non-alcoholic steatohepatitis in adults. Alimentary Pharmacology & Therapeutics. [Internet]. Aug 2011;34(3):274-285. Available from: http://www.ncbi.nlm.nih.gov/pubmed/21623852 [Accessed: Jul 10, 2014]

[2] Ludwig J, Viggiano TR, McGill DB, Oh BJ. Nonalcoholic steatohepatitis: Mayo Clinic experiences with a hitherto unnamed disease. Mayo Clinic Proceedings [Internet]. Jul 1980;55(7):434-438. Available from: http://www.ncbi.nlm.nih.gov/pubmed/7382552 [Accessed: Dec 26, 2016]

[3] Kleiner DE, Brunt EM, Van Natta M, Behling C, Contos MJ, Cummings OW, et al. Design and validation of a histological scoring system for nonalcoholic fatty liver disease. Hepatology [Internet]. Jun 2005;41(6):1313-1321. Available from: http://www.ncbi.nlm.nih.gov/pubmed/15915461 [Accesed: Jun 17, 2015]

[4] Cuadrado A, Orive A, García-Suárez C, Domínguez A, Fernández-Escalante JC, Crespo J, et al. Non-alcoholic steatohepatitis (NASH) and hepatocellular carcinoma. Obesity Surgery [Internet]. Mar 1, 2005;15(3):442-446. Available from: http://www.springerlink.com/index/10.1381/0960892053576596 [Accessed: Dec 26, 2016]

[5] Singh S, Allen AM, Wang Z, Prokop LJ, Murad MH, Loomba R. Fibrosis progression in nonalcoholic fatty liver vs nonalcoholic steatohepatitis: A systematic review and meta-analysis of paired-biopsy studies. Clinical Gastroenterology and Hepatology [Internet]. Apr 2015;13(4):643-54-9-40. Available from: http://linkinghub.elsevier.com/retrieve/pii/S1542356514006028 [Accessed: Dec 26, 2016]

[6] Pais R, Charlotte F, Fedchuk L, Bedossa P, Lebray P, Poynard T, et al. A systematic review of follow-up biopsies reveals disease progression in patients with non-alcoholic fatty liver. Journal of Hepatology [Internet]. Sep 2013;59(3):550-556. Available from: http://www.ncbi.nlm.nih.gov/pubmed/23665288 [Accessed: Apr 23, 2016]

[7] Adams LA, Sanderson S, Lindor KD, Angulo P. The histological course of nonalcoholic fatty liver disease: A longitudinal study of 103 patients with sequential liver biopsies. Journal of Hepatology [Internet]. Jan 2005;42(1):132-138. Available from: http://linkinghub.elsevier.com/retrieve/pii/S0168827804004350 [Accessed: Dec 26, 2016]

[8] Ong JP, Pitts A, Younossi ZM. Increased overall mortality and liver-related mortality in non-alcoholic fatty liver disease. Journal of Hepatology [Internet]. Oct 2008;49(4):608-612. Available from: http://www.ncbi.nlm.nih.gov/pubmed/18682312 [Accessed: Jun 4, 2016]

[9] Stepanova M, Rafiq N, Makhlouf H, Agrawal R, Kaur I, Younoszai Z, et al. Predictors of all-cause mortality and liver-related mortality in patients with non-alcoholic fatty liver disease (NAFLD). Digestive Diseases and Sciences [Internet]. Oct 2013;58(10):3017-3023. Available from: http://www.ncbi.nlm.nih.gov/pubmed/23775317 [Accessed: Jun 4, 2016]

[10] Francque SM, van der Graaff D, Kwanten WJ. Non-alcoholic fatty liver disease and cardiovascular risk: Pathophysiological mechanisms and implications. Journal of Hepatology

[Internet]. Aug 2016;**65**(2):425-443. Available from: http://linkinghub.elsevier.com/retrieve/pii/S0168827816301076 [Accessed: Dec 27, 2016]

[11] Anstee QM, Targher G, Day CP. Progression of NAFLD to diabetes mellitus, cardiovascular disease or cirrhosis. Nature Reviews Gastroenterology & Hepatology [Internet]. Jun 2013;**10**(6):330-344. Available from: http://www.ncbi.nlm.nih.gov/pubmed/23507799 [Accessed: May 17, 2016]

[12] Machado M, Marques-Vidal P, Cortez-Pinto H. Hepatic histology in obese patients undergoing bariatric surgery. Journal of Hepatology [Internet]. Oct 2006;**45**(4):600-606. Available from: http://www.ncbi.nlm.nih.gov/pubmed/16899321 [Accessed: Mar 1, 2016]

[13] Boza C, Riquelme A, Ibañez L, Duarte I, Norero E, Viviani P, et al. Predictors of non-alcoholic steatohepatitis (NASH) in obese patients undergoing gastric bypass. Obesity Surgery [Internet]. Sep 2005;**15**(8):1148-1153. Available from: http://www.ncbi.nlm.nih.gov/pubmed/16197788 [Accessed: Jun 4, 2016]

[14] Fabbrini E, Magkos F. Hepatic steatosis as a marker of metabolic dysfunction. Nutrients [Internet]. Jun 2015;**7**(6):4995-5019. Available from: http://www.pubmedcentral.nih.gov/articlerender.fcgi?artid=4488828&tool=pmcentrez&rendertype=abstract [Accessed: Jun 4, 2016]

[15] Gastaldelli A, Cusi K, Pettiti M, Hardies J, Miyazaki Y, Berria R, et al. Relationship between hepatic/visceral fat and hepatic insulin resistance in nondiabetic and type 2 diabetic subjects. Gastroenterology [Internet]. Aug 2007;**133**(2):496-506. Available from: http://www.ncbi.nlm.nih.gov/pubmed/17681171 [Accessed: Mar 8, 2016]

[16] Kotronen A, Juurinen L, Hakkarainen A, Westerbacka J, Cornér A, Bergholm R, et al. Liver fat is increased in type 2 diabetic patients and underestimated by serum alanine aminotransferase compared with equally obese nondiabetic subjects. Diabetes Care [Internet]. Jan 2008;**31**(1):165-169. Available from: http://www.ncbi.nlm.nih.gov/pubmed/17934148 [Accessed: Jun 4, 2016]

[17] Targher G, Bertolini L, Rodella S, Tessari R, Zenari L, Lippi G, et al. Nonalcoholic fatty liver disease is independently associated with an increased incidence of cardiovascular events in type 2 diabetic patients. Diabetes Care [Internet]. Aug 2007;**30**(8):2119-2121. Available from: http://www.ncbi.nlm.nih.gov/pubmed/17519430 [Accessed: Jun 4, 2016]

[18] Leite NC, Salles GF, Araujo ALE, Villela-Nogueira CA, Cardoso CRL. Prevalence and associated factors of non-alcoholic fatty liver disease in patients with type-2 diabetes mellitus. Liver International [Internet]. Jan 2009;**29**(1):113-119. Available from: http://www.ncbi.nlm.nih.gov/pubmed/18384521 [Accessed: Jun 4, 2016]

[19] Loomba R, Abraham M, Unalp A, Wilson L, Lavine J, Doo E, et al. Association between diabetes, family history of diabetes, and risk of nonalcoholic steatohepatitis and fibrosis. Hepatology [Internet]. Sep 2012;**56**(3):943-951. Available from: http://www.pubmedcentral.nih.gov/articlerender.fcgi?artid=3407289&tool=pmcentrez&rendertype=abstract [Accessed: Jun 4, 2016]

[20] Streba LAM, Vere CC, Rogoveanu I, Streba CT. Nonalcoholic fatty liver disease, meta-bolic risk factors, and hepatocellular carcinoma: An open question. World Journal of Gastroenterology [Internet]. Apr 14, 2015;21(14):4103-4110. Available from: http://www. pubmedcentral.nih.gov/articlerender.fcgi?artid=4394070&tool=pmcentrez&rendertype =abstract [Accessed: Jun 4, 2016]

[21] Marchesini G, Bugianesi E, Forlani G, Cerrelli F, Lenzi M, Manini R, et al. Nonalcoholic fatty liver, steatohepatitis, and the metabolic syndrome. Hepatology [Internet]. Apr 2003;37(4):917-923. Available from: http://www.ncbi.nlm.nih.gov/pubmed/12668987 [Accessed: May 14, 2016]

[22] Doycheva I, Cui J, Nguyen P, Costa EA, Hooker J, Hofflich H, et al. Non-invasive screening of diabetics in primary care for NAFLD and advanced fibrosis by MRI and MRE. Alimentary Pharmacology & Therapeutics [Internet]. Jan 2016;43(1):83-95. Available from: http://www.ncbi.nlm.nih.gov/pubmed/26369383 [Accessed: Jan 31, 2017]

[23] Zhang E, Wartelle-Bladou C, Lepanto L, Lachaine J, Cloutier G, Tang A. Cost-utility anal-ysis of nonalcoholic steatohepatitis screening. European Radiology [Internet]. Nov 21, 2015;25(11):3282-3294. Available from: http://www.ncbi.nlm.nih.gov/pubmed/25994191 [Accessed: Jan 31, 2017]

[24] Chalasani N, Younossi Z, Lavine JE, Diehl AM, Brunt EM, Cusi K, et al. The diagnosis and management of non-alcoholic fatty liver disease: Practice Guideline by the American Association for the Study of Liver Diseases, American College of Gastroenterology, and the American Gastroenterological Association. Hepatology [Internet]. Jun 2012;55(6):2005-2023. Available from: http://www.ncbi.nlm.nih.gov/pubmed/22488764 [Accessed: Feb 1, 2017]

[25] European Association for the Study of the Liver (EASL), European Association for the Study of Diabetes (EASD), European Association for the Study of Obesity (EASO). EASL-EASD-EASO Clinical Practice Guidelines for the management of non-alcoholic fatty liver disease. Journal of Hepatology [Internet]. Jun 2016;64(6):1388-1402. Available from: http://www.ncbi.nlm.nih.gov/pubmed/27062661 [Accessed: Dec 27, 2016]

[26] Angulo P. Nonalcoholic fatty liver disease. The New England Journal of Medicine [Internet]. Apr 18, 2002;346(16):1221-1231. Available from: http://www.ncbi.nlm.nih. gov/pubmed/11961152 [Accessed: Feb 21, 2015]

[27] Tahan V, Canbakan B, Balci H, Dane F, Akin H, Can G, et al. Serum gamma-glutamyltranspep-tidase distinguishes non-alcoholic fatty liver disease at high risk. Hepatogastroenterology [Internet]. Feb 1, 2017;55(85):1433-1438. Available from: http://www.ncbi.nlm.nih.gov/ pubmed/18795706

[28] O'Brien J, Powell LW. Non-alcoholic fatty liver disease: Is iron relevant? Hepatology International [Internet]. Jan 12, 2012;6(1):332-341. Available from: http://www.ncbi.nlm. nih.gov/pubmed/22020821 [Accessed: Feb 1, 2017]

[29] Ravi S, Shoreibah M, Raff E, Bloomer J, Kakati D, Rasheed K, et al. Autoimmune mark-ers do not impact clinical presentation or natural history of steatohepatitis-related

liver disease. Digestive Diseases and Sciences [Internet]. Dec 15, 2015;**60**(12):3788-3793. Available from: http://www.ncbi.nlm.nih.gov/pubmed/26173506 [Accessed: Feb 2, 2017]

[30] Amarapurkar DN, Patel ND. Clinical spectrum and natural history of non-alcoholic steatohepatitis with normal alanine aminotransferase values. Tropical Gastroenterology [Internet]. Feb 2, 2017;**25**(3):130-134. Available from: http://www.ncbi.nlm.nih.gov/pubmed/15682660

[31] Portillo-Sanchez P, Bril F, Maximos M, Lomonaco R, Biernacki D, Orsak B, et al. High prevalence of nonalcoholic fatty liver disease in patients with type 2 diabetes mellitus and normal plasma aminotransferase levels. The Journal of Clinical Endocrinology and Metabolism [Internet]. Jun 2015;**100**(6):2231-2238. Available from: http://www.ncbi.nlm.nih.gov/pubmed/25885947 [Accessed: Feb 2, 2017]

[32] Schwenzer NF, Springer F, Schraml C, Stefan N, Machann J, Schick F. Non-invasive assessment and quantification of liver steatosis by ultrasound, computed tomography and magnetic resonance. Journal of Hepatology [Internet]. Sep 2009;**51**(3):433-445. Available from: http://www.ncbi.nlm.nih.gov/pubmed/19604596 [Accessed: Feb 2, 2017]

[33] Saadeh S, Younossi ZM, Remer EM, Gramlich T, Ong JP, Hurley M, et al. The utility of radiological imaging in nonalcoholic fatty liver disease. Gastroenterology [Internet]. Sep 2002;**123**(3):745-750. Available from: http://www.ncbi.nlm.nih.gov/pubmed/12198701 [Accessed: Feb 2, 2017]

[34] Dasarathy S, Dasarathy J, Khiyami A, Joseph R, Lopez R, McCullough AJ. Validity of real time ultrasound in the diagnosis of hepatic steatosis: A prospective study. Journal of Hepatology [Internet]. Dec 2009;**51**(6):1061-1067. Available from: http://linkinghub.elsevier.com/retrieve/pii/S0168827809005856 [Accessed: Feb 2, 2017]

[35] Noureddin M, Lam J, Peterson MR, Middleton M, Hamilton G, Le T-A, et al. Utility of magnetic resonance imaging versus histology for quantifying changes in liver fat in nonalcoholic fatty liver disease trials. Hepatology [Internet]. Dec 2013;**58**(6):1930-1940. Available from: http://doi.wiley.com/10.1002/hep.26455 [Accessed: Feb 2, 2017]

[36] Raptis DA, Fischer MA, Graf R, Nanz D, Weber A, Moritz W, et al. MRI: The new reference standard in quantifying hepatic steatosis? Gut [Internet]. Jan 2012;**61**(1):117-127. Available from: http://www.ncbi.nlm.nih.gov/pubmed/21997548 [Accessed: Feb 2, 2017]

[37] Sasso M, Beaugrand M, de Ledinghen V, Douvin C, Marcellin P, Poupon R, et al. Controlled attenuation parameter (CAP): A novel VCTE™ guided ultrasonic attenuation measurement for the evaluation of hepatic steatosis: Preliminary study and validation in a cohort of patients with chronic liver disease from various causes. Ultrasound in Medicine and Biology [Internet]. Nov 2010;**36**(11):1825-1835. Available from: http://linkinghub.elsevier.com/retrieve/pii/S0301562910003546 [Accessed: Mar 4, 2017]

[38] Lédinghen V, Vergniol J, Foucher J, Merrouche W, Bail B. Non-invasive diagnosis of liver steatosis using controlled attenuation parameter (CAP) and transient elastography. Liver International [Internet]. Jul 2012;**32**(6):911-918. Available from: http://www.ncbi.nlm.nih.gov/pubmed/22672642 [Accessed: Mar 4, 2017]

[39] Shen F, Zheng R-D, Mi Y-Q, Wang X-Y, Pan Q, Chen G-Y, et al. Controlled attenuation parameter for non-invasive assessment of hepatic steatosis in Chinese patients. World Journal of Gastroenterology [Internet]. Apr 28, 2014;**20**(16):4702. Available from: http://www.ncbi.nlm.nih.gov/pubmed/24782622 [Accessed: Mar 4, 2017]

[40] Kumar M, Rastogi A, Singh T, Behari C, Gupta E, Garg H, et al. Controlled attenuation parameter for non-invasive assessment of hepatic steatosis: Does etiology affect performance? Journal of Gastroenterology and Hepatology [Internet]. Jul 2013;**28**(7):1194-1201. Available from: http://doi.wiley.com/10.1111/jgh.12134 [Accessed: Mar 4, 2017]

[41] Myers RP, Pollett A, Kirsch R, Pomier-Layrargues G, Beaton M, Levstik M, et al. Controlled Attenuation Parameter (CAP): A noninvasive method for the detection of hepatic steatosis based on transient elastography. Liver International [Internet]. Jul 2012;**32**(6):902-910. Available from: http://www.ncbi.nlm.nih.gov/pubmed/22435761 [Accessed: Mar 4, 2017]

[42] Imajo K, Kessoku T, Honda Y, Tomeno W, Ogawa Y, Mawatari H, et al. Magnetic resonance imaging more accurately classifies steatosis and fibrosis in patients with nonalcoholic fatty liver disease than transient elastography. Gastroenterology [Internet]. Mar 2016;**150**(3):626-637.e7. Available from: http://linkinghub.elsevier.com/retrieve/pii/S0016508515017345 [Accessed: Feb 19, 2017]

[43] Chan W-K, Nik Mustapha NR, Mahadeva S. Controlled attenuation parameter for the detection and quantification of hepatic steatosis in nonalcoholic fatty liver disease. Journal of Gastroenterology and Hepatology [Internet]. Jul 2014;**29**(7):1470-1476. Available from: http://www.ncbi.nlm.nih.gov/pubmed/24548002 [Accessed: Mar 4, 2017]

[44] de Lédinghen V, Wong GL-H, Vergniol J, Chan HL-Y, Hiriart J-B, Chan AW-H, et al. Controlled attenuation parameter for the diagnosis of steatosis in non-alcoholic fatty liver disease. Journal of Gastroenterology and Hepatology [Internet]. Apr 2016;**31**(4):848-855. Available from: http://www.ncbi.nlm.nih.gov/pubmed/26514665 [Accessed: Mar 4, 2017]

[45] Karlas T, Petroff D, Sasso M, Fan J-G, Mi Y-Q, de Lédinghen V, et al. Individual patient data meta-analysis of controlled attenuation parameter (CAP) technology for assessing steatosis. Journal of Hepatology [Internet]. May 2017;**66**(5):1022-1230. Available from: http://linkinghub.elsevier.com/retrieve/pii/S0168827816307553 [Accessed: Feb 2, 2017]

[46] Tang A, Desai A, Hamilton G, Wolfson T, Gamst A, Lam J, et al. Accuracy of MR imaging-estimated proton density fat fraction for classification of dichotomized histologic steatosis grades in nonalcoholic fatty liver disease. Radiology [Internet]. Feb 2015;**274**(2):416-425. Available from: http://pubs.rsna.org/doi/10.1148/radiol.14140754 [Accessed: Oct 29, 2017]

[47] Bedogni G, Bellentani S, Miglioli L, Masutti F, Passalacqua M, Castiglione A, et al. The fatty liver index: A simple and accurate predictor of hepatic steatosis in the general population. BMC Gastroenterology [Internet]. Nov 2, 2006;**6**(1):33. Available from: http://bmcgastroenterol.biomedcentral.com/articles/10.1186/1471-230X-6-33 [Accessed: Feb 2, 2017]

[48] Kotronen A, Peltonen M, Hakkarainen A, Sevastianova K, Bergholm R, Johansson LM, et al. Prediction of non-alcoholic fatty liver disease and liver fat using metabolic and genetic factors. Gastroenterology [Internet]. Sep 2009;137(3):865-872. Available from: http://linkinghub.elsevier.com/retrieve/pii/S0016508509009135 [Accessed: Feb 2, 2017]

[49] Lee J-H, Kim D, Kim HJ, Lee C-H, Yang JI, Kim W, et al. Hepatic steatosis index: A simple screening tool reflecting nonalcoholic fatty liver disease. Digestive and Liver Disease [Internet]. Jul 2010;42(7):503-508. Available from: http://linkinghub.elsevier.com/retrieve/pii/S1590865809003363 [Accessed: Feb 2, 2017]

[50] Poynard T, Ratziu V, Naveau S, Thabut D, Charlotte F, Messous D, et al. The diagnostic value of biomarkers (SteatoTest) for the prediction of liver steatosis. Comparative Hepatology Dec 23, 2005;4(1):10. Available from: http://comparative-hepatology.biomed-central.com/articles/10.1186/1476-5926-4-10 [Accessed: Feb 2, 2017]

[51] Cuthbertson DJ, Weickert MO, Lythgoe D, Sprung VS, Dobson R, Shoajee-Moradie F, et al. External validation of the fatty liver index and lipid accumulation product indices, using 1H-magnetic resonance spectroscopy, to identify hepatic steatosis in healthy controls and obese, insulin-resistant individuals. European Journal of Endocrinology [Internet]. Nov 8, 2014;171(5):561-569. Available from: http://www.eje-online.org/cgi/doi/10.1530/EJE-14-0112 [Accessed: Oct 29, 2017]

[52] Calori G, Lattuada G, Ragogna F, Garancini MP, Crosignani P, Villa M, et al. Fatty liver index and mortality: The Cremona study in the 15th year of follow-up. Hepatology [Internet]. Jul 2011;54(1):145-152. Available from: http://doi.wiley.com/10.1002/hep.24356 [Accessed: Mar 4, 2017]

[53] Younossi ZM, Stepanova M, Rafiq N, Makhlouf H, Younoszai Z, Agrawal R, et al. Pathologic criteria for nonalcoholic steatohepatitis: Interprotocol agreement and ability to predict liver-related mortality. Hepatology [Internet]. Jun 2011;53(6):1874-1882. Available from: http://doi.wiley.com/10.1002/hep.24268 [Accessed: Dec 26, 2016]

[54] Angulo P, Kleiner DE, Dam-Larsen S, Adams LA, Bjornsson ES, Charatcharoenwitthaya P, et al. Liver fibrosis, but no other histologic features, is associated with long-term outcomes of patients with nonalcoholic fatty liver disease. Gastroenterology [Internet]. Aug 2015;149(2):389-97.e10. Available from: http://linkinghub.elsevier.com/retrieve/pii/S0016508515005995 [Accessed: Dec 26, 2016]

[55] Angulo P. Long-term mortality in nonalcoholic fatty liver disease: Is liver histology of any prognostic significance? Hepatology [Internet]. Feb 2010;51(2):373-375. Available from: http://doi.wiley.com/10.1002/hep.23521 [Accessed: Feb 7, 2017]

[56] Arulanandan A, Ang B, Bettencourt R, Hooker J, Behling C, Lin GY, et al. Association between quantity of liver fat and cardiovascular risk in patients with nonalcoholic fatty liver disease independent of nonalcoholic steatohepatitis. Clinical Gastroenterology and Hepatology [Internet]. Aug 2015;13(8):1513-20.e1. Available from: http://linkinghub.elsevier.com/retrieve/pii/S1542356515001135 [Accessed: Feb 2, 2017]

[57] Ratziu V, Charlotte F, Heurtier A, Gombert S, Giral P, Bruckert E, et al. Sampling vari-
      ability of liver biopsy in nonalcoholic fatty liver disease. Gastroenterology [Internet]. Jun
      2005;**128**(7):1898-1906. Available from: http://www.ncbi.nlm.nih.gov/pubmed/15940625
      [Accessed: Feb 4, 2017]

[58] Gawrieh S, Knoedler DM, Saeian K, Wallace JR, Komorowski RA. Effects of interventions
      on intra- and interobserver agreement on interpretation of nonalcoholic fatty liver dis-
      ease histology. Annals of Diagnostic Pathology [Internet]. Feb 2011;**15**(1):19-24. Available
      from: http://linkinghub.elsevier.com/retrieve/pii/S1092913410001413 [Accessed: Oct 29,
      2017]

[59] Sumida Y, Nakajima A, Itoh Y. Limitations of liver biopsy and non-invasive diagnostic
      tests for the diagnosis of nonalcoholic fatty liver disease/nonalcoholic steatohepatitis.
      World Journal of Gastroenterology [Internet]. Jan 14, 2014;**20**(2):475-485. Available from:
      http://www.ncbi.nlm.nih.gov/pubmed/24574716 [Accessed: Oct 29, 2017]

[60] Castera L, Vilgrain V, Angulo P. Noninvasive evaluation of NAFLD. Nature Reviews
      Gastroenterology & Hepatology [Internet]. Sep 24, 2013;**10**(11):666-675. Available from:
      http://www.ncbi.nlm.nih.gov/pubmed/24061203 [Accessed: Feb 7, 2017]

[61] Kaswala DH, Lai M, Afdhal NH. Fibrosis assessment in nonalcoholic fatty liver disease
      (NAFLD) in 2016. Digestive Diseases and Sciences [Internet]. May 26, 2016;**61**(5):1356-
      1364. Available from: http://link.springer.com/10.1007/s10620-016-4079-4 [Accessed:
      Feb 8, 2017]

[62] McPherson S, Hardy T, Henderson E, Burt AD, Day CP, Anstee QM. Evidence of NAFLD
      progression from steatosis to fibrosing-steatohepatitis using paired biopsies: Implications
      for prognosis and clinical management. Journal of Hepatology [Internet]. May
      2015;**62**(5):1148-1155. Available from: http://www.ncbi.nlm.nih.gov/pubmed/25477264
      [Accessed: Apr 19, 2016]

[63] Frith J, Day CP, Henderson E, Burt AD, Newton JL. Non-alcoholic fatty liver disease
      in older people. Gerontology [Internet]. Jan 2009;**55**(6):607-613. Available from: http://
      www.ncbi.nlm.nih.gov/pubmed/19690397 [Accessed: May 30, 2016]

[64] Assy N, Kaita K, Mymin D, Levy C, Rosser B, Minuk G. Fatty infiltration of liver in hyper-
      lipidemic patients. Digestive Diseases and Sciences [Internet]. Oct 2000;**45**(10):1929-1934.
      Available from: http://www.ncbi.nlm.nih.gov/pubmed/11117562 [Accessed: May 23, 2016]

[65] Hui AY, Wong VW-S, Chan HL-Y, Liew C-T, Chan JL-Y, Chan FK-L, et al. Histological
      progression of non-alcoholic fatty liver disease in Chinese patients. Alimentary
      Pharmacology & Therapeutics [Internet]. Feb 15, 2005;**21**(4):407-413. Available from:
      http://www.ncbi.nlm.nih.gov/pubmed/15709991 [Accessed: Dec 26, 2016]

[66] McPherson S, Stewart SF, Henderson E, Burt AD, Day CP. Simple non-invasive fibrosis
      scoring systems can reliably exclude advanced fibrosis in patients with non-alcoholic
      fatty liver disease. Gut [Internet]. Sep 1, 2010;**59**(9):1265-1269. Available from: http://gut.
      bmj.com/cgi/doi/10.1136/gut.2010.216077 [Accessed: Dec 26, 2016]

[67] Hossain N, Afendy A, Stepanova M, Nader F, Srishord M, Rafiq N, et al. Independent predictors of fibrosis in patients with nonalcoholic fatty liver disease. Clinical Gastroenterology and Hepatology [Internet]. Nov 2009;7(11):1224-1229.e2. Available from: http://www.ncbi.nlm.nih.gov/pubmed/19559819 [Accessed: Dec 26, 2016]

[68] Yang JD, Abdelmalek MF, Pang H, Guy CD, Smith AD, Diehl AM, et al. Gender and menopause impact severity of fibrosis among patients with nonalcoholic steatohepatitis. Hepatology [Internet]. Apr 2014;59(4):1406-1414. Available from: http://doi.wiley.com/10.1002/hep.26761 [Accessed: Dec 26, 2016]

[69] Klair JS, Yang JD, Abdelmalek MF, Guy CD, Gill RM, Yates K, et al. A longer duration of estrogen deficiency increases fibrosis risk among postmenopausal women with nonalcoholic fatty liver disease. Hepatology [Internet]. Jul 2016;64(1):85-91. Available from: http://doi.wiley.com/10.1002/hep.28514 [Accessed: Dec 26, 2016]

[70] Anstee QM, Day CP. The genetics of nonalcoholic fatty liver disease: Spotlight on PNPLA3 and TM6SF2. Semin Liver Disease [Internet]. Aug 2015;35(3):270-290. Available from: http://www.ncbi.nlm.nih.gov/pubmed/26378644 [Accessed: Jun 21, 2016]

[71] Romeo S, Kozlitina J, Xing C, Pertsemlidis A, Cox D, Pennacchio LA, et al. Genetic variation in PNPLA3 confers susceptibility to nonalcoholic fatty liver disease. Nature Genetics [Internet]. Dec 2008;40(12):1461-1465. Available from: http://www.ncbi.nlm.nih.gov/pubmed/18820647 [Accessed: Jun 21, 2016]

[72] Kawaguchi T, Sumida Y, Umemura A, Matsuo K, Takahashi M, Takamura T, et al. Genetic polymorphisms of the human PNPLA3 gene are strongly associated with severity of nonalcoholic fatty liver disease in Japanese. PLoS One [Internet]. 2012;7(6):e38322. Available from: http://www.ncbi.nlm.nih.gov/pubmed/22719876 [Accessed: Jun 21, 2016]

[73] Liu Y-L, Patman GL, Leathart JBS, Piguet A-C, Burt AD, Dufour J-F, et al. Carriage of the PNPLA3 rs738409 C > G polymorphism confers an increased risk of non-alcoholic fatty liver disease associated hepatocellular carcinoma. Journal of Hepatology [Internet]. Jul 2014;61(1):75-81. Available from: http://www.ncbi.nlm.nih.gov/pubmed/24607626 [Accessed: Dec 27, 2016]

[74] Liu Y-L, Reeves HL, Burt AD, Tiniakos D, McPherson S, Leathart JBS, et al. TM6SF2 rs58542926 influences hepatic fibrosis progression in patients with non-alcoholic fatty liver disease. Nature Communication [Internet]. 2014;5:4309. Available from: http://www.ncbi.nlm.nih.gov/pubmed/24978903 [Accessed: Jun 22, 2016]

[75] Sookoian S, Castaño GO, Scian R, Mallardi P, Fernández Gianotti T, Burgueño AL, et al. Genetic variation in transmembrane 6 superfamily member 2 and the risk of nonalcoholic fatty liver disease and histological disease severity. Hepatology [Internet]. Feb 2015;61(2):515-525. Available from: http://www.ncbi.nlm.nih.gov/pubmed/25302781 [Accessed: Jun 22, 2016]

[76] Donati B, Dongiovanni P, Romeo S, Meroni M, McCain M, Miele L, et al. MBOAT7 rs641738 variant and hepatocellular carcinoma in non-cirrhotic individuals. Science

Report [Internet]. Dec 3, 2017;7(1):4492. Available from: http://www.ncbi.nlm.nih.gov/pubmed/28674415 [Accessed: Oct 29, 2017]

[77] Petta S, Grimaudo S, Cammà C, Cabibi D, Di Marco V, Licata G, et al. IL28B and PNPLA3 polymorphisms affect histological liver damage in patients with non-alcoholic fatty liver disease. Journal of Hepatology [Internet]. Jun 2012;56(6):1356-1362. Available from: http://www.ncbi.nlm.nih.gov/pubmed/22314430 [Accessed: Aug 3, 2015]

[78] Zoppini G, Fedeli U, Gennaro N, Saugo M, Targher G, Bonora E. Mortality from chronic liver diseases in diabetes. American Journal of Gastroenterology [Internet]. Jul 3, 2014;109(7):1020-1025. Available from: http://www.ncbi.nlm.nih.gov/pubmed/24890439 [Accessed: Dec 26, 2016]

[79] Vilar-Gomez E, Martinez-Perez Y, Calzadilla-Bertot L, Torres-Gonzalez A, Gra-Oramas B, Gonzalez-Fabian L, et al. Weight loss through lifestyle modification significantly reduces features of nonalcoholic steatohepatitis. Gastroenterology [Internet]. Aug 2015;149(2):367-378.e5. Available from: http://www.ncbi.nlm.nih.gov/pubmed/25865049 [Accessed: Feb 8, 2017]

[80] Williams CD, Stengel J, Asike MI, Torres DM, Shaw J, Contreras M, et al. Prevalence of non-alcoholic fatty liver disease and nonalcoholic steatohepatitis among a largely middle-aged population utilizing ultrasound and liver biopsy: A prospective study. Gastroenterology [Internet]. Jan 2011;140(1):124-131. Available from: http://linkinghub.elsevier.com/retrieve/pii/S0016508510014162 [Accessed: Mar 2, 2016]

[81] Loria P, Marchesini G, Nascimbeni F, Ballestri S, Maurantonio M, Carubbi F, et al. Cardiovascular risk, lipidemic phenotype and steatosis. A comparative analysis of cirrhotic and non-cirrhotic liver disease due to varying etiology. Atherosclerosis [Internet]. Jan 2014;232(1):99-109. Available from: http://www.ncbi.nlm.nih.gov/pubmed/24401223 [Accessed: Jun 4, 2016]

[82] Jiang ZG, Tapper EB, Connelly MA, Pimentel CFMG, Feldbrügge L, Kim M, et al. Steatohepatitis and liver fibrosis are predicted by the characteristics of very low density lipoprotein in nonalcoholic fatty liver disease. Liver International [Internet]. Aug 2016;36(8):1213-1220. Available from: http://doi.wiley.com/10.1111/liv.13076 [Accessed: Dec 26, 2016]

[83] Targher G, Bertolini L, Scala L, Cigolini M, Zenari L, Falezza G, et al. Associations between serum 25-hydroxyvitamin D3 concentrations and liver histology in patients with non-alcoholic fatty liver disease. Nutrition, Metabolism & Cardiovascular Diseases [Internet]. Sep 2007;17(7):517-524. Available from: http://linkinghub.elsevier.com/retrieve/pii/S0939475306001086 [Accessed: Dec 28, 2016]

[84] Iruzubieta P, Terán Á, Crespo J, Fábrega E. Vitamin D deficiency in chronic liver disease. World Journal of Hepatology [Internet]. Dec 27, 2014;6(12):901. Available from: http://www.ncbi.nlm.nih.gov/pubmed/25544877 [Accessed: Dec 26, 2016]

[85] Hsu CC, Kowdley KV. The effects of alcohol on other chronic liver diseases. Clinical Liver Disease [Internet]. Aug 2016;20(3):581-594. Available from: http://linkinghub.elsevier.com/retrieve/pii/S1089326116300137 [Accessed: Dec 28, 2016]

[86] Ajmera VH, Terrault NA, Harrison SA. Is moderate alcohol use in non-alcoholic fatty liver disease good or bad? a critical review. Hepatology [Internet]. Jun 2017;65(6): 2090-2099. Available from: http://www.ncbi.nlm.nih.gov/pubmed/28100008 [Accessed: Feb 18, 2017]

[87] 2015-2020 Dietary Guidelines: health.gov [Internet]. 2015. Available from: https://health.gov/dietaryguidelines/2015/guidelines/ [Accessed: Feb 18, 2017]

[88] Kang L, Sebastian BM, Pritchard MT, Pratt BT, Previs SF, Nagy LE. Chronic ethanol-induced insulin resistance is associated with macrophage infiltration into adipose tissue and altered expression of adipocytokines. Alcoholism: Clinical and Experimental Research [Internet]. Sep 2007;31(9):1581-1588. Available from: http://doi.wiley.com/10.1111/j.1530-0277.2007.00452.x [Accessed: Feb 18, 2017]

[89] Conigrave KM, Hu BF, Camargo CA, Stampfer MJ, Willett WC, Rimm EB. A prospective study of drinking patterns in relation to risk of type 2 diabetes among men. Diabetes [Internet]. Oct 2001;50(10):2390-2395. Available from: http://www.ncbi.nlm.nih.gov/pubmed/11574424 [Accessed: Feb 18, 2017]

[90] Pischon T, Girman CJ, Rifai N, Hotamisligil GS, Rimm EB. Association between dietary factors and plasma adiponectin concentrations in men. American Journal of Clinical Nutrition [Internet]. Apr 2005;81(4):780-786. Available from: http://www.ncbi.nlm.nih.gov/pubmed/15817852 [Accessed: Feb 18, 2017]

[91] Davies MJ, Baer DJ, Judd JT, Brown ED, Campbell WS, Taylor PR. Effects of moderate alcohol intake on fasting insulin and glucose concentrations and insulin sensitivity in postmenopausal women: A randomized controlled trial. Journal of the American Medical Association [Internet]. May 15, 2002;287(19):2559-2562. Available from: http://www.ncbi.nlm.nih.gov/pubmed/12020337 [Accessed: Feb 18, 2017]

[92] Dunn W, Sanyal AJ, Brunt EM, Unalp-Arida A, Donohue M, McCullough AJ, et al. Modest alcohol consumption is associated with decreased prevalence of steatohepatitis in patients with non-alcoholic fatty liver disease (NAFLD). Journal of Hepatology [Internet]. Aug 2012;57(2):384-391. Available from: http://linkinghub.elsevier.com/retrieve/pii/S0168827812002796 [Accessed: Feb 18, 2017]

[93] Kwon HK, Greenson JK, Conjeevaram HS. Effect of lifetime alcohol consumption on the histological severity of non-alcoholic fatty liver disease. Liver International [Internet]. Jan 2014;34(1):129-135. Available from: http://doi.wiley.com/10.1111/liv.12230 [Accessed: Feb 18, 2017]

[94] Ascha MS, Hanounch IA, Lopez R, Tamimi TA-R, Feldstein AF, Zein NN. The incidence and risk factors of hepatocellular carcinoma in patients with nonalcoholic steatohepatitis. Hepatology [Internet]. Jun 2010;51(6):1972-1978. Available from: http://doi.wiley.com/10.1002/hep.23527 [Accessed: Dec 27, 2016]

[95] Wieckowska A, Zein NN, Yerian LM, Lopez AR, McCullough AJ, Feldstein AE. In vivo assessment of liver cell apoptosis as a novel biomarker of disease severity in nonalcoholic fatty liver disease. Hepatology [Internet]. Jul 2006;44(1):27-33. Available from: http://doi.wiley.com/10.1002/hep.21223 [Accessed: Feb 18, 2017]

[96] Feldstein AE, Wieckowska A, Lopez AR, Liu Y-C, Zein NN, McCullough AJ. Cytokeratin-18 fragment levels as noninvasive biomarkers for nonalcoholic steatohepatitis: A multicenter validation study. Hepatology [Internet]. Oct 2009;50(4):1072-1078. Available from: http://doi.wiley.com/10.1002/hep.23050 [Accessed: Feb 18, 2017]

[97] Feldstein AE, Alkhouri N, De Vito R, Alisi A, Lopez R, Nobili V. Serum cytokeratin-18 fragment levels are useful biomarkers for nonalcoholic steatohepatitis in children. The American Journal of Gastroenterology [Internet]. Sep 11, 2013;108(9):1526-1531. Available from: http://www.nature.com/doifinder/10.1038/ajg.2013.168 [Accessed: Feb 18, 2017]

[98] Cusi K, Chang Z, Harrison S, Lomonaco R, Bril F, Orsak B, et al. Limited value of plasma cytokeratin-18 as a biomarker for NASH and fibrosis in patients with non-alcoholic fatty liver disease. Journal of Hepatology [Internet]. Jan 2014;60(1):167-174. Available from: http://linkinghub.elsevier.com/retrieve/pii/S0168827813005965 [Accessed: Feb 18, 2017]

[99] Yesilova Z, Yaman H, Oktenli C, Ozcan A, Uygun A, Cakir E, et al. Systemic markers of lipid peroxidation and antioxidants in patients with nonalcoholic fatty liver disease. The American Journal of Gastroenterology [Internet]. Apr 2005;100(4):850-855. Available from: http://www.ncbi.nlm.nih.gov/pubmed/15784031 [Accessed: Oct 23, 2017]

[100] Chalasani N, Deeg MA, Crabb DW. Systemic levels of lipid peroxidation and its metabolic and dietary correlates in patients with nonalcoholic steatohepatitis. The American Journal of Gastroenterology [Internet]. Aug 2004;99(8):1497-1502. Available from: http://www.nature.com/doifinder/10.1111/j.1572-0241.2004.30159.x [Accessed: Oct 23, 2017]

[101] Jayakumar S, Harrison SA, Loomba R. Noninvasive markers of fibrosis and inflammation in nonalcoholic fatty liver disease. Current Hepatology Reports [Internet]. Jun 21, 2016;15(2):86-95. Available from: http://www.ncbi.nlm.nih.gov/pubmed/27795938 [Accessed: Feb 18, 2017]

[102] Dixon JB, Bhathal PS, O'Brien PE. Nonalcoholic fatty liver disease: Predictors of non-alcoholic steatohepatitis and liver fibrosis in the severely obese. Gastroenterology [Internet]. Jul 2001;121(1):91-100. Available from: http://www.ncbi.nlm.nih.gov/pubmed/11438497 [Accessed: Oct 30, 2017]

[103] Poynard T, Ratziu V, Charlotte F, Messous D, Munteanu M, Imbert-Bismut F, et al. Diagnostic value of biochemical markers (NashTest) for the prediction of non alcoholo steato hepatitis in patients with non-alcoholic fatty liver disease. BMC Gastroenterology [Internet]. Nov 10, 2006;6(1):34. Available from: http://bmcgastroenterol.biomedcentral.com/articles/10.1186/1471-230X-6-34 [Accessed: Oct 30, 2017]

[104] Hyysalo J, Männistö VT, Zhou Y, Arola J, Kärjä V, Leivonen M, et al. A population-based study on the prevalence of NASH using scores validated against liver histology. Journal of Hepatology [Internet]. Apr 2014;60(4):839-846. Available from: http://linkinghub.elsevier.com/retrieve/pii/S0168827813008738 [Accessed: Oct 30, 2017]

[105] Anty R, Iannelli A, Patouraux S, Bonnafous S, Lavallard VJ, Senni-Buratti M, et al. A new composite model including metabolic syndrome, alanine aminotransferase and

cytokeratin-18 for the diagnosis of non-alcoholic steatohepatitis in morbidly obese patients. Alimentary Pharmacology & Therapeutics [Internet]. Dec 2010;**32**(11-12):1315-1322. Available from: http://doi.wiley.com/10.1111/j.1365-2036.2010.04480.x [Accessed: Oct 30, 2017]

[106] Younossi ZM, Page S, Rafiq N, Birerdinc A, Stepanova M, Hossain N, et al. A biomarker panel for non-alcoholic steatohepatitis (NASH) and NASH-related fibrosis. Obesity Surgery [Internet]. Apr 8, 2011;**21**(4):431-439. Available from: http://link.springer.com/10.1007/s11695-010-0204-1 [Accessed: Oct 30, 2017]

[107] Feldstein AE, Lopez R, Tamimi TA-R, Yerian L, Chung Y-M, Berk M, et al. Mass spectrometric profiling of oxidized lipid products in human nonalcoholic fatty liver disease and nonalcoholic steatohepatitis. Hepatology [Internet]. Oct 2010;**51**(10):3046-3054. Available from: http://www.ncbi.nlm.nih.gov/pubmed/20631297 [Accessed: Oct 30, 2017]

[108] Bell LN, Theodorakis JL, Vuppalanchi R, Saxena R, Bemis KG, Wang M, et al. Serum proteomics and biomarker discovery across the spectrum of nonalcoholic fatty liver disease. Hepatology [Internet]. Jan 2010;**51**(1):111-120. Available from: http://www.ncbi.nlm.nih.gov/pubmed/19885878 [Accessed: Oct 29, 2017]

[109] Barr J, Vázquez-Chantada M, Alonso C, Pérez-Cormenzana M, Mayo R, Galán A, et al. Liquid chromatography–mass spectrometry-based parallel metabolic profiling of human and mouse model serum reveals putative biomarkers associated with the progression of nonalcoholic fatty liver disease. Journal of Proteome Research [Internet]. Sep 3, 2010;**9**(9):4501-4512. Available from: http://www.ncbi.nlm.nih.gov/pubmed/20684516 [Accessed: Feb 18, 2017]

[110] Iruzubieta P, Arias-Loste MT, Barbier-Torres L, Martinez-Chantar ML, Crespo J. The need for biomarkers in diagnosis and prognosis of drug-induced liver disease: Does metabolomics have any role? BioMed Research International [Internet]. 2015;**2015**:1-8. Available from: http://www.ncbi.nlm.nih.gov/pubmed/26824035 [Accessed: Feb 18, 2017]

[111] Safaei A, Arefi Oskouie A, Mohebbi SR, Rezaei-Tavirani M, Mahboubi M, Peyvandi M, et al. Metabolomic analysis of human cirrhosis, hepatocellular carcinoma, non-alcoholic fatty liver disease and non-alcoholic steatohepatitis diseases. Gastroenterology and Hepatology from Bed to Bench [Internet]. 2016;**9**(3):158-173. Available from: http://www.ncbi.nlm.nih.gov/pubmed/27458508 [Accessed: Feb 18, 2017]

[112] Barr J, Caballería J, Martínez-Arranz I, Domínguez-Díez A, Alonso C, Muntané J, et al. Obesity-dependent metabolic signatures associated with nonalcoholic fatty liver disease progression. Journal of Proteome Research [Internet]. Apr 6, 2012;**11**(4):2521-2532. Available from: http://www.ncbi.nlm.nih.gov/pubmed/22364559 [Accessed: Feb 18, 2017]

[113] Alonso C, Fernández-Ramos D, Varela-Rey M, Martínez-Arranz I, Navasa N, Van Liempd SM, et al. Metabolomic identification of subtypes of nonalcoholic steatohepatitis. Gastroenterology [Internet]. 2017;**152**(6):1449-1461.e7. Available from: http://linkinghub.elsevier.com/retrieve/pii/S0016508517300720 [Accessed: Mar 5, 2017]

[114]   Tan Y, Ge G, Pan T, Wen D, Gan J. A pilot study of serum microRNAs panel as potential
        biomarkers for diagnosis of nonalcoholic fatty liver disease. PLoS One [Internet]. Aug
        20, 2014;9(8):e105192. Available from: http://www.ncbi.nlm.nih.gov/pubmed/25141008
        [Accessed: Oct 29, 2017]

[115]   Shah AG, Lydecker A, Murray K, Tetri BN, Contos MJ, Sanyal AJ, et al. Comparison of
        noninvasive markers of fibrosis in patients with nonalcoholic fatty liver disease. Clinical
        Gastroenterology and Hepatology [Internet]. Oct 2009;7(10):1104-1112. Available from:
        http://www.ncbi.nlm.nih.gov/pubmed/19523535 [Accessed: Oct 26, 2017]

[116]   Musso G, Gambino R, Cassader M, Pagano G. Meta-analysis: Natural history of non-
        alcoholic fatty liver disease (NAFLD) and diagnostic accuracy of non-invasive tests for
        liver disease severity. Annals of Medicine [Internet]. Dec 2, 2011;43(8):617-649. Available
        from: http://www.ncbi.nlm.nih.gov/pubmed/21039302 [Accessed: Feb 18, 2017]

[117]   Sandrin L, Fourquet B, Hasquenoph J-M, Yon S, Fournier C, Mal F, et al. Transient elas-
        tography: A new noninvasive method for assessment of hepatic fibrosis. Ultrasound
        in Medicine and Biology [Internet]. Dec 2003;29(12):1705-1713. Available from: http://
        www.ncbi.nlm.nih.gov/pubmed/14698338 [Accessed: Feb 19, 2017]

[118]   Petta S, Di Marco V, Cammà C, Butera G, Cabibi D, Craxì A. Reliability of liver stiff-
        ness measurement in non-alcoholic fatty liver disease: The effects of body mass index.
        Aliment Pharmacol Ther [Internet]. Jun 2011;33(12):1350-1360. Available from: http://
        doi.wiley.com/10.1111/j.1365-2036.2011.04668.x [Accessed: Feb 19, 2017]

[119]   Myers RP, Pomier-Layrargues G, Kirsch R, Pollett A, Duarte-Rojo A, Wong D, et al.
        Feasibility and diagnostic performance of the FibroScan XL probe for liver stiffness mea-
        surement in overweight and obese patients. Hepatology [Internet]. Jan 2012;55(1):199-
        208. Available from: http://www.ncbi.nlm.nih.gov/pubmed/21898479 [Accessed: Feb
        19, 2017]

[120]   Castera L, Pawlotsky J-M. Noninvasive diagnosis of liver fibrosis in patients with
        chronic hepatitis C. MedGenMed [Internet]. Nov 9, 2005;7(4):39. Available from: http://
        www.ncbi.nlm.nih.gov/pubmed/16614661 [Accessed: Feb 19, 2017]

[121]   Pathik P, Ravindra S, Ajay C, Prasad B, Jatin P, Prabha S. Fibroscan versus simple
        noninvasive screening tools in predicting fibrosis in high-risk nonalcoholic fatty liver
        disease patients from Western India. Annals of Gastroenterology [Internet]. Apr-Jun
        2017;28(2):281-286. Available from: http://www.ncbi.nlm.nih.gov/pubmed/25830783

[122]   Yoneda M, Fujita K, Inamori M, Nakajima A, Tamano M, Hiraishi H, et al. Transient elas-
        tography in patients with non-alcoholic fatty liver disease (NAFLD). Gut [Internet]. Apr 5,
        2007;56(9):1330-1331. Available from: http://www.ncbi.nlm.nih.gov/pubmed/17470477
        [Accessed: Feb 19, 2017]

[123]   Cassinotto C, Boursier J, de Lédinghen V, Lebigot J, Lapuyade B, Cales P, et al. Liver
        stiffness in nonalcoholic fatty liver disease: A comparison of supersonic shear imaging,
        FibroScan, and ARFI with liver biopsy. Hepatology [Internet]. Jun 2016;63(6):1817-1827.
        Available from: http://doi.wiley.com/10.1002/hep.28394 [Accessed: Feb 19, 2017]

[124] Lupsor M, Badea R, Stefanescu H, Grigorescu M, Serban A, Radu C, et al. Performance of unidimensional transient elastography in staging non-alcoholic steatohepatitis. Journal of Gastrointestinal and Liver Diseases [Internet]. Mar 2010;19(1):53-60. Available from: http://www.ncbi.nlm.nih.gov/pubmed/20361076 [Accessed: Feb 19, 2017]

[125] Yoneda M, Yoneda M, Mawatari H, Fujita K, Endo H, Iida H, et al. Noninvasive assessment of liver fibrosis by measurement of stiffness in patients with nonalcoholic fatty liver disease (NAFLD). Digestive and Liver Disease [Internet]. May 2008;40(5):371-378. Available from: http://www.ncbi.nlm.nih.gov/pubmed/18083083 [Accessed: Feb 19, 2017]

[126] Kumar R, Rastogi A, Sharma MK, Bhatia V, Tyagi P, Sharma P, et al. Liver stiffness measurements in patients with different stages of nonalcoholic fatty liver disease: Diagnostic performance and clinicopathological correlation. Digestive Diseases and Sciences [Internet]. Jan 12, 2013;58(1):265-274. Available from: http://link.springer.com/10.1007/s10620-012-2306-1 [Accessed: Feb 19, 2017]

[127] Lin X-F, Shi K-Q, You J, Liu W-Y, Luo Y-W, Wu F-L, et al. Increased risk of colorectal malignant neoplasm in patients with nonalcoholic fatty liver disease: A large study. Molecular Biology Reports [Internet]. May 22, 2014;41(5):2989-2997. Available from: http://www.ncbi.nlm.nih.gov/pubmed/24449368 [Accessed: Mar 7, 2017]

[128] Wong VW-S, Vergniol J, Wong GL-H, Foucher J, Chan HL-Y, Le Bail B, et al. Diagnosis of fibrosis and cirrhosis using liver stiffness measurement in nonalcoholic fatty liver disease. Hepatology [Internet]. Feb 2010;51(2):454-462. Available from: http://www.ncbi.nlm.nih.gov/pubmed/20101745 [Accessed: Feb 19, 2017]

[129] Nobili V, Vizzutti F, Arena U, Abraldes JG, Marra F, Pietrobattista A, et al. Accuracy and reproducibility of transient elastography for the diagnosis of fibrosis in pediatric nonalcoholic steatohepatitis. Hepatology [Internet]. Aug 2008;48(2):442-448. Available from: http://www.ncbi.nlm.nih.gov/pubmed/18563842 [Accessed: Mar 8, 2017]

[130] de Lédinghen V, Wong VW-S, Vergniol J, Wong GL-H, Foucher J, Chu SH-T, et al. Diagnosis of liver fibrosis and cirrhosis using liver stiffness measurement: Comparison between M and XL probe of FibroScan®. Journal of Hepatology [Internet]. Apr 2012;56(4):833-839. Available from: http://www.ncbi.nlm.nih.gov/pubmed/22173167 [Accessed: Feb 19, 2017]

[131] Wong VW-S, Vergniol J, Wong GL-H, Foucher J, Chan AW-H, Chermak F, et al. Liver stiffness measurement using XL probe in patients with nonalcoholic fatty liver disease. The American Journal of Gastroenterology [Internet]. Dec 2, 2012;107(12):1862-1871. Available from: http://www.ncbi.nlm.nih.gov/pubmed/23032979 [Accessed: Feb 19, 2017]

[132] Palmeri ML, Wang MH, Rouze NC, Abdelmalek MF, Guy CD, Moser B, et al. Noninvasive evaluation of hepatic fibrosis using acoustic radiation force-based shear stiffness in patients with nonalcoholic fatty liver disease. Journal of Hepatology [Internet]. Sep 2011;55(3):666-672. Available from: http://linkinghub.elsevier.com/retrieve/pii/S0168827811000079 [Accessed: Feb 19, 2017]

[133] Liu H, Fu J, Hong R, Liu L, Li F. Acoustic radiation force impulse elastography for the non-invasive evaluation of hepatic fibrosis in non-alcoholic fatty liver disease patients:

A systematic review & meta-analysis. PLoS One [Internet]. Jul 1, 2015;**10**(7):e0127782. Available from: http://dx.plos.org/10.1371/journal.pone.0127782 [Accessed: Feb 19, 2017]

[134] Talwalkar JA, Yin M, Fidler JL, Sanderson SO, Kamath PS, Ehman RL. Magnetic resonance imaging of hepatic fibrosis: Emerging clinical applications. Hepatology [Internet]. Dec 27, 2007;**47**(1):332-342. Available from: http://www.ncbi.nlm.nih.gov/pubmed/18161879 [Accessed: Feb 19, 2017]

[135] Yin M, Glaser KJ, Talwalkar JA, Chen J, Manduca A, Ehman RL. Hepatic MR elastography: Clinical performance in a series of 1377 consecutive examinations. Radiology [Internet]. Jan 2016;**278**(1):114-124. Available from: http://pubs.rsna.org/doi/10.1148/radiol.2015142141 [Accessed: Feb 19, 2017]

[136] Gallego-Durán R, Cerro-Salido P, Gomez-Gonzalez E, Pareja MJ, Ampuero J, Rico MC, et al. Imaging biomarkers for steatohepatitis and fibrosis detection in non-alcoholic fatty liver disease. Scientific Reports [Internet]. Aug 12, 2016;**6**:31421. Available from: http://www.ncbi.nlm.nih.gov/pubmed/27514671 [Accessed: Dec 26, 2016]

[137] Pavlides M, Banerjee R, Tunnicliffe EM, Kelly C, Collier J, Wang LM, et al. Multiparametric magnetic resonance imaging for the assessment of non-alcoholic fatty liver disease severity. Liver International [Internet]. Jul 2017;**37**(7):1065-1073. Available from: http://www.ncbi.nlm.nih.gov/pubmed/27778429 [Accessed: Oct 29, 2017]

[138] Evans CDJ, Oien KA, MacSween RNM, Mills PR. Non-alcoholic steatohepatitis: A common cause of progressive chronic liver injury? Journal of Clinical Pathology [Internet]. Sep 2002;**55**(9):689-692. Available from: http://www.ncbi.nlm.nih.gov/pubmed/12195000 [Accessed: Dec 26, 2016]

[139] Harrison SA, Torgerson S, Hayashi PH. The natural history of nonalcoholic fatty liver disease: A clinical histopathological study. The American Journal of Gastroenterology [Internet]. Sep 2003;**98**(9):2042-2047. Available from: http://www.ncbi.nlm.nih.gov/pubmed/14499785 [Accessed: Dec 26, 2016]

[140] Fassio E, Alvarez E, Domínguez N, Landeira G, Longo C. Natural history of nonalcoholic steatohepatitis: A longitudinal study of repeat liver biopsies. Hepatology [Internet]. Oct 2004;**40**(4):820-826. Available from: http://doi.wiley.com/10.1002/hep.20410 [Accessed: Dec 26, 2016]

[141] Ekstedt M, Franzén LE, Mathiesen UL, Thorelius L, Holmqvist M, Bodemar G, et al. Long-term follow-up of patients with NAFLD and elevated liver enzymes. Hepatology [Internet]. Oct 2006;**44**(4):865-873. Available from: http://doi.wiley.com/10.1002/hep.21327 [Accessed: Dec 26, 2016]

[142] Hamaguchi E, Takamura T, Sakurai M, Mizukoshi E, Zen Y, Takeshita Y, et al. Histological course of nonalcoholic fatty liver disease in Japanese patients: Tight glycemic control, rather than weight reduction, ameliorates liver fibrosis. Diabetes Care [Internet]. Feb 1, 2010;**33**(2):284-286. Available from: http://care.diabetesjournals.org/cgi/doi/10.2337/dc09-0148 [Accessed: Dec 26, 2016]

[143] Wong VW-S, Wong GL-H, Choi PC-L, Chan AW-H, Li MK-P, Chan H-Y, et al. Disease progression of non-alcoholic fatty liver disease: A prospective study with paired liver biopsies at 3 years. Gut [Internet]. Jul 1, 2010;59(7):969-974. Available from: http://gut. bmj.com/cgi/doi/10.1136/gut.2009.205088 [Accessed: Dec 26, 2016]

[144] Chan W-K, Ida NH, Cheah P-L, Goh K-L. Progression of liver disease in non-alcoholic fatty liver disease: A prospective clinicopathological follow-up study. Journal of Digestive Diseases [Internet]. Oct 2014;15(10):545-552. Available from: http://www.ncbi. nlm.nih.gov/pubmed/25060399 [Accessed: Dec 26, 2016]

[145] Fracanzani AL, Valenti L, Bugianesi E, Andreoletti M, Colli A, Vanni E, et al. Risk of severe liver disease in nonalcoholic fatty liver disease with normal aminotransferase levels: A role for insulin resistance and diabetes. Hepatology [Internet]. Sep 2008;48(3):792-798. Available from: http://doi.wiley.com/10.1002/hep.22429 [Accessed: Feb 20, 2017]

[146] Goh GB-B, Pagadala MR, Dasarathy J, Unalp-Arida A, Sargent R, Hawkins C, et al. Clinical spectrum of non-alcoholic fatty liver disease in diabetic and non-diabetic patients. BBA Clinical [Internet]. Jun 2015;3:141-145. Available from: http://linkinghub. elsevier.com/retrieve/pii/S221464741400018X [Accessed: Feb 20, 2017]

[147] Bazick J, Donithan M, Neuschwander-Tetri BA, Kleiner D, Brunt EM, Wilson L, et al. Clinical model for NASH and advanced fibrosis in adult patients with diabetes and NAFLD: Guidelines for referral in NAFLD. Diabetes Care [Internet]. Jul 2015;38(7):1347-1355. Available from: http://care.diabetesjournals.org/lookup/doi/10.2337/dc14-1239 [Accessed: Feb 20, 2017]

[148] Motamed N, Sohrabi M, Ajdarkosh H, Hemmasi G, Maadi M, Sayeedian FS, et al. Fatty liver index vs waist circumference for predicting non-alcoholic fatty liver disease. World Journal of Gastroenterology [Internet]. Mar 14, 2016;22(10):3023-3030. Available from: http://www.wjgnet.com/1007-9327/full/v22/i10/3023.htm [Accessed: Feb 21, 2017]

[149] DeFilippis AP, Blaha MJ, Martin SS, Reed RM, Jones SR, Nasir K, et al. Nonalcoholic fatty liver disease and serum lipoproteins: The multi-ethnic study of atherosclerosis. Atherosclerosis [Internet]. Apr 2013;227(2):429-436. Available from: http://www.ncbi. nlm.nih.gov/pubmed/23419204 [Accessed: Feb 21, 2017]

[150] Marchesini G, Marzocchi R. Metabolic syndrome and NASH. Clinical Liver Disease [Internet]. Feb 2007;11(1):105-117, ix. Available from: http://www.ncbi.nlm.nih.gov/ pubmed/17544974 [Accessed: Aug 3, 2015]

[151] Ekstedt M, Hagström H, Nasr P, Fredrikson M, Stål P, Kechagias S, et al. Fibrosis stage is the strongest predictor for disease-specific mortality in NAFLD after up to 33 years of follow-up. Hepatology [Internet]. May 2015;61(5):1547-1554. Available from: http:// doi.wiley.com/10.1002/hep.27368 [Accessed: Dec 26, 2016]

[152] Sanyal A, Poklepovic A, Moyneur E, Barghout V. Population-based risk factors and resource utilization for HCC: US perspective. Current Medical Research and Opinion

[Internet]. Sep 29, 2010;**26**(9):2183-2191. Available from: http://www.tandfonline.com/doi/full/10.1185/03007995.2010.506375 [Accessed: Dec 27, 2016]

[153] Maeda S, Kamata H, Luo J-L, Leffert H, Karin M. IKKbeta couples hepatocyte death to cytokine-driven compensatory proliferation that promotes chemical hepatocarcinogenesis. Cell [Internet]. Jul 1, 2005;**121**(7):977-990. Available from: http://linkinghub.elsevier.com/retrieve/pii/S0092867405003946 [Accessed: Feb 21, 2017]

[154] Adams LA, Lymp JF, St Sauver J, Sanderson SO, Lindor KD, Feldstein A, et al. The natural history of nonalcoholic fatty liver disease: A population-based cohort study. Gastroenterology [Internet]. Jul 2005;**129**(1):113-121. Available from: http://www.ncbi.nlm.nih.gov/pubmed/16012941 [Accessed: May 3, 2016]

[155] Chitturi S, Abeygunasekera S, Farrell GC, Holmes-Walker J, Hui JM, Fung C, et al. NASH and insulin resistance: Insulin hypersecretion and specific association with the insulin resistance syndrome. Hepatology [Internet]. Feb 2002;**35**(2):373-379. Available from: http://doi.wiley.com/10.1053/jhep.2002.30692 [Accessed: Feb 21, 2017]

[156] Pagano G, Pacini G, Musso G, Gambino R, Mecca F, Depetris N, et al. Nonalcoholic steatohepatitis, insulin resistance, and metabolic syndrome: Further evidence for an etiologic association. Hepatology [Internet]. Feb 2002;**35**(2):367-372. Available from: http://doi.wiley.com/10.1053/jhep.2002.30690 [Accessed: Feb 21, 2017]

[157] DeFronzo RA, Tobin JD, Andres R. Glucose clamp technique: A method for quantifying insulin secretion and resistance. American Journal of Physiology [Internet]. Sep 1979;**237**(3):E214-E223. Available from: http://www.ncbi.nlm.nih.gov/pubmed/382871 [Accessed: Dec 27, 2016]

[158] Matthews DR, Hosker JP, Rudenski AS, Naylor BA, Treacher DF, Turner RC. Homeostasis model assessment: Insulin resistance and beta-cell function from fasting plasma glucose and insulin concentrations in man. Diabetologia [Internet]. Jul 1985;**28**(7):412-419. Available from: http://www.ncbi.nlm.nih.gov/pubmed/3899825 [Accessed: Dec 27, 2016]

[159] Armstrong MJ, Gaunt P, Aithal GP, Barton D, Hull D, Parker R, et al. Liraglutide safety and efficacy in patients with non-alcoholic steatohepatitis (LEAN): A multicentre, double-blind, randomised, placebo-controlled phase 2 study. Lancet (London, England) [Internet]. Feb 13, 2016;**387**(10019):679-690. Available from: http://linkinghub.elsevier.com/retrieve/pii/S014067361500803X [Accessed: Mar 6, 2017]

[160] Belfort R, Harrison SA, Brown K, Darland C, Finch J, Hardies J, et al. A placebo-controlled trial of pioglitazone in subjects with nonalcoholic steatohepatitis. The New England Journal of Medicine [Internet]. Nov 30, 2006;**355**(22):2297-2307. Available from: http://www.ncbi.nlm.nih.gov/pubmed/17135584 [Accessed: Mar 6, 2017]

[161] Cusi K, Orsak B, Bril F, Lomonaco R, Hecht J, Ortiz-Lopez C, et al. Long-term pioglitazone treatment for patients with nonalcoholic steatohepatitis and prediabetes or Type 2 diabetes mellitus. Annals of Internal Medicine [Internet]. Sep 6, 2016;**165**(5):305. Available from: http://www.ncbi.nlm.nih.gov/pubmed/27322798 [Accessed: Mar 6, 2017]

[162] Sanyal AJ, Chalasani N, Kowdley KV, McCullough A, Diehl AM, Bass NM, et al. Pioglitazone, vitamin E, or placebo for nonalcoholic steatohepatitis. The New England Journal of Medicine [Internet]. May 6, 2010;362(18):1675-1685. Available from: http://www.ncbi.nlm.nih.gov/pubmed/20427778 [Accessed: Mar 6, 2017]

[163] Aithal GP, Thomas JA, Kaye PV, Lawson A, Ryder SD, Spendlove I, et al. Randomized, placebo-controlled trial of pioglitazone in nondiabetic subjects with nonalcoholic steatohepatitis. Gastroenterology [Internet]. Oct 2008;135(4):1176-1184. Available from: http://linkinghub.elsevier.com/retrieve/pii/S0016508508011013 [Accessed: Mar 6, 2017]

[164] García-Monzón C, Lo Iacono O, Crespo J, Romero-Gómez M, García-Samaniego J, Fernández-Bermejo M, et al. Increased soluble CD36 is linked to advanced steatosis in nonalcoholic fatty liver disease. European Journal of Clinical Investigation [Internet]. Jan 2014;44(1):65-73. Available from: http://doi.wiley.com/10.1111/eci.12192 [Accessed: Dec 26, 2016]

[165] Fernández-Friera L, Ibáñez B, Fuster V. Imaging subclinical atherosclerosis: Is it ready for prime time? A review. Journal of Cardiovascular Translational Research [Internet]. Oct 14, 2014;7(7):623-634. Available from: http://link.springer.com/10.1007/s12265-014-9582-4 [Accessed: Dec 27, 2016]

[166] Robsahm TE, Aagnes B, Hjartåker A, Langseth H, Bray FI, Larsen IK. Body mass index, physical activity, and colorectal cancer by anatomical subsites: A systematic review and meta-analysis of cohort studies. European Journal of Cancer Prevention [Internet]. Nov 2013;22(6):492-505. Available from: http://content.wkhealth.com/linkback/openurl?sid=WKPTLP:landingpage&an=00008469-201311000-00002 [Accessed: Mar 7, 2017]

[167] Kaminski MF, Polkowski M, Kraszewska E, Rupinski M, Butruk E, Regula J. A score to estimate the likelihood of detecting advanced colorectal neoplasia at colonoscopy. Gut [Internet]. Jul 2014;63(7):1112-1119. Available from: http://gut.bmj.com/lookup/doi/10.1136/gutjnl-2013-304965 [Accessed: Mar 7, 2017]

[168] Peeters PJHL, Bazelier MT, Leufkens HGM, de Vries F, De Bruin ML. The risk of colorectal cancer in patients with Type 2 diabetes: Associations with treatment stage and obesity. Diabetes Care [Internet]. Mar 2015;38(3):495-502. Available from: http://www.ncbi.nlm.nih.gov/pubmed/25552419 [Accessed: Mar 7, 2017]

[169] Aune D, Greenwood DC, Chan DSM, Vieira R, Vieira AR, Navarro Rosenblatt DA, et al. Body mass index, abdominal fatness and pancreatic cancer risk: A systematic review and non-linear dose-response meta-analysis of prospective studies. Annals of Oncology [Internet]. Apr 1, 2012;23(4):843-852. Available from: https://academic.oup.com/annonc/article-lookup/doi/10.1093/annonc/mdr398 [Accessed: Mar 7, 2017]

[170] Rose DP, Vona-Davis L. Biochemical and molecular mechanisms for the association between obesity, chronic inflammation, and breast cancer. Biofactors [Internet]. Jan 2014;40(1):1-12. Available from: http://doi.wiley.com/10.1002/biof.1109 [Accessed: Mar 7, 2017]

[171] Schmid D, Ricci C, Behrens G, Leitzmann MF. Adiposity and risk of thyroid cancer: A systematic review and meta-analysis. Obesity Reviews [Internet]. Dec 2015;**16**(12):1042-1054. Available from: http://www.ncbi.nlm.nih.gov/pubmed/26365757 [Accessed: Mar 7, 2017]

[172] Sørensen HT, Mellemkjaer L, Jepsen P, Thulstrup AM, Baron J, Olsen JH, et al. Risk of cancer in patients hospitalized with fatty liver: A Danish cohort study. Journal of Clinical Gastroenterology [Internet]. Apr 2003;**36**(4):356-359. Available from: http://www.ncbi.nlm.nih.gov/pubmed/12642745 [Accessed: Mar 7, 2017]

[173] Bilici A, Ozguroglu M, Mihmanli I, Turna H, Adaletli I. A case-control study of non-alcoholic fatty liver disease in breast cancer. Medical Oncology [Internet]. 2007;**24**(4):367-371. Available from: http://www.ncbi.nlm.nih.gov/pubmed/17917083 [Accessed: Mar 7, 2017]

[174] Stadlmayr A, Aigner E, Steger B, Scharinger L, Lederer D, Mayr A, et al. Nonalcoholic fatty liver disease: An independent risk factor for colorectal neoplasia. Journal of Internal Medicine [Internet]. Jul 2011;**270**(1):41-49. Available from: http://www.ncbi.nlm.nih.gov/pubmed/21414047 [Accessed: Mar 7, 2017]

[175] Wong VW-S, Wong GL-H, Tsang SW-C, Fan T, Chu WC-W, Woo J, et al. High prevalence of colorectal neoplasm in patients with non-alcoholic steatohepatitis. Gut [Internet]. Jun 1, 2011;**60**(6):829-836. Available from: http://www.ncbi.nlm.nih.gov/pubmed/21339204 [Accessed: Dec 27, 2016]

[176] Hwang ST, Cho YK, Park JH, Kim HJ, Park Il D, Sohn II C, et al. Relationship of non-alcoholic fatty liver disease to colorectal adenomatous polyps. Journal of Gastroenterology and Hepatology [Internet]. Mar 2010;**25**(3):562-567. Available from: http://www.ncbi.nlm.nih.gov/pubmed/20074156 [Accessed: Mar 7, 2017]

[177] Kim S, Keku TO, Martin C, Galanko J, Woosley JT, Schroeder JC, et al. Circulating levels of inflammatory cytokines and risk of colorectal adenomas. Cancer Research [Internet]. Jan 1, 2008;**68**(1):323-328. Available from: http://www.ncbi.nlm.nih.gov/pubmed/18172326 [Accessed: Mar 7, 2017]

[178] Machado MV, Gonçalves S, Carepa F, Coutinho J, Costa A, Cortez-Pinto H. Impaired renal function in morbid obese patients with nonalcoholic fatty liver disease. Liver International [Internet]. Feb 2012;**32**(2):241-248. Available from: http://doi.wiley.com/10.1111/j.1478-3231.2011.02623.x [Accessed: Feb 21, 2017]

[179] Targher G, Chonchol MB, Byrne CD. CKD and nonalcoholic fatty liver disease. American Journal of Kidney Diseases [Internet]. Oct 2014;**64**(4):638-652. Available from: http://www.ncbi.nlm.nih.gov/pubmed/25085644 [Accessed: Feb 21, 2017]

[180] Choudhary NS, Saraf N, Kumar N, Rai R, Saigal S, Gautam D, et al. Nonalcoholic fatty liver is not associated with incident chronic kidney disease. European Journal of Gastroenterology & Hepatology [Internet]. Dec 2015;**28**(4):1. Available from: http://www.ncbi.nlm.nih.gov/pubmed/26636408 [Accessed: Feb 21, 2017]

[181] Musso G, Gambino R, Tabibian JH, Ekstedt M, Kechagias S, Hamaguchi M, et al. Association of non-alcoholic fatty liver disease with chronic kidney disease: A systematic review and meta-analysis. PLOS Medicine [Internet]. Jul 22, 2014;11(7):e1001680. Available from: http://dx.plos.org/10.1371/journal.pmed.1001680 [Accessed: Feb 21, 2017]

[182] Musso G, Cassader M, Olivetti C, Rosina F, Carbone G, Gambino R. Association of obstructive sleep apnoea with the presence and severity of non-alcoholic fatty liver disease. A systematic review and meta-analysis. Obesity Reviews [Internet]. May 2013;14(5):417-431. Available from: http://doi.wiley.com/10.1111/obr.12020 [Accessed: Feb 21, 2017]

[183] Minville C, Hilleret M-N, Tamisier R, Aron-Wisnewsky J, Clement K, Trocme C, et al. Nonalcoholic fatty liver disease, nocturnal hypoxia, and endothelial function in patients with sleep apnea. Chest [Internet]. Mar 1, 2014;145(3):525-533. Available from: http://linkinghub.elsevier.com/retrieve/pii/S0012369215343646 [Accessed: Feb 21, 2017]

[184] Sookoian S, Pirola CJ. Obstructive sleep apnea is associated with fatty liver and abnormal liver enzymes: A meta-analysis. Obesity Surgery [Internet]. Nov 7, 2013;23(11):1815-1825. Available from: http://www.ncbi.nlm.nih.gov/pubmed/23740153 [Accessed: Jun 4, 2016]

[185] Drager LF, Jun JC, Polotsky VY. Metabolic consequences of intermittent hypoxia: Relevance to obstructive sleep apnea. Best Practice & Research: Clinical Endocrinology & Metabolism [Internet]. Oct 2010;24(5):843-851. Available from: http://linkinghub.elsevier.com/retrieve/pii/S1521690X10001119 [Accessed: Feb 21, 2017]

[186] Targher G, Lonardo A, Rossini M. Nonalcoholic fatty liver disease and decreased bone mineral density: Is there a link? Journal of Endocrinological Investigation [Internet]. Aug 24, 2015;38(8):817-825. Available from: http://link.springer.com/10.1007/s40618-015-0315-6 [Accessed: Dec 27, 2016]

[187] Miele L, Vallone S, Cefalo C, La Torre G, Di Stasi C, Vecchio FM, et al. Prevalence, characteristics and severity of non-alcoholic fatty liver disease in patients with chronic plaque psoriasis. Journal of Hepatology [Internet]. Oct 2009;51(4):778-786. Available from: http://www.ncbi.nlm.nih.gov/pubmed/19664838 [Accessed: Dec 27, 2016]

[188] Cerda C, Pérez Ayuso RM, Riquelme A, Soza A, Villaseca P, Sir-Petermann T, et al. Nonalcoholic fatty liver disease in women with polycystic ovary syndrome. Journal of Hepatology [Internet]. Sep 2007;47(3):412-417. Available from: http://linkinghub.elsevier.com/retrieve/pii/S0168827807002899 [Accessed: Dec 27, 2016]

[189] Xu L, Ma H, Miao M, Li Y. Impact of subclinical hypothyroidism on the development of non-alcoholic fatty liver disease: A prospective case control study. Journal of Hepatology [Internet]. Nov 2012;57(5):1153-1154. Available from: http://www.ncbi.nlm.nih.gov/pubmed/22940010 [Accessed: Jun 4, 2016]

[190] Adams LA, Feldstein A, Lindor KD, Angulo P. Nonalcoholic fatty liver disease among patients with hypothalamic and pituitary dysfunction. Hepatology [Internet]. Apr

2004;39(4):909-914. Available from: http://www.ncbi.nlm.nih.gov/pubmed/15057893 [Accessed: Jun 4, 2016]

[191] Barbonetti A, Caterina Vassallo MR, Cotugno M, Felzani G, Francavilla S, Francavilla F. Low testosterone and non-alcoholic fatty liver disease: Evidence for their independent association in men with chronic spinal cord injury. The Journal of Spinal Cord Medicine [Internet]. Feb 25, 2016;1-7. Available from: http://www.ncbi.nlm.nih.gov/pubmed/25614040 [Accessed: Jun 4, 2016]

[192] Morlán-Coarasa MJ, Arias-Loste MT, Ortiz-García de la Foz V, Martínez-García O, Alonso-Martín C, Crespo J, et al. Incidence of non-alcoholic fatty liver disease and metabolic dysfunction in first episode schizophrenia and related psychotic disorders: A 3-year prospective randomized interventional study. Psychopharmacology (Berlin) [Internet]. Dec 12, 2016;233(23-24):3947-3952. Available from: http://link.springer.com/10.1007/s00213-016-4422-7 [Accessed: Dec 26, 2016]

5

Intra-Abdominal Hypertension and Abdominal Compartment Syndrome in Liver Diseases

Hiroteru Kamimura, Tomoyuki Sugano,
Ryoko Horigome, Naruhiro Kimura,
Masaaki Takamura, Hirokazu Kawai,
Satoshi Yamagiwa and Shuji Terai

Abstract

Intra-abdominal hypertension (IAH) is defined as an intra-abdominal pressure (IAP) above 12 mmHg. Abdominal compartment syndrome (ACS) is defined as an IAP above 20 mmHg with evidence of organ failure. Moreover, IAH/ACS is a condition that can cause acute renal failure, respiratory failure, circulatory disease, gastrointestinal dysfunction, and liver failure due to elevated IAP. The incidence of IAH/ACS increases in the more critically ill patient and is associated with significantly increased morbidity and mortality. Ascites, blood, or tumors increase IAP. In liver cirrhosis, massive ascites is often encountered. Hence, preventing IAH/ACS conditions may improve outcomes of patients with liver disease.

Keywords: intra-abdominal hypertension (IAH), abdominal compartment syndrome (ACS), hepatorenal syndrome (HRS)

1. Introduction

The pressure within the abdominal cavity is normally a little higher than the atmospheric pressure to less than 0 mmHg. Certain physiological conditions such as morbid obesity and pregnancy may be associated with chronic IAP elevations. However, even small increases in intra-abdominal pressure can have adverse effects on renal function, cardiac output, hepatic blood flow, respiratory mechanics, splanchnic perfusion, and intracranial pressure. IAP is approximately 5–7 mmHg in critically ill adults.

Wendt et al. firstly described oliguria in the presence of elevated intra-abdominal pressure in 1876 [1]. In 1947, Bradley published a seminal study of the renal effects of elevated IAP in humans [2]. Despite these early descriptions of the adverse effects of IAH, physicians are not careful about the significance of increased abdominal pressure.

Until recently, patients with ACS were not infrequently managed in the intensive care unit and typically presented with a tense distended abdomen, increased peak inspiratory airway pressure, severe hypercapnia, hypotension, and oliguria. Abdominal ascites occurs typically at the end stage of liver failure. Massive ascites also influences IAP and causes oliguria and acute kidney injury. Commonly, we recognize this symptom and confused it with hepatorenal syndrome (HRS). In such patients, we should take into account the elevation of renal paren-chymal and renal vein pressures, as they are likely the mechanisms of renal impairment. Note that IAH/ACS and HRS are occurring simultaneously. Recently, Matsumoto et al. reported that renal vein dilation predicts poor outcome in patients with refractory cirrhotic ascites [3].

2. Pathophysiology of ACS

The pathology of IAH/ACS is perfusion imbalance in multiple organs: compression of the portal system in the abdominal cavity, compression of the inferior vena cava system in ret-roperitoneal organs, compression of the diaphragm in the intrathoracic organ, and perfusion dysfunction of the brain circulation through increase of intrathoracic pressure [4].

The perfusion imbalance in the upper body originated from the abdominal cavity, which causes circulation impairment and further increased intrathoracic cavity pressure and retroperitoneal cavity. This imbalance presents a functional disorder that substantially affects multiple organs.

ACS is similar to the compartment syndrome in muscular diseases. It is a circulatory disease caused by internal pressure of organs sectioned in a small wall of the compliance anatomically [5]. The normal IAP ranges from sub-atmospheric level to 0 mmHg. Certain physiological conditions, such as morbid obesity and pregnancy, may be associated with chronic IAP elevations. Moreover, IAH is defined as an IAP above 12 mmHg. ACS is defined as an IAP above 20 mmHg with evi-dence of organ failure [6]. IAP is the steady state of pressure concealed within the abdominal cavity. The normal IAP for critically ill patients are 5–7 mmHg range. Once, IAP have increased, patients become the state of IAH. IAH is recognized sustained IAP greater than to 12 mmHg. IAH may also be subclassified according to the duration of symptoms into one of the four groups. This fulminant example of IAH commonly leads to rapid development of ACS. With its development over a protracted time course, the abdominal wall adapts and progressively distends in response to increasing IAP, allowing time for the body to adapt physiologically. The clinical consideration of IAH subtypes is useful in prescribing patients at risk for ACS (**Table 1**) [6].

Primary ACS is characterized by the presence of acute or subacute IAH of relatively brief duration occurring as a result of an intra-abdominal cause such as severe acute pancreatitis, abdominal trauma, ruptured abdominal aortic aneurysm, and liver transplantation [7].

Secondary ACS is characterized by the presence of subacute or chronic IAH that develops mas-sive fluid resuscitation such as an extra-abdominal cause such as sepsis, capillary leak, burns [8].

Classification of IAH		
Hyperacute IAH	Elevated IAP for seconds	Secondary to physical activity, coughing, laughing, sneezing, straining, or defecation
Acute IAH	Elevated IAP that develops over hours and can lead to rapid development of ACS	Secondary to trauma or intra-abdominal hemorrhage
Subacute IAH	Elevated IAP that develops over days and can also lead to ACS	Medical patients
Chronic IAH	Elevated IAP that develops over months or years.	Pregnancy, morbid obesity, intra-abdominal tumor, ascites

IAH, intra-abdominal hypertension; ACS, abdominal compartment syndrome.

Table 1. Classification of intra-abdominal hypertension.

Grading of IAH	
Grade I	IAP 12-15 mmHg
Grade II	IAP 16-20 mmHg
Grade III	IAP 21-21 mmHg
Grade IV	IAP > 25 mmHg

Table 2. Grading of intra-abdominal hypertension.

The World Society of Abdominal Compartment Syndrome classified IAH into grade I–IV and ACS (**Table 2**) [9].

Burch et al. suggested that most patients with grade III and all patients with grade IV should undergo abdominal decompression [10].

3. ACS results in non-abdominal organ failure

3.1. Cardiovascular

Due to the increased intrathoracic pressure, indirect measures of cardiac filling such as central venous pressure and pulmonary artery occlusion pressure give inaccurate results and can be increased despite profound intravascular volume depletion. The decrease in cardiac output caused by intra-abdominal hypertension is therefore exacerbated by hypovolemia [11].

3.2. Respiratory

Respiratory distress and failure: Initial signs of ACS include elevated peak airway pressures in intubated patients with decreased tidal volumes. The ensuing increase in intrathoracic pressure and hypoxic pulmonary vasoconstriction can lead to pulmonary hypertension [12].

3.3. Neurological

Intracranial perfusion pressure is decreased by increase in intracranial pressure (ICP) caused by venal perfusion defect, including renal failure. For increased ICP, decompressive laparotomy has been shown to reduce intractable elevated ICP in patients with IAH, and compression of the ureters is not thought to contribute to renal dysfunction, as the insertion of ureteric stents does not result in an improvement in urine output [13].

4. Intra-abdominal organ failure in ACS

4.1. Renal function disorder

ACS is characterized by marked reduction in glomerular filtration rate (GFR) and renal plasma flow in the absence of other causes of renal failure. Moreover, changes in cardiac output, direct compression of the renal vessels or renal parenchyma with diminished renal blood flow, increase in renal vascular resistance, and distribution of blood from the renal cortex to the medulla are reported the mechanisms of renal dysfunction [14]. Bradley et al. are the first to report that animals become anuric with an IAP of 30 mmHg [2]. Additional factors that cause IAP to reach ACS range include reduction in cardiac output and elevated levels of catecholamines [15]. Renin, angiotensin, and inflammatory cytokines may also come into play, further worsening renal function.

4.2. Liver function disorder

Diebel et al. reported that the portal vein (PV) pressure decreased experimentally in 65% of patients with an IAP of 40 mmHg, and liver tissue microcirculation quantity decreases to 71% [16].

Liver dysfunction occurs due to decrease PV flow because of IAH. Furthermore, with cardiac dysfunction, liver ischemia becomes worse. Persistent IAP decrease the mean arterial blood pressure in the superior mesenteric artery (SMA) and PV flow by 50% [17].

Rasmussen et al. reported that an IAP of 25 mm Hg results in a 66% decrease in PV blood flow and a 6.5-fold increase in portal/hepatic vascular resistance compared to baseline levels [18].

Furthermore, in studies evaluating the effects of increased IAP on hepatocyte, the characteristics of the sinusoid should be expected to elucidate hepatic dysfunction from increased IAP.

4.3. Gastrointestinal functional disorder

To determine the possibility of bacterial translocation (BT), of which there is failure of the mucous membrane barrier mechanism caused by decline in blood circulation in mucous membranes, pH in the mucous membrane declined as well. Besides, this phenomenon is regarded as the cause of multiple organ dysfunction syndrome (MODS) after ACS, but there is no direct proof. Even if the IAP is at 20 mmHg, blood flow to the intestinal mucosa decreases to 28%

experimentally in 61% of the baseline value of 40 mmHg [16]. In MODS, there is gastrointestinal mucous membrane acidosis of which the IAP is expected to be at 10 mmHg is derived from ACS.

5. Diagnosis of ACS

There are various methods of measuring intermittent IAP, such as invasive (direct, i.e., needle puncture of the abdomen during peritoneal dialysis or laparoscopy) and noninvasive (indirect, i.e., transduction of intravesicular or "bladder," gastric, colonic or uterine pressure via the balloon catheter). Noninvasive measurement of bladder internal pressure and intragastric

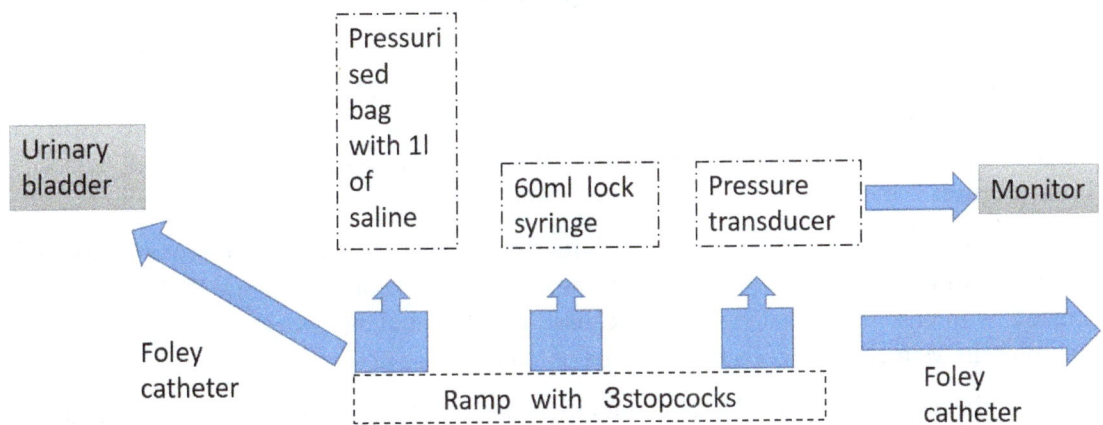

Figure 1. Measurement of intra-abdominal pressure using bladder pressure measurements.

pressure are recommended. The internal bladder pressure are commonly related to IAP measured directly in the range of 5–70 mmHg [6].

Intrabladder pressure monitoring estimated for IAP can be obtained either via a closed transducer technique or the closed Foley Manometer technique, which seems safe and does not alter the risk of UTI in patients with critical illness [19] (**Figure 1**).

6. ACS treatment

Discussions on IAP to become the adaptation standard of decompression is divided, but more than 25 mmHg is assumed to be a tentative adaptation standard clinically. However, recently, reports on gastrointestinal disorder due to impairment of IAP in the lower abdominal cavity need to be considered. The World Society of the Abdominal Compartment Syndrome suggested a management algorithm for IAH/ACS [20].

An early indication of the open abdomen technique has been shown to reduce mortality [21]. Chen et al. reported that laparoscopy can be used as a safe alternative for ACS decompression [22].

The World Society of the Abdominal Compartment Syndrome has noted that correct fluid therapy and perfusion support during resuscitation form the cornerstone of medical management in patients with abdominal hypertension [23].

Pharmacologic therapy is less effective than drainage procedures. Agustí et al. reported that dobutamine restores intestinal mucosal blood flow in a porcine model of intra-abdominal hyperpressure [24].

If a patient experiences decompensation, ACS should be re-examined as a potential cause.

7. Possible involvement of IAH/ACS and HRS

We reported an autopsy case with HRS and ACS diagnosed with a clinical and histopathological consideration of liver and kidney diseases. Further clinical studies are needed to improve the management of renal failure in patients with acute liver failure and advanced liver cirrhosis (**Figures 2** and **3**) [25].

HRS was originally described in 1863 by Flint as an association between liver disease and oliguric renal failure in the absence of significant renal histological change [26]. HRS is recognized by intense intrarenal vasospasm caused by the imbalance between vasodilatory and vasoconstrictive mediators seen in end stage of liver disease [27].

Although the precise role of IAH in HRS remains incompletely understood, it can be argued that diminished glomerular perfusion due to venous congestion results in further decline of GFR.

Cade et al. reported significant increases in urine flow rate and creatinine clearance after reduction in IAP from 22 to 10 mmHg with paracentesis in patients with cirrhosis [28]. Moreover,

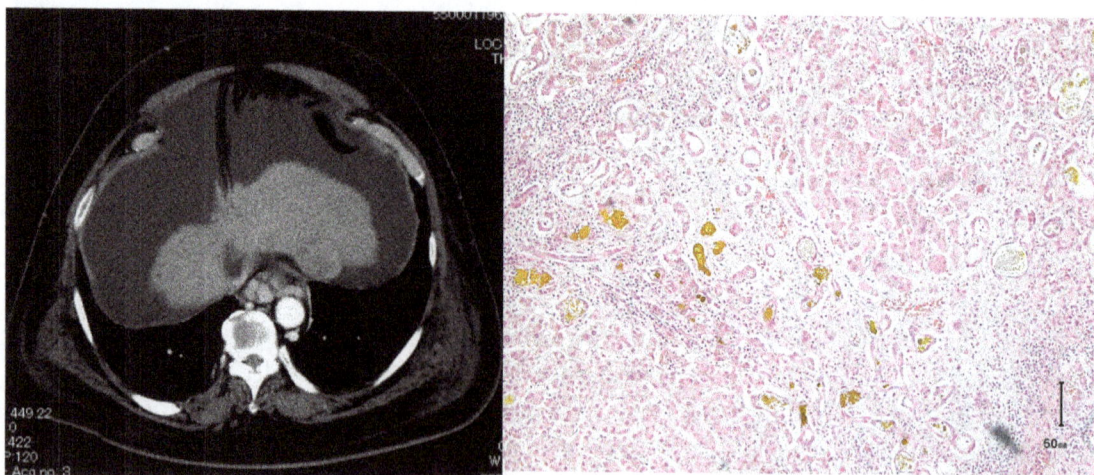

Figure 2. Liver: end-stage liver cirrhosis. Microscopic findings showed hepatic sinusoidal dilation due to portal hypertension and severe jaundice.

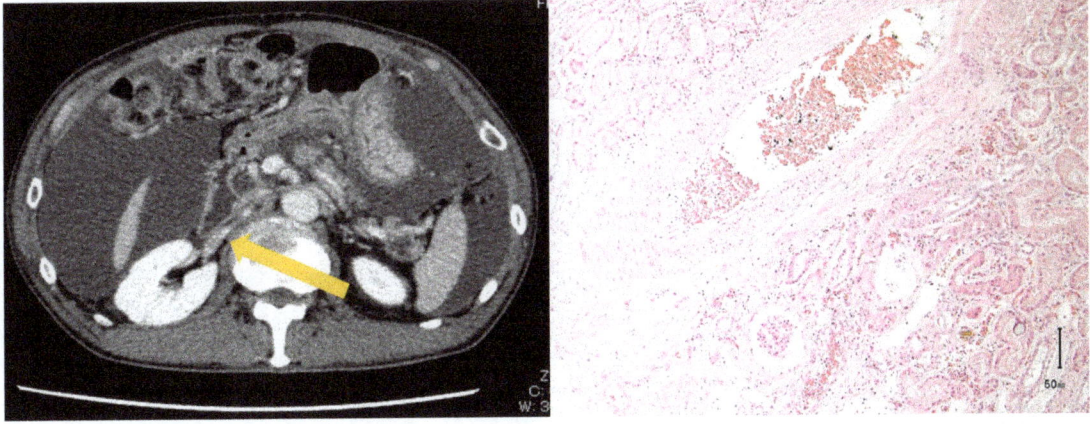

Figure 3. Kidney: microscopic findings showed swelling in the renal tubules. There was no change in the glomerulus and collecting tubule and no renal fibrosis. CT the right renal vein was compressed by massive ascites (arrow).

compression of renal vein is suggested to be vital in the development renal dysfunction. IAH is the significant pathological mechanism and independent risk factor in the occurrence and development of HRS [29]. Further, attempts should be made to decrease IAP following surgical decompression, large-volume paracentesis (LVP), and appropriate diuretic drug.

8. Drug strategy for ACS

Several methods are reported to control refractory abdominal ascites in end-stage liver cirrhosis, such as avoidance of non-steroidal anti-inflammatory drugs [30], dietary sodium restriction [31], diuretic, LVP, cell-free and concentrated ascites reinfusion therapy [32], transjugular intrahepatic portosystemic shunt [33], and peritoneovenous shunt [34].

IAH is defined as an IAP above 12 mmHg. Hence, abdominal ascites in early stage of liver cirrhosis should be treated and early stage of ascites in outpatient should be managed immediately. Outpatients with clinically apparent ascites will require diuretic therapy in addition to dietary sodium restriction. Diuretic therapy typically consists of treatment regimen for cirrhotic ascites such as combination of oral spironolactone and furosemide. Recently, aquaporin-2 is a vasopressin-regulated water channel expressed in the renal collecting duct. Urine aquaporin-2 is considered a marker of collecting duct responsiveness to tolvaptan. In Japan, on September 2013, tolvaptan was approved (in doses up to 7.5 mg/day) for treating patients with ascites who showed an inadequate response to conventional diuretics [35].

9. Conclusion

Massive ascites also influences IAP and causes oliguria and acute kidney injury (AKI). Commonly, we recognize this symptom at the stage of end stage of liver cirrhosis. This symptom has the possible involvement with HRS. In such patients, we should take into account the elevation of renal parenchymal and renal vein pressures, as they are likely the mechanisms of renal impairment. Note that IAH/ACS and HRS are occurring simultaneously. Hepatologists should consider IAH and ACS in end-stage liver cirrhosis.

Acknowledgements

The authors would like to thank Takao Tsuchida in the Division of Gastroenterology and Hepatology at the Niigata University for his excellent assistance in histological analyses.

Funding

This work was supported by a Grant-in-Aid for Research Activity Start-up 17H06691 from the Ministry of Education, Culture, Sports, Science and Technology (MEXT) to Hiroteru Kamimura.

Author details

Hiroteru Kamimura*, Tomoyuki Sugano, Ryoko Horigome, Naruhiro Kimura, Masaaki Takamura, Hirokazu Kawai, Satoshi Yamagiwa and Shuji Terai

*Address all correspondence to: hiroteruk@med.niigata-u.ac.jp

Division of Gastroenterology and Hepatology, Niigata University Graduate School of Medical and Dental Sciences, Niigata, Japan

References

[1] Wendt E. Ueber den einfluss des intraabdominalenn druckes auf die absonderungsge-schwindigkeit des harnes. Archives of Physiology and Heilkunde. 1876;57:527

[2] Bradley SE, Bradley GP. The effect of increased intra-abdominal pressure on renal function in man. The Journal of Clinical Investigation. 1947;26:1010-1022

[3] Matsumoto N, Ogawa M, Kumagawa M, Watanabe Y, Hirayama M, Miura T, Nakagawara H, Matsuoka S, Moriyama M, Fujikawa H. Renal vein dilation predicts poor outcome in patients with refractory cirrhotic ascites. Hepatology Research. 2018;48:E117-E125

[4] Cheatham ML, White MW, Sagraves SG, Johnson JL, Block EF. Abdominal perfusion pressure: A superior parameter in the assessment of intra-abdominal hypertension. The Journal of Trauma 2000;49:621-626

[5] Campano D, Robaina JA, Kusnezov N, Dunn JC, Waterman BR. Surgical management for chronic exertional compartment syndrome of the leg: A systematic review of the literature. Arthroscopy. 2016;32:1478-1486

[6]   Malbrain ML, Cheatham ML, Kirkpatrick A, Sugrue M, Parr M, De Waele J, Balogh Z, Leppäniemi A, Olvera C, Ivatury R, D'Amours S, Wendon J, Hillman K, Johansson K, Kolkman K, Wilmer A. Results from the international conference of experts on intra-abdominal hypertension and abdominal compartment syndrome. I. Definitions. Intensive Care Medicine. 2006;**32**:1722-1732

[7]   Cosgriff N, Moore EE, Sauaia A, Kenny-Moynihan M, Burch JM, Galloway B. Predicting life-threatening coagulopathy in the massively transfused trauma patient: Hypothermia and acidoses revisited. The Journal of Trauma. 1997;**42**:857-861

[8]   Aspesi M, Gamberoni C, Severgnini P, Colombo G, Chiumello D, Minoja G, Tulli G, Malacrida R, Pelosi P, Chiaranda M. The abdominal compartment syndrome. Clinical relevance. Minerva Anestesiologica. 2002;**68**:138-146

[9]   Malbrain ML, Deeren D, De Potter TJ. Intra-abdominal hypertension in the critically ill: It is time to pay attention. Current Opinion in Critical Care; 2005;**11**:156-171

[10] Burch JM, Moore EE, Moore FA, Franciose R. The abdominal compartment syndrome. The Surgical Clinics of North America. 1996;**76**:833-842

[11] Ridings PC, Bloomfield GL, Blocher CR, Sugerman HJ. Cardiopulmonary effects of raised intra-abdominal pressure before and after intravascular volume expansion. The Journal of Trauma. 1995;**39**:1071-1075

[12] Cullen DJ, Coyle JP, Teplick R, Long MC. Cardiovascular, pulmonary, and renal effects of massively increased intra-abdominal pressure in critically ill patients. Critical Care Medicine. 1989;**17**:118-121

[13] Constantini S, Cotev S, Rappaport ZH, Pomeranz S, Shalit MN. Intracranial pressure monitoring after elective intracranial surgery. A retrospective study of 514 consecutive patients. Journal of Neurosurgery. Oct 1988;**69**(4):540-544

[14] Mohmand H, Goldfarb S. Renal dysfunction associated with intra-abdominal hypertension and the abdominal compartment syndrome. Journal of the American Society of Nephrology. Apr 2011;**22**(4):615-621

[15] Mikami O, Fujise K, Matsumoto S, Shingu K, Ashida M, Matsuda T. High intra-abdominal pressure increases plasma catecholamine concentrations during pneumoperitoneum for laparoscopic procedures. Archives of Surgery. 1998;**133**:39-43

[16] Diebel LN, Dulchavsky SA, Brown WJ. Splanchnic ischemia and bacterial translocation in the abdominal compartment syndrome. The Journal of Trauma. 1997;**43**:852-855

[17] Mogilner J, Sukhotnik I, Brod V, Hayari L, Coran AG, Shiloni E, Eldar S, Bitterman H. Effect of elevated intra-abdominal pressure on portal vein and superior mesenteric artery blood flow in a rat. Journal of Laparoendoscopic & Advanced Surgical Techniques. Part A. 2009;**19**(Suppl 1):S59-S62

[18] Rasmussen IB, Berggren U, Arvidsson D, Ljungdahl M, Haglund U. Effects of pneumoperitoneum on splanchnic hemodynamics: An experimental study in pigs. The European Journal of Surgery. 1995;**161**:819-826

[19] Desie N, Willems W, De laet I, Dits H, Van Regenmorte N, Schoonheydt K, Van De Vyvere M, Malbrain M. Intra-abdominal pressure measurement using the Foley manometer does not increase the risk for urinary tract infection in critically ill patients. Annals of Intensive Care. 2012;**2**(Suppl 1):S10

[20] Kirkpatrick AW, Roberts DJ, De Waele J, Jaeschke R, Malbrain ML, De Keulenaer B, Duchesne J, Bjorck M, Leppaniemi A, Ejike JC, Sugrue M, Cheatham M, Ivatury R, Ball CG, Reintam Blaser A, Regli A, Balogh ZJ, D'Amours S, Debergh D, Kaplan M, Kimball E, Olvera C. Pediatric guidelines sub-Committee for the World Society of the abdominal compartment syndrome. Intra-abdominal hypertension and the abdominal compartment syndrome: Updated consensus definitions and clinical practice guidelines from the world Society of the Abdominal Compartment Syndrome. Intensive Care Medicine. 2013;**39**:1190-1206

[21] Madigan M, Kemp C, Johnson J, Cotton B. Secondary abdominal compartment syndrome after severe extremity injury. The Journal of Trauma. 2008;**64**:280-285

[22] Chen RJ, Fang JF, Lin BC, Kao JL. Laparoscopic decompression of abdominal compartment syndrome after blunt hepatic trauma. Surgical Endoscopy. 2000;**14**:966-967

[23] Regli A, De Keulenaer B, De Laet I, Roberts D, Dabrowski W, Malbrain ML. Fluid therapy and perfusional considerations during resuscitation in critically ill patients with intra-abdominal hypertension. Anaesthesiology Intensive Therapy. 2015;**47**:45-53

[24] Agusti M, Elizalde JI, Adalia R, Cifuentes A, Fontanals J, Taura P. Dobutamine restores intestinal mucosal blood flow in a porcine model of intra-abdominal hyperpressure. Critical Care Medicine. 2000;**28**:467-472

[25] Kamimura H, Watanabe T, Sugano T, Nakajima N, Yokoyama J, Kamimura K, Tsuchiya A, Takamura M, Kawai H, Kato T, Watanabe G, Yamagiwa S, Terai S. A case of Hepatorenal syndrome and abdominal compartment syndrome with high renal congestion. American Journal of Case Reports. 2017;**18**:1000-1004

[26] Flint A. Clinical report on hydroperitoneum, based on an analysis of 46 cases. The American Journal of the Medical Sciences. 1863;**45**:306-309

[27] Gines P, Guevara M, Arroyo V, Rodes J. Hepatorenal syndrome. Lancet. 2003;**362**:1819-1827

[28] Cade R, Wagemaker H, Vogel S, Mars D, Hood-Lewis D, Privette M, Peterson J, Schlein E, Hawkins R, Raulerson D, et al. Hepatorenal syndrome. Studies of the effect of vascular volume and intraperitoneal pressure on renal and hepatic function. The American Journal of Medicine. 1987;**82**:427-438

[29] Bloomfield GL, Blocher CR, Fakhry IF, Sica DA, Sugerman HJ. Elevated intra-abdominal pressure increases plasma renin activity and aldosterone levels. The Journal of Trauma. 1997;**42**:997-1004

[30] Arroyo V, Ginés P, Rimola A, Gaya L. Renal function abnormalities, prostaglandins, and effects of nonsteroidal anti-inflammatory drugs in cirrhosis with ascites. An overview with emphasis on pathogenesis. The American Journal of Medicine. 1986;**81**:104-122

[31] Runyon BA, Montano AA, Akriviadis EA, Antillon MR, Irving MA, McHutchison JG. The serum-ascites albumin gradient is superior to the exudate-transudate concept in the differential diagnosis of ascites. Annals of Internal Medicine. 1992;**117**:215-220

[32] Inoue N, Yamazaki Z, Oda T, Sugiura M, Wada T. Treatment of intractable ascites by continuous reinfusion of the sterilized, cell-free and concentrated ascitic fluid. Transactions – American Society for Artificial Internal Organs. 1977;**23**:699-702

[33] Ginès P, Arroyo V, Vargas V, Planas R, Casafont F, Panés J, Hoyos M, Viladomiu L, Rimola A, Morillas R, et al. Paracentesis with intravenous infusion of albumin as compared with peritoneovenous shunting in cirrhosis with refractory ascites. The New England Journal of Medicine. 1991;**325**:829-835

[34] Park JS, Won JY, Park SI, Park SJ, Lee DY. Percutaneous peritoneovenous shunt creation for the treatment of benign and malignant refractory ascites. Journal of Vascular and Interventional Radiology. 2001;**12**:1445-1448

[35] Sakaida I, Terai S, Kurosaki M, Yasuda M, Okada M, Bando K, Fukuta Y. Effectiveness and safety of tolvaptan in liver cirrhosis patients with edema:Interim results of post-marketing surveillance of tolvaptan in liver cirrhosis (START study). Hepatology Research. Oct 2017;**47**(11):1137-1146

6

Role of Lipid Droplet Proteins in the Development of NAFLD and Hepatic Insulin Resistance

Kaori Minehira and Philippe Gual

Abstract

NAFLD is diagnosed, when the liver fat exceeds more than 5% of liver weight. Inside of hepatocytes, these fats are stored in cytosolic lipid droplets. The lipid droplets can be formed from a bud, vesicles of the lipid bilayer, which lines at a vicinity of the endoplasmic reticulum (ER). On the surface of droplets, there are several structural/ functional proteins such as lipid droplet proteins, lipogenic enzymes, and lipases. Interestingly, the lipid droplet proteins seem to have great impact on a development of NAFLD. Some proteins can interact with transcriptional factors such as SREBP1c and PPAR-alpha/gamma, and some proteins strongly impact a mitochondrial structure. As a result, the lipid droplet proteins highly influence lipid handling and fatty acid oxidation in hepatocytes. This chapter will elucidate our recent understanding of the role of each lipid droplet protein in fatty liver formation and in hepatic insulin resistance. Existing information on genetically modified animals as well as on human NAFLD was reviewed on Perilipin families, CIDE proteins, Seipin, and PNPLAs. Finally, the chapter will discuss how the lipid droplet proteins could potentially lead/protect from hepatic insulin resistance via abnormal accumulation of ceramides and diacylglycerols, autophagy, ER stress, and oxidative stress.

Keywords: perilipin, CIDE proteins, insulin sensitivity, mitochondrial oxidation, autophagy, ER stress

1. Introduction

Liver can store a certain amount of excess glucose as a form of glycogen. A part of the stored glycogen can then be retransformed into glucose (so-called gluconeogenesis) during a fasting condition to leave the liver. Contrary to the glucose, an excess lipid is not normally stored in the liver. However, in a pathological case, excess lipid storage can be observed in hepatocytes, which is called hepatic steatosis. Hepatic steatosis could be diagnosed in different grades according to histological observation (Grade 1: 5–33% lipid invasion in hepatocytes, Grade 2: 33–66%, and Grade 3: >66%). Up to 90% of obese patients could have the hepatic steatosis, and the presence is linked to several metabolic dysfunctions such as insulin resistance, oxidative stress, endoplasmic reticulum (ER) stress, and mitochondrial dysfunctions [1–3]. As a result, hepatic steatosis often leads to abnormal gluconeogenesis, which is a typical phenotype of type 2 diabetes. To better prevent such metabolic dysfunctions, scientists have been actively investigating mechanisms by which hepatic lipids impact metabolic functions.

2. Lipid droplet structure

When excess fat is present in a liver, these fats are stored intracellularly in cytosolic lipid droplet compartment. Today, an origin of a lipid droplet biosynthesis has not been understood completely. Walther and Farese suggested different models of the lipid droplet biosynthesis [4]. Most accepted lipid droplet biosynthesis model is that triglyceride (TG) accumulated at the ER membranes forms a bud, a vesicle of the lipid bilayer [5]. On ER membranes, phospholipids are added onto the surface of growing lipid droplets. Secondary, lipid droplets could increase their size via lipid droplet fusion. Finally, a matured lipid droplet is formed consisting TG and cholesterol esters in a core, coated by a membrane monolayer of phospholipids and sphingomyelin (**Figure 1A**). On the surface and/or vicinity of droplets, there are several structural/functional proteins such as lipid

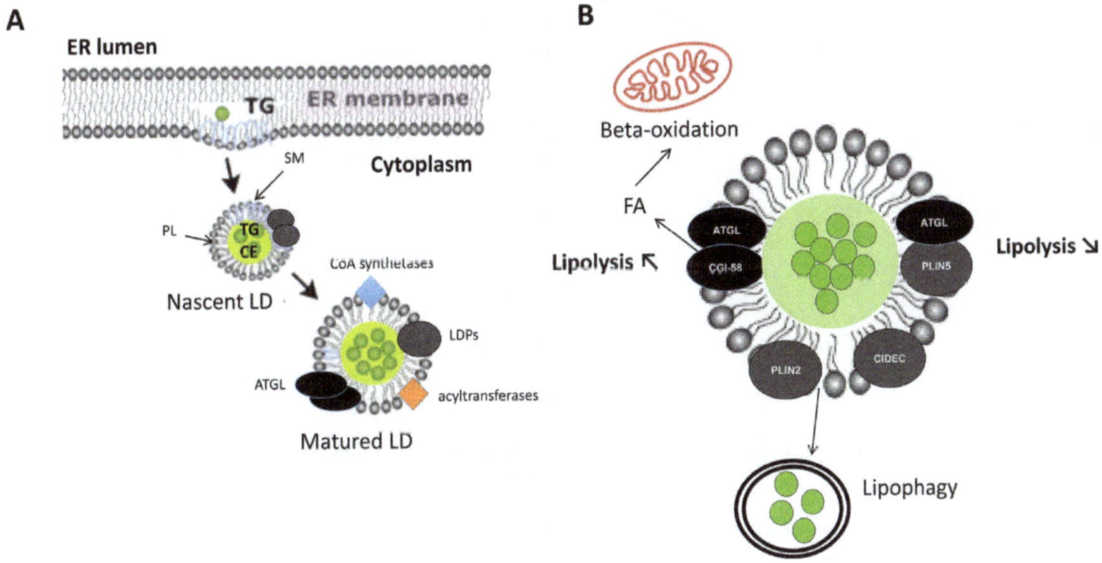

Figure 1. Lipid droplet formation. (A) Formation of nascent lipid droplet (LD) with lipid droplet proteins (LDPs), (B) lipid droplet biology.

droplet proteins, lipogenic enzymes, and lipases (**Figure 1B**). Enzymes required for lipid droplet synthesis are also located in the ER. This strategic enzyme location helps to form, stabilize, and degrade lipid droplets when necessary. Hydrolysis of lipid is highly regulated by different enzymes such as adipose triglyceride lipase (ATGL), hormone-sensitive lipase (HSL), and monoglyceride lipase (MGL). ATGL is responsible for the hydrolysis of triglyceride, followed by HSL, which cleaves one molecule of fatty acid from diacylglycerol, and finally hydrolysis is completed by MGL. In hepatocytes, ATGL interacts both lipid droplet protein, perilipin 5 (PLIN5) and comparative gene identification-58 (CGI-58). When ATGL interacts with PLIN5, this decreases lipolysis; however, if ATGL interacts with CGI-58, this increases lipolysis [6]. Therefore, lipid droplet proteins play a key role regulating a fate of cellular lipid storage (**Table 1**).

LD protein	Expression cites	Observed functions	Reported interactions with other genes/proteins
PLIN1 (perilipin A)	WAT, cardiac muscle liposarcoma, BAT	LD stability, control of hormone-induced lipolysis	ATGL, CGI58, [97, 98], SREBP1c [19], CIDEC [15]
PLIN2 (ADRP, adipophilin)	Liver, WAT, mammary gland, macrophages, sebocytes, ubiquitous expression	LD stability, adipocytes differentiation, VLDL lipidation	PPAR alpha, gamma [21, 99, 100], delta [101] hepatic von Hippel-Lindau protein [102]
PLIN3 (TIP47)	Ubiquitous expression, skeletal muscle, neutrophils, sebocytes	LD stability, PGE$_2$ production, intracellular trafficking	Mannose-6-phosphate receptor [9]
PLIN4 (S3-12)	WAT, skeletal muscle	LD stability, adipocytes differentiation	PLIN5 [32]
PLIN5 (OXPAT, LSDP5, MLDP)	Skeletal muscle, BAT, heart, liver, beta-cells	LD stability, fat oxidation, mitochondrial recruitment	PPARalpha [60], delta [103], CIG58, ATGL [6], ABHD5 [104]
PLPNA3 (Adiponutrin)	WAT, liver, skeletal muscle, pancreas	Triglyceride and retinyl palmitate esterase activity	SREBP1c [105]
PLPNA2 (ATGL)	Adipose tissue	Lipolysis	SIRT1 [106], PLIN5 [6], PLIN1 [33, 97]
CIDEA	Adipose tissue, liver	Lipogenesis	SREBP1c [41, 42]
CIDEB	Adipose tissue	Contributes to lipogenesis, lipidation of VLDL, hepatitis virus assembly	HCV NS58 protein [107]
CIDEC (FSP27)	Adipose tissue, liver	LD stability, LF fusion, lipid transfer	PPAR alpha, gamma [42, 45]
SEIPIN (BCSL)	Adipose tissue, liver, brain, testis	Maturation of LD, lipolysis	

Table 1. Lipid droplet proteins.

3. Lipid droplet protein families

Lipid droplet proteins were discovered in the 1990s in phospholipid monolayer of lipid droplet [7–9]. At that time, each lipid droplet proteins had a different nomenclature. In 2010, it was suggested to uniform their names as the "perilipin family protein: PAT protein" [10]. PAT was named after the three proteins: PLIN1 (Perilipin), PLIN2 (Adipose differentiation-related protein; ADRP), and PLIN3 (Tail-interacting protein of 47 kDa; TIP47). All PLIN families contain a conserved domain called PAT domain [11] with an exception of PLIN4 that only contains long 11-mer repeat motifs [12]. The expression of these proteins and their functions are slightly different, and their exact roles for each cell type have not been yet completely understood. Interestingly, their expression depends on a size of lipid droplets (small lipid droplets: PLIN3, PLIN4, PLIN5; medium lipid droplets: PLIN2; and large lipid droplet: PLIN1).

3.1. PLIN1

PLIN1 was one of the first lipid droplet protein identified in adipocytes [13, 14], and its expression is mainly observed in matured adipocytes. During a differentiation of premature adipocytes, PLIN2 plays a major role to lipidate small lipid droplets. Once lipid droplet gains enough size, PLIN1 replaces PLIN2 to stabilize large lipid-rich lipid droplets and helps to mature adipocytes. PLIN1 also interacts with cell-death-inducing DNA-fragmentation-factor 45-like effector (CIDE)-C for a lipid droplets fusion process [15]. Among different reported functions of PLIN1 in adipocytes, the most well-characterized role of PLIN1 is a control of lipolysis. PLIN1 co-localizes with ATGL and CGI-58 on a surface of lipid droplets at a basal condition. Upon a lipolytic stimulation, PLIN1 is phosphorylated and CGI-58 is released and activates ATGL for a lipolysis. In hepatocytes, PLIN1 is not expressed in normal healthy liver, but its expression is observed in steatotic hepatocytes [16–18]. During a formation of hepatic steatosis, the expression of PLIN1 is synchronized with sterol regulatory element-binding protein (SREBP)-1c, a key regulator of de novo lipogenesis [19]. As a result, both genes could strongly contribute to accelerate the pathogenesis of hepatic steatosis [20].

3.2. PLIN2

PLIN2 was originally named as adipose differentiation-related protein due to its high expression during an adipocyte differentiation [8]. PLIN2 is ubiquitously expressed and its expression in the liver is high among other lipid droplet proteins [21]. Chronic alcohol consumption stimulates de novo lipogenesis and induces hepatic steatosis together with an upregulation of PLIN2 [22]. Hepatocellular ballooning and oxidative injury were also observed under such condition [18]. Magne et al. observed in human NAFLD patients that PLIN2 polymorphism (ser1Pro) was linked to a decreased VLDL levels [23].

A recent study demonstrated that the PLIN2 and PLIN3 double-knockout in hepatocytes induced insulin resistance [24]. In addition, the overexpression of PLIN2 in rat skeletal muscle resulted in an accumulation of TG in muscle without insulin resistance [25]. However, general deletion of PLIN2 in mice also showed a protective role against hepatic steatosis and insulin resistance (discussed in a later paragraph, **Table 2**). The exact impacts of PLIN2 modification on insulin resistance have not yet been fully elucidated.

LD proteins	Up or downregulation	Outcomes
PLIN1	**Downregulation** KO mice [61] KO mice [62]	Body fat↓, fat oxidation↑ Lipolysis↑, cardiac steatosis↑, cardiac hypertrophy
PLIN2	**Downregulation** ASO [63, 64] KO—alcohol diet [66] KO—high fat diet [65] Liver specific KO—methionine-choline deficient diet [95] Lep (ob/ob)/Plin2 double KO mice [108] KO–high fat diet [109]	Hepatic steatosis↓ (ceramide-, DAG↓), IR ↓ Hepatic steatosis↓ (ceramide↓), IR ↓, glucose tolerance- Hepatic steatosis↓, body fat↓, adipose inflammation↓ Hepatic steatosis↓, hepatic inflammation↓, fibrosis↓ VLDL secretion ↑ Hepatic steatosis ↓, IR↓ (liver, muscle) Hepatic steatosis ↓VLDL -
PLIN3	**Downregulation** ASO [67]	Hepatic steatosis ↓ IR↓
PLIN4	**Downregulation** KO [32]	Cardiac steatosis↓
PLIN5	**Downregulation** KO [38] KO [40] **Upregulation** Adenovirus [68]	Lack of lipid droplet in heart, ROS↑, heart mal function, Hepatic steatosis ↓, mitochondrial oxidative capacity↑, lipotoxic injury Hepatic steatosis ↑ IR-
PLPNA3	**Downregulation** KO [55, 56] **Upregulation** G allele knock-in Ref. [57]	Hepatic steatosis - Hepatic steatosis ↑
PLPNA2	**Downregulation** KO [69] Liver-specific KO [70]	Steatosis in different organs↑, IR↓ Hepatic steatosis ↑ (DAG↓), IR -
CIDEC	**Downregulation** KO [47, 110] KO in ob/ob by shRNA [46] ASO [111] **Upregulation** Adenovirus [46]	Hepatic steatosis ↓, IR↓ Hepatic steatosis ↓, IR↓ Hepatic steatosis ↓, body fat↓, IR↓ Hepatic steatosis↑
SEIPIN	**Downregulation** Adipose-specific KO [112] KO [49] **Upregulation** Transgenic mice overexpressing a short isoform of human BSCL2 in adipose [113]	Hepatic steatosis↑, IR↑, adipocyte hypertrophy and progressive lipodystrophy Hepatic steatosis↑, IR↑ Hepatic steatosis↑, IR↑, white adipose tissue ↓, lipolysis ↑

Abbreviations: KO; knockout, ASO; antisense oligonucleotide, IR; insulin resistance.

Table 2. Experimental modification of lipid droplet protein and the effect on steatosis.

3.3. PLIN3

PLIN3 was originally named tail-interacting protein of 47 kDa and ubiquitously expressed among tissues. PLIN3 is localized at the cytosol and lipid droplet [9, 26]. It is also implicated in intracellular trafficking of lysosomal enzymes [9]. Four-helix bundle in PLIN3 has been suggested to contribute to fatty acid binding and lipid droplet recruitment [9]. PLIN2 and PLIN3 share similar functions, and both proteins cannot bind CGI-58 and, therefore, influence lipolysis [27]. Co-expression of PLIN2 and PLIN3 has been reported in many tissues; however, a distinct role of PLIN3 has not been clearly identified. Interestingly, PLIN3 expression was also observed in stellate cells in the liver [17]. Lipopolysaccharide treatment also predominantly stimulated PLIN3 expression in HL-60-derived neutrophils [28]. Knockdown of PLIN3 via siRNA decreased a lipid droplet formation as well as PGE_2 secretion. This observation was unique to PLIN3, and PLIN2 was not detected under such conditions. This implies that PLIN3 might be implicated in a lipid droplet formation related to conditions with cellular stresses.

Another unique observation to PLIN3 was that mice lacking mTORC2 (mammalian target of rapamycin complex) activity in skeletal muscle showed increased fat mass and PLIN3 [29]. This was due to an increased AMPK activity. mTORC plays an important role in insulin signaling. However, the implication of PLIN3 in insulin resistance has not yet been addressed.

3.4. PLIN4

PLIN4 was originally called S3–12 and is the only PAT protein that does not contain the PAT domain. Its molecular weight is three times higher than other PAT proteins. The protein has been shown to present at cytosol and lipid droplets [30]. Its expression was induced during adipogenesis [31]. PLIN4-KO mice present no phenotypic changes in adipose tissues, whereas TG content in heart tissues was significantly reduced [32]. PLIN5 expression was also decreased under such condition. Given close location of PLIN4 and PLIN5 in chromosome 19 in human, it was suggested a potential transcriptional interference between two genes. PLIN4 remains the least studied PAT protein, and further investigations are required to understand PLIN4 roles in lipid droplet physiology.

3.5. PLIN5

PLIN5 was discovered by different researchers simultaneously and named as myocardial lipid droplet protein (MDLP), OXPAT, or lipid storage droplet protein 5 (LSDP5) [33, 34]. This was due to a high expression of PLIN5 in heart and other oxidative tissues such as skeletal muscle and liver. PLIN5 expression is also reported in pancreatic beta cells and hepatic stellate cells [35, 36]. A unique feature with PLIN5 is that mitochondria are physically recruited to lipid droplets expressing high PLIN5 (**Figure 2**) [37, 38]. Its expression is regulated by PPAR-alpha, and most importantly, PLIN5 plays roles in regulating cellular fat oxidation. PLIN5 stabilizes lipid droplets by sequestrating fatty acids, and because PLIN5 can recruit mitochondria to lipid droplet surface, it facilitates to release fatty acids to mitochondria for the oxidation [39]. Given its gatekeeper roles on the lipid oxidation, it has been suggested that PLIN5 could protect cardiac myocytes and hepatocytes from oxidative stress [38, 40]. PLIN5 leads several modifications on the lipid metabolism as well as insulin sensitivity, and details are discussed in a separate paragraph.

AML12 cells

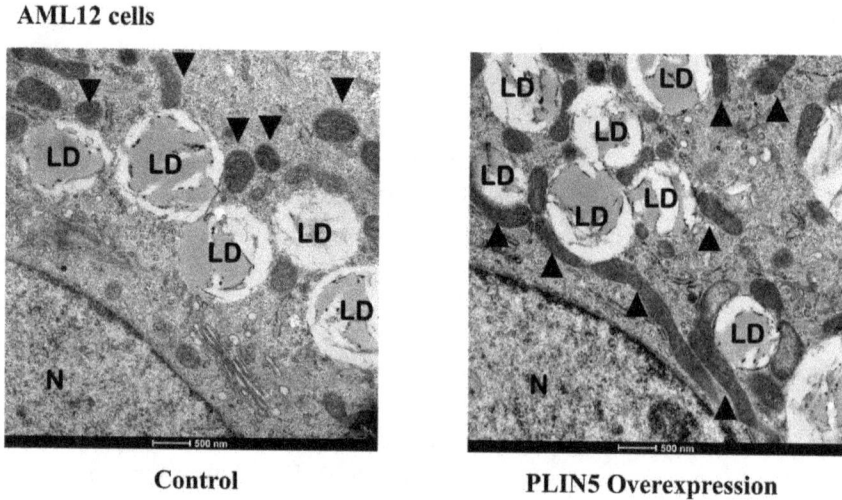

Control   PLIN5 Overexpression

Figure 2. Electron microscopy image of hepatocyte overexpressing PLIN5. When PLIN5 is overexpressed, mitochondria (closed triangle) is highly recruited toward lipid droplets (LD). N: nucleus.

3.6. CIDE proteins

Cell-death-inducing DNA fragmentation-factor 45-like effector (CIDE) proteins have also been found on a lipid droplet surface. CIDEA expression is controlled by SREBP-1c and found in a fatty liver [41, 42]. CIDEB is constitutively expressed in a liver and plays a role in VLDL production [43, 44]. Interestingly, it has been reported that CIDEB and PLIN2 exert opposite functions for a control of VLDL lipidation [44]. CIDEC, is also named as fat-specific protein 27 (FSP27), found as a cofactor of PLIN1 for lipid droplet fusion in adipocytes [15]. CIDEC is regulated by PPAR-alpha/gamma [42, 45]. Like CIDEA, hepatic CIDEC was induced in leptin-deficient *ob/ob* mice. It has also been demonstrated that CIDEC overexpression induces steatosis, whereas knockdown of CIDEC alleviates hepatic fat accumulation in *ob/ob* mice lacking hepatic PPARγ [46]. Effect of CIDEC on mitochondrial activity and insulin sensitivity is an active research field of today [15, 47, 48]. Toy et al. demonstrated that white adipocytes from CIDEC KO mice had accelerated mitochondrial activities and increased proteins and size, leading to brown adipocyte characteristics.

3.7. SEIPIN

SEIPIN is highly expressed in brain, testis, and adipose tissue. Mutations in SEIPIN are known as Berardinelli-Seip congenital lipodystrophy (BSCL), a rare recessive disorder characterized by near absence of adipose tissue accompanied by a severe insulin resistance [49]. Several studies convincingly demonstrated that SEIPIN plays a crucial role in adipogenesis, lipid droplet homeostasis and lipolysis. It is also well known that human BSCL patients and mice lacking SEIPIN develop diabetes and severe hepatic steatosis. Interestingly, our previous studies demonstrated that SEIPIN expression seems to be dependent on lipid droplet size (**Figure 3**), and the low SEIPIN expresser had an impaired gluconeogenesis in NAFLD patients (personal observation).

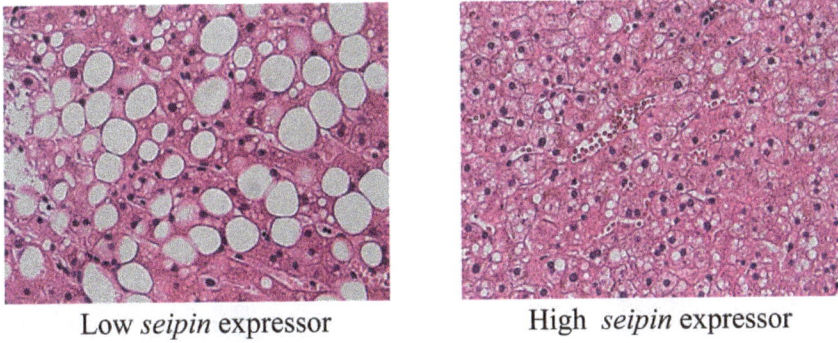

Low *seipin* expressor   High *seipin* expressor

Figure 3. Liver histology from NAFLD patients.

3.8. PNPLA3 and PNPLA2

Patatin-like phospholipase domain-containing protein 3 (PNPLA3), also called adiponutrin, was consistently associated with NAFLD in GWAS observations [50, 51]. The single nucleotide polymorphism (SNP) in PNPLA3 was identified as a major determinant of hepatic fat content from exome-wide association studies. This is the rs738409 C > G SNP encoding for the isoleucine to methionine substitution [50]. PNPLA3 is expressed in the retina, hepatic stellate cells, and hepatocytes and localized in the endoplasmic reticulum and at a surface of lipid droplets. A mechanism by which PNPLA3 leads the hepatic steatosis phenotype has not been clearly understood. PNPLA3 has a triglyceride and retinylpalmitate esterase activity [52–54], suggesting a possible link to hepatic fat accumulation. However, PNPLA3 knockout mice did not develop hepatic steatosis [55, 56]. Mice having Pnpla3i148m knock-in recently showed increased hepatic steatosis [57]. The role of PNPLA3 in the development of NAFLD still remains elusive.

PNPLA2 is known as adipose triglyceride transfer protein (ATGL) and is expressed on lipid droplet surface at a basal condition. Its activity is strongly influenced by PLINs [25]. As shown in **Figure 1**, ATGL is the first enzyme hydrolyzing neutral lipids.

4. Expression of lipid droplet proteins in human NAFLD

Lipid droplet proteins are highly expressed in human NAFLD. PLIN1, PLIN2, and PLIN3 were upregulated in NAFLD [18, 58, 59]. And the distribution of PLINs seems to depend on the lipid droplet size [17, 18]. PLIN2 was also observed in stellate cells [18, 59]. We have compared the expression of different lipid droplet proteins in human NAFLD. The steatosis was judged by a histological assessment showing four different grades (S0 < S1 < S2 < S3). Despite a similar BMI among different groups, the gene expression of lipid droplet proteins increased depending on the degree of steatosis (**Figure 4A**). When compared the livers from patients with or without type 2 diabetes who had a similar degree of hepatic steatosis (S3), the expressions of lipid droplet proteins were significantly lower in diabetic patients than in nondiabetic individuals (**Figure 4B**). This result implies possible link between lipid droplet proteins and hepatic insulin signaling.

A

B

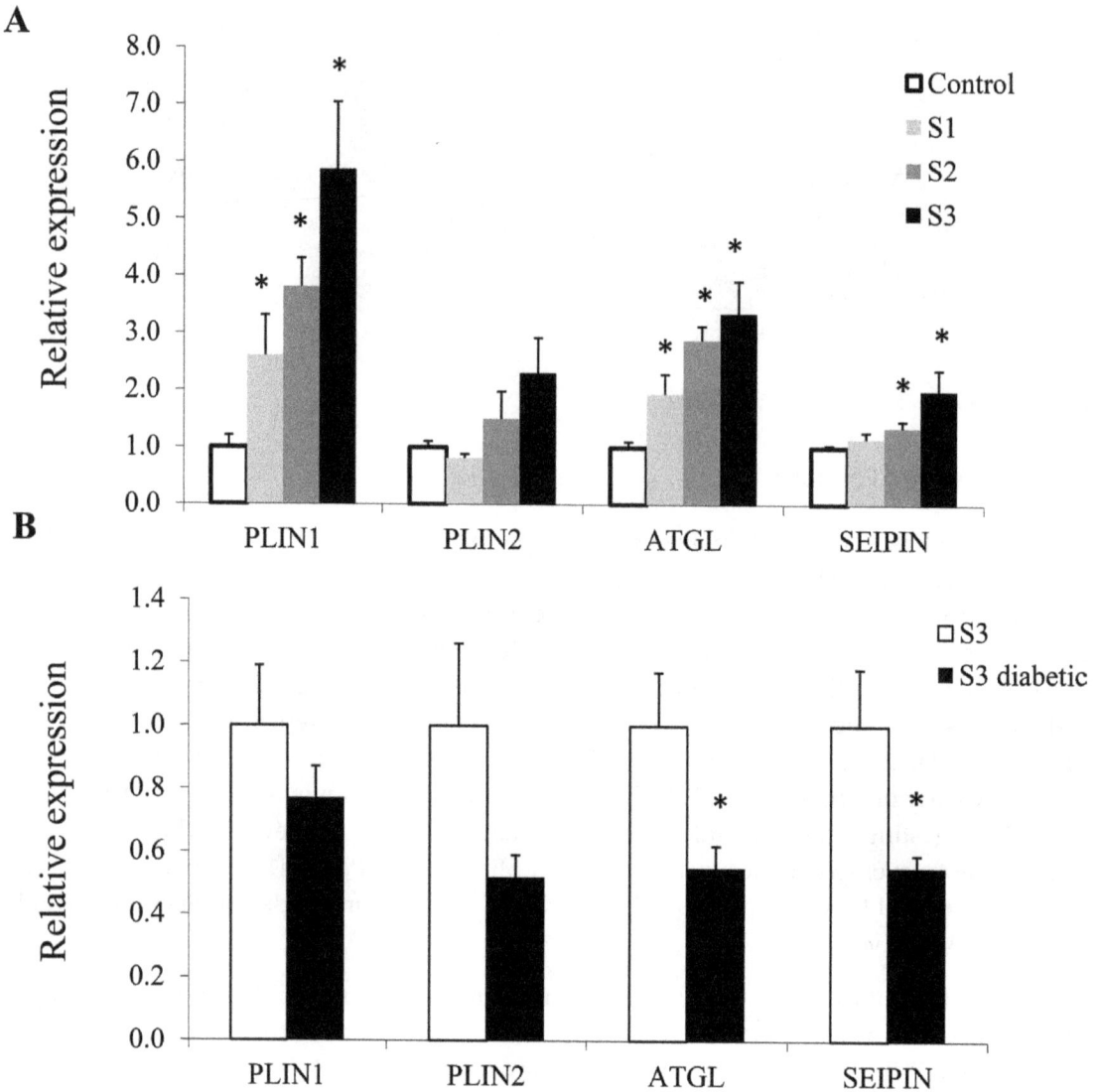

Figure 4. Expression of lipid droplet proteins in human NAFLD. NAFLD patients were separated into 5 groups depending on their degree of fatty liver. Gene expression of lipid droplets genes were analysed and compared among groups. (A) NALFD non diabetic, (B) Comparison of S3 NAFLD patients with or without type 2 diabetes.

5. Experimental modification of lipid droplet proteins and TG accumulation in hepatocytes

It has been shown that modifications on the lipid droplet proteins have striking impacts on lipid droplet biology. Hepatic cell line AML-12 is used to study the effect of downregulation of SEIPIN gene. Downregulation of the gene markedly altered lipid droplets size distributions and increased smaller droplets size, suggesting a default in lipid droplet maturation (**Figure 5**). When PLIN5 was knocked down in hepatocytes, the TG content dramatically

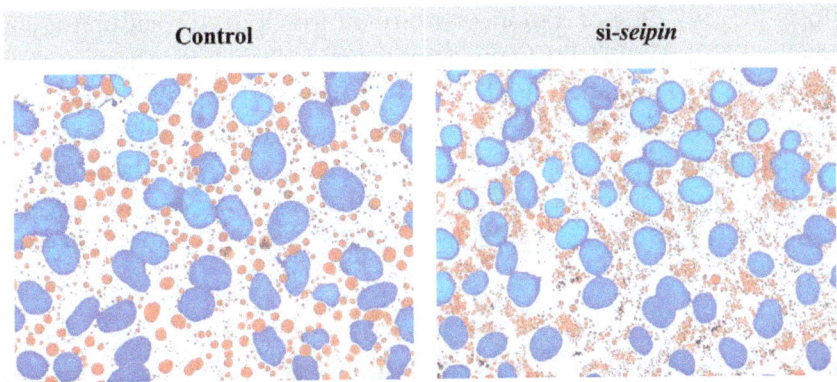

Figure 5. Lipid droplet morphology when SEIPIN was downregulated. Downregulation of SEIPIN by siRNA resulted in a fractionation of lipid droplets.

decreased due to accelerated lipolysis and beta-oxidation [60]. PPAR-alpha was required for the PLIN5-induced beta-oxidation. On the contrary, the overexpression of PLIN5 leads a significant increase in cellular TG. Therefore, modifications on lipid droplets proteins govern intracellular TG content in hepatocytes, although the mechanisms and phenotypes (lipid droplet size and/or localization) might be depending on a type of lipid droplet proteins involved.

6. Experimental modification of lipid droplet proteins in mice

Table 2 displays animals with genetic modifications in lipid droplet proteins and their effect on steatosis and metabolism (**Table 2**). PLIN1 KO mice present reduced body fat as well as fat oxidation judged by respiratory quotient [61]. Another research group also studied the PLIN1 KO mice and found increased lipolysis and cardiac hypertrophy [62]. PLIN2 null mice studied by different scientific groups consistently demonstrated a protection against diet-induced obesity, fatty liver, and alcohol-induced fatty accompanied by an improved insulin sensitivity [63–66]. Similar results were obtained in mice treated by PLIN2 antisense oligonucleotide, demonstrating improved insulin sensitivity [64]. PLIN3 downregulation was studied by using antisense oligonucleotide (ASO) in C57BL/6 J mice fed high fat diet. The reduction in PLIN3 significantly decreased hepatic fat content and improved glucose tolerance as well as insulin sensitivity in liver, adipose, and skeletal muscle [67]. Chen et al. generated PLIN4 KO mice [32], which showed no major modification in body weight and fat mass. Interestingly, only cardiac TG content was significantly reduced. The KO mice did not alter any gene expression involved in glucose and lipid metabolism. PLIN5 KO mice also developed cardiac dysfunction. The PLIN5 KO animal displayed reduced hepatic steatosis with increased mitochondrial proliferation, lipotoxic injury in the hepatocytes [40]. Interestingly, overexpression of PLIN5 by use of adenovirus technology demonstrated a development of severe hepatic steatosis without a sign of hepatic insulin resistance [68].

Although a strong link between PNPLA3 and hepatic steatosis has been demonstrated in GWAS studies [50], absence of PNPLA3 gene did not influence TG hydrolysis, nor did hepatic steatosis [55, 56]. One of a pioneer study on the lipid droplet biology and insulin resistance was the PNPLA2/ATGL KO mice published in 2006 [69]. Mice with global ATGL deletion induced TG accumulation in all tissues [69]. Surprisingly, despite the severe steatosis, the mice exhibit enhanced glucose tolerance and insulin sensitivity. Later on, Wu et al. studied the effect of liver-specific deletion of ATGL [70]. The liver-specific KO mice progressively developed a severe form of hepatic steatosis; however, the hepatic DAG content was 50-fold lower and had comparable plasma glucose, TG, and cholesterol levels to those of controls.

CIDEC/FSP27 downregulation was studied in Fsp27−/− and ob/ob × Fsp27−/− mice [46, 47], demonstrating decreased hepatic steatosis and insulin resistance. These animals are resistant to diet-induced obesity, dyslipidemia. Deletion of SEIPIN, as seen in BSCL patients, leads to severe form of hepatic steatosis accompanied by insulin resistance [49].

7. NAFLD and insulin resistance, implication of lipid droplet proteins

It has been widely accepted that increased TG content in ectopic organs, especially in the liver and skeletal muscle, induces insulin resistance [71–73]. Despite strong evidences demonstrating the link, there are also a few studies to show that hepatic steatosis can be dissociated from

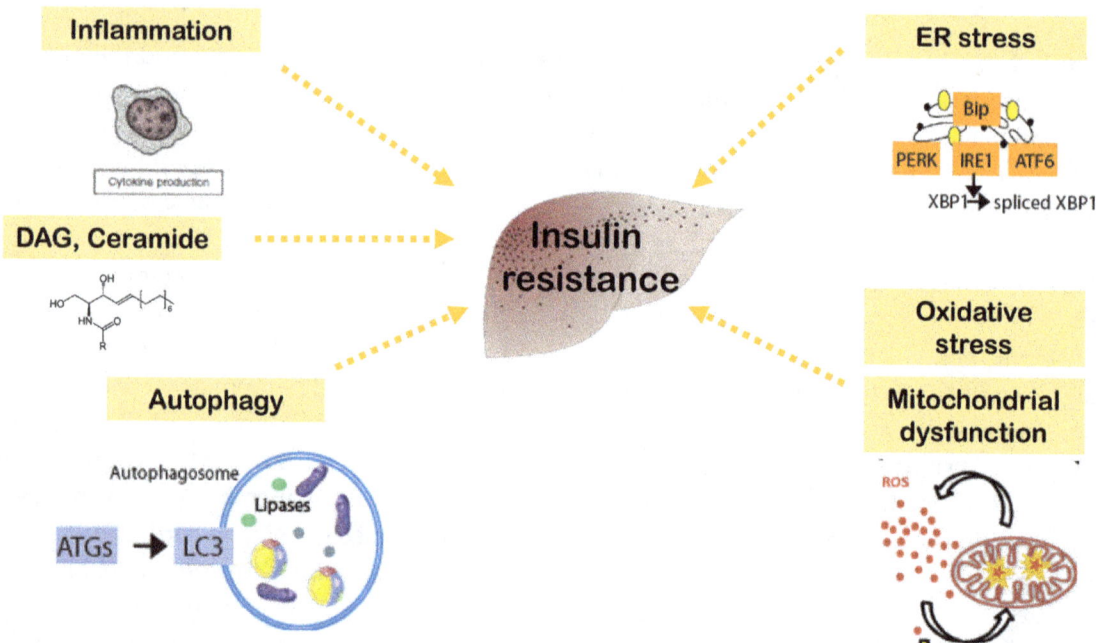

Figure 6. Different events leading hepatic insulin resistance in NAFLD. In human NAFLD, increased diacylglycerols (DAG) and ceramides are often observed. Under such conditions, autophagy is frequently decreased, leading to a disturbed lipid handling as well as increased ER stress and oxidative stress. These factors are known to induce insulin resistance.

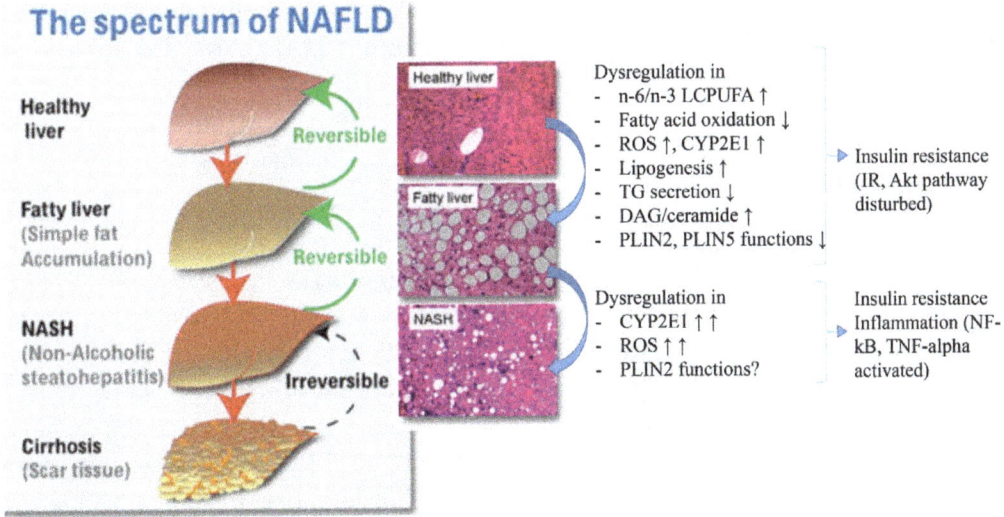

Figure 7. Dysregulated factors during steatosis and NASH development. Hepatic steatosis has many dysregulation in lipid metabolism, leading to insulin resistance. As a result of accelerated cellular damages due to oxidative stress and ER stress, inflammation is installed and NASH development starts.

insulin resistance such as liver-specific microsomal TG transfer protein (MTP) knockout mice [74]. While it is not physiological context at all, it may help to understand the contribution of each gene to the development of hepatic steatosis and insulin resistance at a molecular level. In a steatotic liver from the MTP knockout mice, we had identified upregulations of different lipid droplet proteins such as PLIN5, PLIN2, and SEIPIN. We then hypothesized that the upregulation of these genes was not deleterious in terms of hepatic insulin sensitivity. Indeed, the overexpression of these lipid droplet proteins always induced TG accumulation in hepatocytes; however, none of these *in vitro* models developed apparent insulin resistance. If true, what mechanisms possibly explain the development of hepatic insulin resistance in NAFLD? Different theories are briefly introduced below (**Figures 6** and **7**).

8. Ceramide/Diacylglycerol theory

In a steatotic liver, different lipid species are accumulated such as diacylglycerol (DAG) and ceramide. It was postulated that the accumulation of DAG and/or ceramide induced insulin resistance [75]. However, some of the models of NAFLD present increased hepatic DAG and ceramide without insulin resistance. Interestingly, a recent study demonstrated that the abnormal compartmentalization of these lipid intermediates, rather than total lipid content, is what might truly interfere with the insulin sensitivity [76]. This might support some inconsistent results from various mouse models studied by modulating PLINs (**Table 2**). DAG induces PKC epsilon translocation to the plasma membrane, inhibiting the intracellular kinase domain of the insulin receptor [77, 78]. In the case of PLIN5 overexpressed liver that was dissociated from hepatic insulin resistance, we did not observe the PKC epsilon translocation to the plasma membrane despite significant increase in DAG (personal observation). Accumulation of ceramides in the plasma membrane has also been demonstrated to disturb insulin signaling [79], and we have only observed significant increase in some of ceramides. As the PLIN-induced hepatic steatosis might depend on the type of PLIN proteins, each phenotype of hepatic steatosis needs to be finely studied. Therefore, the link between DAG/ceramide and hepatic insulin resistance in NAFLD requires more scientific investigations on each specific PLIN protein modification.

9. Autophagy theory

Selective autophagy process for a degradation of intracellular lipids is called lipophagy. The lipophagy is an additional mechanism that contributes to lipid droplet breakdown, and PLIN2 has been shown to play a role in this process [80, 81]. Autophagy is also involved in delivering fatty acids to lipid droplets for a lipolysis and mitochondrial oxidation [82, 83]. Inhibition of autophagy has been shown to accelerate lipid accumulation and impair beta-oxidation in the liver [84, 85]. Interestingly, *atg7* inhibition via shRNA in a mouse liver resulted in an impairment of autophagy system together with an impaired insulin signaling and an induced ER stress [85]. These effects were completely reversed when a downstream target *atg5* was blocked. This strongly supports an idea that autophagy plays one of a key role in insulin signaling pathway. How the lipophagy and lipid droplet proteins are involved in the insulin resistance are still open questions.

10. ER stress theory

Hepatic ER deals with redox regulation, glucose deprivation, protein synthesis, VLDL assembly and secretion, and cholesterol biosynthesis. It has been suggested that ER stress is implicated in insulin resistance, inflammation, and lipotoxicity, which are frequently observed in NAFLD patients [86]. Recently, Akoumi et al. tested a hypothesis that palmitate might induce ER stress by disturbing lipid droplet formation in cytosol and lead to an abnormal accumulation of lipid in an ER compartment. They found in cardiomyoblast cell line that palmitate-induced ER stress was associated with an abnormal storage of DAGs located in the ER. Concomitantly, significant degradation of PLIN2 but not PLIN3 or PLIN5 was observed, suggesting a potential scenario of PLIN2 as a protector/regulator of ER stress. Pharmacological ER stress also demonstrated a role of PLIN2 in ER stress-induced lipogenesis [87]. Author suggested that the presence (or induction) of PLIN2 during the ER stress might protect hepatocytes by storing lipids in a cytosolic compartment. It was a very tentative hypothesis; however, it was not supported at least in *Saccharomyces cerevisiae* that an absence of lipid droplet formation did not affect cell viability during ER stress [88]. There are still many remaining questions to be answered in the field of ER stress and the role of lipid droplet proteins. Their implication on metabolic disease such as NAFLD is one of a key aspect to be further investigated.

11. Oxidative stress theory

Reactive oxygen species (ROS) is produced in a highly regulated manner in multiple organelles such as the ER and mitochondria. ROS is produced as a result of oxidative protein folding and mitochondrial respiration. NAFLD, especially NASH (nonalcoholic steatohep-atitis), has been strongly linked with the biomarkers of oxidative stress [89, 90]. In a case of NAFLD development, beta-oxidation can be abnormally stimulated due to an excess fat accumulation, which surcharges mitochondrial system for the oxidation. As a result, abnormal ROS production at complex I of the mitochondrial electron-transport chain is induced, leading to the mitochondrial oxidative damage. Under such condition, the redox imbalance, lower antioxidant potential, and an enhanced free-radical activity lead to a sig-nificant reduction in systemic antioxidant capacity of plasma [91]. These conditions are indeed considered as a trigger of "second hit," which then induces NASH. Cytochrome P450 E12 (CYP2E1), a member of the cytochrome P450 mixed-function oxidase system, has been found as a marker of NASH, which distinguishes NASH from hepatic steatosis [92]. The induction of liver microsomal CYP2E1 contributes as a major free-radical source that aggravates oxidative stress in NASH. In addition to ROS production, cytokine is produced progressing a fatty liver to NASH. A depletion of n-3 long-chain polyunsaturated fatty acids (LCPUFA) was also found in NAFLD/NASH. n-3 LCPUFA has been shown to highly influence signaling pathway in a liver and contributes to NAFLD development [93, 94]. The n-3 LCPUFA downregulates sterol regulatory element-binding protein-1 (SRBBP-1), there-fore inhibiting *de novo* lipogenesis. It could also act as a ligand activators of PPAR-alpha, therefore stimulating fatty acid oxidation. The decreased n-3 LCPUFA and increased ratio of n-6/n-3 LCPUFA were reported in NAFLD/NASH patients. These conditions acceler-ate high oxidative stress and hepatocellular injury. Interestingly, Fujii et al. demonstrated in NAFLD/NASH patients that PLIN2 seemed preferentially expressed in droplets of bal-looned hepatocytes. The presence of PLIN2-positive ballooned hepatocytes was indeed correlated with inflammation [18]. Indeed, liver-specific knockout of PLIN2 in mice had reduced hepatic inflammation [95]. The role of PLIN2 on hepatic inflammation in NAFLD/NASH needs further investigation.

As indicated previously, PLIN5 has strong interactions with mitochondrial functions. Zheng et al. studied myocardium from PLIN5-deficient mice and found that the ROS production and malondialdehyde levels, a marker for oxidative stress, were significantly increased [96]. In this model, the phosphorylation of PI3K and Akt, which was induced by ischemia/reperfu-sion injury, was greatly reduced by PLIN5 deletion in the myocardium. It remains an open question whether the PLIN5 may have an impact on NASH development by interfering with the ROS production.

12. Conclusion

Research on lipid droplet proteins and lipid droplet biology has gained strong insights dur-ing the last decades. Most of the lipid droplet proteins are induced in NAFLD and required for a normal adipogenesis. Given specific expression patterns and roles of lipid droplet proteins, the phenotypes lead by experimental modifications of the lipid droplets proteins displayed diverse patterns. Further research is required to clarify their roles in NAFLD, spe-cially by focusing on interactions of different lipid droplet proteins and other functional proteins, lipid droplet localization, interaction with mitochondria as well as fatty acid compositions in the droplets. Their roles in mitochondrial physiology are a particular importance to understand how lipid droplet protein could influence hepatic energy metabolism and insulin signaling.

Author details

Kaori Minehira[1]* and Philippe Gual[2]

*Address all correspondence to: kaori.minehiracastelli@rd.nestle.com

1 Nestlé Institute of Health Sciences, Lausanne, Switzerland

2 Université Côte d'Azur, INSERM, U1065, C3M, Team 8, Chronic liver diseases associated with obesity and alcohol, Nice, France

References

[1] de Alwis NM, Day CP. Non-alcoholic fatty liver disease: The mist gradually clears. Journal of Hepatology. 2008;48(Suppl 1):S104-S112

[2] Kaser S, Ebenbichler CF, Tilg H. Pharmacological and non-pharmacological treatment of non-alcoholic fatty liver disease. International Journal of Clinical Practice. 2010; 64(7):968-983

[3] Byrne CD, Targher GNAFLD. A multisystem disease. Journal of Hepatology. 2015; 62(1 Suppl):S47-S64

[4] Farese RV Jr, Walther TC. Lipid droplets finally get a little R-E-S-P-E-C-T. Cell. 2009; 139(5):855-860

[5] Tan JS, Seow CJ, Goh VJ, Silver DL. Recent advances in understanding proteins involved in lipid droplet formation, growth and fusion. Journal of Genetics and Genomics. 2014;41(5):251-259

[6] Wang H, Bell M, Sreenivasan U, Hu H, Liu J, Dalen K, et al. Unique regulation of adipose triglyceride lipase (ATGL) by perilipin 5, a lipid droplet-associated protein. The Journal of Biological Chemistry. 2011;286(18):15707-15715

[7] Greenberg AS, Egan JJ, Wek SA, Garty NB, Blanchette-Mackie EJ, Londos C. Perilipin, a major hormonally regulated adipocyte-specific phosphoprotein associated with the periphery of lipid storage droplets. The Journal of Biological Chemistry. 1991;266(17): 11341-11346

[8] Jiang HP, Serrero G. Isolation and characterization of a full-length cDNA coding for an adipose differentiation-related protein. Proceedings of the National Academy of Sciences of the United States of America. 1992;89(17):7856-7860

[9] Diaz E, Pfeffer SR. TIP47: A cargo selection device for mannose 6-phosphate receptor trafficking. Cell. 1998;**93**(3):433-443

[10] Kimmel AR, Brasaemle DL, McAndrews-Hill M, Sztalryd C, Londos C. Adoption of PERILIPIN as a unifying nomenclature for the mammalian PAT-family of intracellular lipid storage droplet proteins. Journal of Lipid Research. 2010;**51**(3):468-471

[11] Miura S, Gan JW, Brzostowski J, Parisi MJ, Schultz CJ, Londos C, et al. Functional conservation for lipid storage droplet association among Perilipin, ADRP, and TIP47 (PAT)-related proteins in mammals, drosophila, and Dictyostelium. The Journal of Biological Chemistry. 2002;**277**(35):32253-32257

[12] Itabe H, Yamaguchi T, Nimura S, Sasabe N. Perilipins: A diversity of intracellular lipid droplet proteins. Lipids in Health and Disease. 2017;**16**(1):83

[13] Brasaemle DL, Rubin B, Harten IA, Gruia-Gray J, Kimmel AR, Londos C. Perilipin a increases triacylglycerol storage by decreasing the rate of triacylglycerol hydrolysis. The Journal of Biological Chemistry. 2000;**275**(49):38486-38493

[14] Blanchette-Mackie EJ, Dwyer NK, Barber T, Coxey RA, Takeda T, Rondinone CM, et al. Perilipin is located on the surface layer of intracellular lipid droplets in adipocytes. Journal of Lipid Research. 1995;**36**(6):1211-1226

[15] Sun Z, Gong J, Wu H, Xu W, Wu L, Xu D, et al. Perilipin1 promotes unilocular lipid droplet formation through the activation of Fsp27 in adipocytes. Nature Communications. 2013;**4**:1594

[16] Caldwell SH, Ikura Y, Iezzoni JC, Liu Z. Has natural selection in human populations produced two types of metabolic syndrome (with and without fatty liver)? Journal of Gastroenterology and Hepatology. 2007;**22**(Suppl 1):S11-S19

[17] Straub BK, Stoeffel P, Heid H, Zimbelmann R, Schirmacher P. Differential pattern of lipid droplet-associated proteins and de novo perilipin expression in hepatocyte steatogenesis. Hepatology. 2008;**47**(6):1936-1946

[18] Fujii H, Ikura Y, Arimoto J, Sugioka K, Iezzoni JC, Park SH, et al. Expression of perilipin and adipophilin in nonalcoholic fatty liver disease; relevance to oxidative injury and hepatocyte ballooning. Journal of Atherosclerosis and Thrombosis. 2009;**16**(6):893-901

[19] Takahashi Y, Shinoda A, Furuya N, Harada E, Arimura N, Ichi I, et al. Perilipin-mediated lipid droplet formation in adipocytes promotes sterol regulatory element-binding protein-1 processing and triacylglyceride accumulation. PLoS One. 2013;**8**(5):e64605

[20] Beier JI, McClain CJ. Mechanisms and cell signaling in alcoholic liver disease. Biological Chemistry. 2010;**391**(11):1249-1264

[21] Motomura W, Inoue M, Ohtake T, Takahashi N, Nagamine M, Tanno S, et al. Up-regulation of ADRP in fatty liver in human and liver steatosis in mice fed with high fat diet. Biochemical and Biophysical Research Communications. 2006;**340**(4):1111-1118

[22] Carr RM, Dhir R, Yin X, Agarwal B, Ahima RS. Temporal effects of ethanol consumption on energy homeostasis, hepatic steatosis, and insulin sensitivity in mice. Alcoholism, Clinical and Experimental Research. 2013;**37**(7):1091-1099

[23] Magne J, Aminoff A, Perman Sundelin J, Mannila MN, Gustafsson P, Hultenby K, et al. The minor allele of the missense polymorphism Ser251Pro in perilipin 2 (PLIN2) disrupts an alpha-helix, affects lipolysis, and is associated with reduced plasma triglyceride concentration in humans. The FASEB Journal. 2013;**27**(8):3090-3099

[24] Bell M, Wang H, Chen H, McLenithan JC, Gong DW, Yang RZ, et al. Consequences of lipid droplet coat protein downregulation in liver cells: Abnormal lipid droplet metabolism and induction of insulin resistance. Diabetes. 2008;**57**(8):2037-2045

[25] Coleman RA, Mashek DG. Mammalian triacylglycerol metabolism: Synthesis, lipolysis, and signaling. Chemical Reviews. 2011;**111**(10):6359-6386

[26] Lu X, Gruia-Gray J, Copeland NG, Gilbert DJ, Jenkins NA, Londos C, et al. The murine perilipin gene: The lipid droplet-associated perilipins derive from tissue-specific, mRNA splice variants and define a gene family of ancient origin. Mammalian Genome. 2001;**12**(9):741-749

[27] Patel S, Yang W, Kozusko K, Saudek V, Savage DB. Perilipins 2 and 3 lack a carboxy-terminal domain present in perilipin 1 involved in sequestering ABHD5 and suppressing basal lipolysis. Proceedings of the National Academy of Sciences of the United States of America. 2014;**111**(25):9163-9168

[28] Nose F, Yamaguchi T, Kato R, Aiuchi T, Obama T, Hara S, et al. Crucial role of perilipin-3 (TIP47) in formation of lipid droplets and PGE2 production in HL-60-derived neutrophils. PLoS One. 2013;**8**(8):e71542

[29] Kleinert M, Parker BL, Chaudhuri R, Fazakerley DJ, Serup A, Thomas KC, et al. mTORC2 and AMPK differentially regulate muscle triglyceride content via Perilipin 3. Molecular Metabolism. 2016;**5**(8):646-655

[30] Wolins NE, Skinner JR, Schoenfish MJ, Tzekov A, Bensch KG, Bickel PE. Adipocyte protein S3-12 coats nascent lipid droplets. The Journal of Biological Chemistry. 2003;**278**(39):37713-37721

[31] Nimura S, Yamaguchi T, Ueda K, Kadokura K, Aiuchi T, Kato R, et al. Olanzapine promotes the accumulation of lipid droplets and the expression of multiple perilipins in human adipocytes. Biochemical and Biophysical Research Communications. 2015;**467**(4):906-912

[32] Chen W, Chang B, Wu X, Li L, Sleeman M, Chan L. Inactivation of Plin4 downregulates Plin5 and reduces cardiac lipid accumulation in mice. American Journal of Physiology. Endocrinology and Metabolism. 2013;**304**(7):E770-E779

[33] Yamaguchi T, Matsushita S, Motojima K, Hirose F, Osumi TMLDP. A novel PAT family protein localized to lipid droplets and enriched in the heart, is regulated by peroxisome proliferator-activated receptor alpha. The Journal of Biological Chemistry. 2006;**281**(20):14232-14240

[34] Dalen KT, Dahl T, Holter E, Arntsen B, Londos C, Sztalryd C, et al. LSDP5 is a PAT protein specifically expressed in fatty acid oxidizing tissues. Biochimica et Biophysica Acta. 2007;**1771**(2):210-227

[35] Trevino MB, Machida Y, Hallinger DR, Garcia E, Christensen A, Dutta S, et al. Perilipin 5 regulates islet lipid metabolism and insulin secretion in a cAMP-dependent manner: Implication of its role in the postprandial insulin secretion. Diabetes. 2015;**64**(4): 1299-1310

[36] Lin J, Chen A. Perilipin 5 restores the formation of lipid droplets in activated hepatic stellate cells and inhibits their activation. Laboratory Investigation. 2016;**96**(7):791-806

[37] Bosma M, Minnaard R, Sparks LM, Schaart G, Losen M, de Baets MH, et al. The lipid droplet coat protein perilipin 5 also localizes to muscle mitochondria. Histochemistry and Cell Biology. 2012;**137**(2):205-216

[38] Kuramoto K, Okamura T, Yamaguchi T, Nakamura TY, Wakabayashi S, Morinaga H, et al. Perilipin 5, a lipid droplet-binding protein, protects heart from oxidative burden by sequestering fatty acid from excessive oxidation. The Journal of Biological Chemistry. 2012;**287**(28):23852-23863

[39] Wang H, Sreenivasan U, Hu H, Saladino A, Polster BM, Lund LM, et al. Perilipin 5, a lipid droplet-associated protein, provides physical and metabolic linkage to mitochondria. Journal of Lipid Research. 2011;**52**(12):2159-2168

[40] Wang C, Zhao Y, Gao X, Li L, Yuan Y, Liu F, et al. Perilipin 5 improves hepatic lipotoxicity by inhibiting lipolysis. Hepatology. 2015;**61**(3):870-882

[41] Wang R, Kong X, Cui A, Liu X, Xiang R, Yang Y, et al. Sterol-regulatory-element-binding protein 1c mediates the effect of insulin on the expression of Cidea in mouse hepatocytes. The Biochemical Journal. 2010;**430**(2):245-254

[42] Zhou L, Xu L, Ye J, Li D, Wang W, Li X, et al. Cidea promotes hepatic steatosis by sensing dietary fatty acids. Hepatology. 2012;**56**(1):95-107

[43] Li JZ, Ye J, Xue B, Qi J, Zhang J, Zhou Z, et al. Cideb regulates diet-induced obesity, liver steatosis, and insulin sensitivity by controlling lipogenesis and fatty acid oxidation. Diabetes. 2007;**56**(10):2523-2532

[44] Li X, Ye J, Zhou L, Gu W, Fisher EA, Li P. Opposing roles of cell death-inducing DFF45-like effector B and perilipin 2 in controlling hepatic VLDL lipidation. Journal of Lipid Research. 2012;**53**(9):1877-1889

[45] Xu MJ, Cai Y, Wang H, Altamirano J, Chang B, Bertola A, et al. Fat-specific protein 27/CIDEC promotes development of alcoholic Steatohepatitis in mice and humans. Gastroenterology. 2015;**149**(4):1030-1041 e6

[46] Matsusue K, Kusakabe T, Noguchi T, Takiguchi S, Suzuki T, Yamano S, et al. Hepatic steatosis in leptin-deficient mice is promoted by the PPARgamma target gene Fsp27. Cell Metabolism. 2008;**7**(4):302-311

[47] Toh SY, Gong J, Du G, Li JZ, Yang S, Ye J, et al. Up-regulation of mitochondrial activity and acquirement of brown adipose tissue-like property in the white adipose tissue of fsp27 deficient mice. PLoS One. 2008;**3**(8):e2890

[48] Gong J, Sun Z, Wu L, Xu W, Schieber N, Xu D, et al. Fsp27 promotes lipid droplet growth by lipid exchange and transfer at lipid droplet contact sites. The Journal of Cell Biology. 2011;**195**(6):953-963

[49] Dollet L, Magre J, Cariou B, Prieur X. Function of seipin: New insights from Bscl2/seipin knockout mouse models. Biochimie. 2014;**96**:166-172

[50] Romeo S, Kozlitina J, Xing C, Pertsemlidis A, Cox D, Pennacchio LA, et al. Genetic variation in PNPLA3 confers susceptibility to nonalcoholic fatty liver disease. Nature Genetics. 2008;**40**(12):1461-1465

[51] Kitamoto T, Kitamoto A, Yoneda M, Hyogo H, Ochi H, Nakamura T, et al. Genome-wide scan revealed that polymorphisms in the PNPLA3, SAMM50, and PARVB genes are associated with development and progression of nonalcoholic fatty liver disease in Japan. Human Genetics. 2013;**132**(7):783-792

[52] He S, McPhaul C, Li JZ, Garuti R, Kinch L, Grishin NV, et al. A sequence variation (I148M) in PNPLA3 associated with nonalcoholic fatty liver disease disrupts triglyceride hydrolysis. The Journal of Biological Chemistry. 2010;**285**(9):6706-6715

[53] Pingitore P, Pirazzi C, Mancina RM, Motta BM, Indiveri C, Pujia A, et al. Recombinant PNPLA3 protein shows triglyceride hydrolase activity and its I148M mutation results in loss of function. Biochimica et Biophysica Acta. 2014;**1841**(4):574-580

[54] Pirazzi C, Valenti L, Motta BM, Pingitore P, Hedfalk K, Mancina RM, et al. PNPLA3 has retinyl-palmitate lipase activity in human hepatic stellate cells. Human Molecular Genetics. 2014;**23**(15):4077-4085

[55] Basantani MK, Sitnick MT, Cai L, Brenner DS, Gardner NP, Li JZ, et al. Pnpla3/Adiponutrin deficiency in mice does not contribute to fatty liver disease or metabolic syndrome. Journal of Lipid Research. 2011;**52**(2):318-329

[56] Chen W, Chang B, Li L, Chan L. Patatin-like phospholipase domain-containing 3/adiponutrin deficiency in mice is not associated with fatty liver disease. Hepatology. 2010;**52**(3):1134-1142

[57] Smagris E, BasuRay S, Li J, Huang Y, Lai KM, Gromada J, et al. Pnpla3I148M knockin mice accumulate PNPLA3 on lipid droplets and develop hepatic steatosis. Hepatology. 2015;**61**(1):108-118

[58] Pawella LM, Hashani M, Eiteneuer E, Renner M, Bartenschlager R, Schirmacher P, et al. Perilipin discerns chronic from acute hepatocellular steatosis. Journal of Hepatology. 2014;**60**(3):633-642

[59] Straub BK, Gyoengyoesi B, Koenig M, Hashani M, Pawella LM, Herpel E, et al. Adipophilin/perilipin-2 as a lipid droplet-specific marker for metabolically active cells and diseases associated with metabolic dysregulation. Histopathology. 2013;**62**(4):617-631

[60] Li H, Song Y, Zhang LJ, Gu Y, Li FF, Pan SY, et al. LSDP5 enhances triglyceride storage in hepatocytes by influencing lipolysis and fatty acid beta-oxidation of lipid droplets. PLoS One. 2012;**7**(6):e36712

[61] Beylot M, Neggazi S, Hamlat N, Langlois D, Forcheron F. Perilipin 1 ablation in mice enhances lipid oxidation during exercise and does not impair exercise performance. Metabolism. 2012;**61**(3):415-423

[62] Liu S, Geng B, Zou L, Wei S, Wang W, Deng J, et al. Development of hypertrophic cardiomyopathy in perilipin-1 null mice with adipose tissue dysfunction. Cardiovascular Research. 2015;**105**(1):20-30

[63] Varela GM, Antwi DA, Dhir R, Yin X, Singhal NS, Graham MJ, et al. Inhibition of ADRP prevents diet-induced insulin resistance. American Journal of Physiology. Gastrointestinal and Liver Physiology. 2008;**295**(3):G621-G628

[64] Imai Y, Varela GM, Jackson MB, Graham MJ, Crooke RM, Ahima RS. Reduction of hepatosteatosis and lipid levels by an adipose differentiation-related protein antisense oligonucleotide. Gastroenterology. 2007;**132**(5):1947-1954

[65] McManaman JL, Bales ES, Orlicky DJ, Jackman M, MacLean PS, Cain S, et al. Perilipin-2-null mice are protected against diet-induced obesity, adipose inflammation, and fatty liver disease. Journal of Lipid Research. 2013;**54**(5):1346-1359

[66] Carr RM, Peralta G, Yin X, Ahima RS. Absence of perilipin 2 prevents hepatic steatosis, glucose intolerance and ceramide accumulation in alcohol-fed mice. PLoS One. 2014;**9**(5):e97118

[67] Carr RM, Patel RT, Rao V, Dhir R, Graham MJ, Crooke RM, et al. Reduction of TIP47 improves hepatic steatosis and glucose homeostasis in mice. American Journal of Physiology. Regulatory, Integrative and Comparative Physiology. 2012;**302**(8):R996-1003

[68] Trevino MB, Mazur-Hart D, Machida Y, King T, Nadler J, Galkina EV, et al. Liver Perilipin 5 expression worsens Hepatosteatosis but not insulin resistance in high fat-fed mice. Molecular Endocrinology. 2015;**29**(10):1414-1425

[69] Haemmerle G, Lass A, Zimmermann R, Gorkiewicz G, Meyer C, Rozman J, et al. Defective lipolysis and altered energy metabolism in mice lacking adipose triglyceride lipase. Science. 2006;**312**(5774):734-737

[70] JW Wu, Wang SP, Alvarez F, Casavant S, Gauthier N, Abed L, et al. Deficiency of liver adipose triglyceride lipase in mice causes progressive hepatic steatosis. Hepatology. 2011;**54**(1):122-132

[71] Rasouli N, Molavi B, Elbein SC, Kern PA. Ectopic fat accumulation and metabolic syndrome. Diabetes, Obesity & Metabolism. 2007;**9**(1):1-10

[72] Boden G. Interaction between free fatty acids and glucose metabolism. Current Opinion in Clinical Nutrition and Metabolic Care. 2002;**5**(5):545-549

[73] Kovacs P, Stumvoll M. Fatty acids and insulin resistance in muscle and liver. Best Practice & Research. Clinical Endocrinology & Metabolism. 2005;**19**(4):625-635

[74] Minehira K, Young SG, Villanueva CJ, Yetukuri L, Oresic M, Hellerstein MK, et al. Blocking VLDL secretion causes hepatic steatosis but does not affect peripheral lipid stores or insulin sensitivity in mice. Journal of Lipid Research. 2008;**49**(9):2038-2044

[75] Petersen MC, Shulman GI. Roles of diacylglycerols and ceramides in hepatic insulin resistance. Trends in Pharmacological Sciences. 2017;**38**(7):649-665

[76] Cantley JL, Yoshimura T, Camporez JP, Zhang D, Jornayvaz FR, Kumashiro N, et al. CGI-58 knockdown sequesters diacylglycerols in lipid droplets/ER-preventing diacyl-glycerol-mediated hepatic insulin resistance. Proceedings of the National Academy of Sciences of the United States of America. 2013;**110**(5):1869-1874

[77] Samuel VT, Liu ZX, Wang A, Beddow SA, Geisler JG, Kahn M, et al. Inhibition of protein kinase Cepsilon prevents hepatic insulin resistance in nonalcoholic fatty liver disease. The Journal of Clinical Investigation. 2007;**117**(3):739-745

[78] Dries DR, Gallegos LL, Newton AC. A single residue in the C1 domain sensitizes novel protein kinase C isoforms to cellular diacylglycerol production. The Journal of Biological Chemistry. 2007;**282**(2):826-830

[79] Lipina C, Hundal HS. Sphingolipids: Agents provocateurs in the pathogenesis of insulin resistance. Diabetologia. 2011;**54**(7):1596-1607

[80] Singh R, Kaushik S, Wang Y, Xiang Y, Novak I, Komatsu M, et al. Autophagy regulates lipid metabolism. Nature. 2009;**458**(7242):1131-1135

[81] Tsai TH, Chen E, Li L, Saha P, Lee HJ, Huang LS, et al. The constitutive lipid droplet protein PLIN2 regulates autophagy in liver. Autophagy. 2017;**13**(7):1130-1144

[82] Rambold AS, Cohen S, Lippincott-Schwartz J. Fatty acid trafficking in starved cells: Regulation by lipid droplet lipolysis, autophagy, and mitochondrial fusion dynamics. Developmental Cell. 2015;**32**(6):678-692

[83] Shpilka T, Elazar Z. Lipid droplets regulate autophagosome biogenesis. Autophagy. 2015;**11**(11):2130-2131

[84] Shpilka T, Welter E, Borovsky N, Amar N, Mari M, Reggiori F, et al. Lipid droplets and their component triglycerides and steryl esters regulate autophagosome biogenesis. The EMBO Journal. 2015;**34**(16):2117-2131

[85] Yang L, Li P, Fu S, Calay ES, Hotamisligil GS. Defective hepatic autophagy in obesity promotes ER stress and causes insulin resistance. Cell Metabolism. 2010;**11**(6):467-478

[86] Ashraf NU, Sheikh TA. Endoplasmic reticulum stress and oxidative stress in the patho-genesis of non-alcoholic fatty liver disease. Free Radical Research. 2015;**49**(12):1405-1418

[87] Lee JS, Mendez R, Heng HH, Yang ZQ, Zhang K, Pharmacological ER. Stress promotes hepatic lipogenesis and lipid droplet formation. American Journal of Translational Research. 2012;**4**(1):102-113

[88] Fei W, Wang H, Fu X, Bielby C, Yang H. Conditions of endoplasmic reticulum stress stimulate lipid droplet formation in *Saccharomyces cerevisiae*. The Biochemical Journal. 2009;**424**(1):61-67

[89] Koek GH, Liedorp PR, Bast A. The role of oxidative stress in non-alcoholic steatohepa-titis. Clinica Chimica Acta. 2011;**412**(15-16):1297-1305

[90] Videla LA, Rodrigo R, Orellana M, Fernandez V, Tapia G, Quinones L, et al. Oxidative stress-related parameters in the liver of non-alcoholic fatty liver disease patients. Clinical Science (London, England). 2004;**106**(3):261-268

[91] Videla LA, Rodrigo R, Araya J, Poniachik J. Insulin resistance and oxidative stress interdependency in non-alcoholic fatty liver disease. Trends in Molecular Medicine. 2006;**12**(12):555-558

[92] Hennig EE, Mikula M, Goryca K, Paziewska A, Ledwon J, Nesteruk M, et al. Extracellular matrix and cytochrome P450 gene expression can distinguish steatohepatitis from ste-atosis in mice. Journal of Cellular and Molecular Medicine. 2014;**18**(9):1762-1772

[93] Valenzuela R, Videla LA. The importance of the long-chain polyunsaturated fatty acid n-6/n-3 ratio in development of non-alcoholic fatty liver associated with obesity. Food & Function. 2011;**2**(11):644-648

[94] Videla LA, Rodrigo R, Araya J, Poniachik J. Oxidative stress and depletion of hepatic long-chain polyunsaturated fatty acids may contribute to nonalcoholic fatty liver dis-ease. Free Radical Biology & Medicine. 2004;**37**(9):1499-1507

[95] Najt CP, Senthivinayagam S, Aljazi MB, Fader KA, Olenic SD, Brock JR, et al. Liver-specific loss of perilipin 2 alleviates diet-induced hepatic steatosis, inflammation, and fibrosis. American Journal of Physiology. Gastrointestinal and Liver Physiology. 2016;**310**(9):G726-G738

[96] Zheng P, Xie Z, Yuan Y, Sui W, Wang C, Gao X, et al. Plin5 alleviates myocardial isch-aemia/reperfusion injury by reducing oxidative stress through inhibiting the lipolysis of lipid droplets. Scientific Reports. 2017;**7**:42574

[97] Zechner R, Kienesberger PC, Haemmerle G, Zimmermann R, Lass A. Adipose triglyc-eride lipase and the lipolytic catabolism of cellular fat stores. Journal of Lipid Research. 2009;**50**(1):3-21

[98] Yamaguchi T, Omatsu N, Morimoto E, Nakashima H, Ueno K, Tanaka T, et al. CGI-58 facilitates lipolysis on lipid droplets but is not involved in the vesiculation of lipid drop-lets caused by hormonal stimulation. Journal of Lipid Research. 2007;**48**(5):1078-1089

[99] Dalen KT, Ulven SM, Arntsen BM, Solaas K, Nebb HI. PPARalpha activators and fast-ing induce the expression of adipose differentiation-related protein in liver. Journal of Lipid Research. 2006;**47**(5):931-943

[100] Mishra R, Emancipator SN, Miller C, Kern T, Simonson MS. Adipose differentiation-related protein and regulators of lipid homeostasis identified by gene expression pro-filing in the murine db/db diabetic kidney. American Journal of Physiology. Renal Physiology. 2004;**286**(5):F913-F921

[101] Suzuki K, Takahashi K, Nishimaki-Mogami T, Kagechika H, Yamamoto M, Itabe H. Docosahexaenoic acid induces adipose differentiation-related protein through acti-vation of retinoid x receptor in human choriocarcinoma BeWo cells. Biological & Pharmaceutical Bulletin. 2009;**32**(7):1177-1182

[102] Rankin EB, Rha J, Selak MA, Unger TL, Keith B, Liu Q, et al. Hypoxia-inducible factor 2 regulates hepatic lipid metabolism. Molecular and Cellular Biology. 2009;29(16): 4527-4538

[103] Bindesboll C, Berg O, Arntsen B, Nebb HI, Dalen KT. Fatty acids regulate perilipin5 in muscle by activating PPARdelta. Journal of Lipid Research. 2013;54(7):1949-1963

[104] Granneman JG, Moore HP, Mottillo EP, Zhu Z. Functional interactions between Mldp (LSDP5) and Abhd5 in the control of intracellular lipid accumulation. The Journal of Biological Chemistry. 2009;284(5):3049-3057

[105] Huang Y, He S, Li JZ, Seo YK, Osborne TF, Cohen JC, et al. A feed-forward loop amplifies nutritional regulation of PNPLA3. Proceedings of the National Academy of Sciences of the United States of America. 2010;107(17):7892-7897

[106] Sathyanarayan A, Mashek MT, Mashek DG. ATGL promotes autophagy/lipophagy via SIRT1 to control hepatic lipid droplet catabolism. Cell Reports. 2017;19(1):1-9

[107] Cai H, Yao W, Li L, Li X, Hu L, Mai R, et al. Cell-death-inducing DFFA-like effector B contributes to the assembly of hepatitis C virus (HCV) particles and interacts with HCV NS5A. Scientific Reports. 2016;6:27778

[108] Chang BH, Li L, Saha P, Chan L. Absence of adipose differentiation related protein upregulates hepatic VLDL secretion, relieves hepatosteatosis, and improves whole body insulin resistance in leptin-deficient mice. Journal of Lipid Research. 2010;51(8):2132-2142

[109] Chang BH, Li L, Paul A, Taniguchi S, Nannegari V, Heird WC, et al. Protection against fatty liver but normal adipogenesis in mice lacking adipose differentiation-related protein. Molecular and Cellular Biology. 2006;26(3):1063-1076

[110] Zhou L, Park SY, Xu L, Xia X, Ye J, Su L, et al. Insulin resistance and white adipose tissue inflammation are uncoupled in energetically challenged Fsp27-deficient mice. Nature Communications. 2015;6:5949

[111] Langhi C, Arias N, Rajamoorthi A, Basta J, Lee RG, Baldan A. Therapeutic silencing of fat-specific protein 27 improves glycemic control in mouse models of obesity and insulin resistance. Journal of Lipid Research. 2017;58(1):81-91

[112] Liu L, Jiang Q, Wang X, Zhang Y, Lin RC, Lam SM, et al. Adipose-specific knockout of SEIPIN/BSCL2 results in progressive lipodystrophy. Diabetes. 2014;63(7):2320-2331

[113] Cui X, Wang Y, Meng L, Fei W, Deng J, Xu G, et al. Overexpression of a short human seipin/BSCL2 isoform in mouse adipose tissue results in mild lipodystrophy. American Journal of Physiology. Endocrinology and Metabolism. 2012;302(6):E705-E713

7

Hepatic Trauma

Ali Ibrahim Yahya

Abstract

Liver is the second most common solid organ frequently injured by blunt trauma and could be the commonest organ injured by penetrating trauma. The injury can be mild and goes undetected or detected and treated conservatively. It can be severe where the liver wounds can bleed until death. Once the patients with liver injury are resuscitated, the degree of liver injury can be evaluated using ultrasound scan and computed tomography imaging. If the patient is stable, diagnostic peritoneal lavage is very helpful when the imaging facilities are not available. Non-operative treatment of liver trauma has been proven to be valuable in 80% of patients with grade I, II, III and IV (grade I—mild injury; grade II—moderate injury; grade III and IV—severe liver injury). Laparotomy is mandatory if the patient's condition is unstable. By using the explorative laparotomy technique, the grade of liver injury is assessed, and accordingly the procedure is performed including suturing, ligation of the bleeding vessel, segmental resection, perihepatic packing, and so on. Morbidity and mortality of liver injury can be minimized with early diagnosis and appropriate management.

Keywords: liver injury, non-operative treatment, grading of liver injury, perihepatic packing

1. Introduction to surgical anatomy of liver

The liver is situated at the right upper quadrant of the abdomen, extending from the 5th intercostal space at the mid-clavicular line to the 10th costal margin, with a length of about 13 cm which is called the liver span. It weighs 1500 g and is the largest intra-abdominal organ, receiving 1.5 L of blood flow per minute. It is surrounded by a membrane called Glisson's capsule. It has two lobes—right and left—separated by falciform ligament, two fissures anteriorly where the ligamentum teres is attached, posterior fissure where the ligamentum venosum is attached and the third fissure on the right lobe called porta hepatis where the hepatic triad enters the liver.

1.1. Surfaces of the liver

The liver has diaphragmatic surface which is related to chest cage. Visceral surfaces are related to the following structures: right kidney, right adrenal gland, gall bladder, duodenum and hepatic flexure.

Its surface is attached to the diaphragm by a falciform ligament, right and left triangular ligament and coronary ligament.

The liver is composed of eight segments. Each lobe is composed of four segments. Each segment has its own artery, vein and duct and can be resected separately without interfering with the other segments.

Cantlie line is an imaginary line that goes from the gall bladder fossa to inferior vena cava.

The liver is composed of hepatic plates. Each plate is composed of hepatocytes, sinusoids and Kupffer cells.

1.2. Vascular supply of liver

Hepatic artery comes from the coeliac axis and divides into the right and left. It supplies 25% of blood to the liver, and portal vein supplies 75% of blood to the liver tissues. The portal vein is formed by superior mesenteric vein and splenic vein behind the neck of the pancreas.

1.2.1. Hepatic veins

There are three large hepatic veins, which drain the hepatic parenchyma of the liver lobes into the inferior vena cava.

1.2.2. Nerve supply

Parasympathetic nerve from the right vagus via coelic plexus, left vagus to porta hepatis, and sympathetic nerve along the blood vessels.

Function of the liver:

1. Bile production and secretion.

2. Detoxification of toxins.

3. Protein synthesis.

4. Production of heparin, bile pigments.

5. Storage of glycogen.

6. Erythropoiesis in infants.

Epidemiology of liver trauma:

Liver is the second most common abdominal organ that can get injured by blunt trauma [1, 26] and is the most common cause of death in abdominal trauma—100% mortality if untreated or missed from examination. Blunt abdominal trauma is more fatal than penetrating trauma. Before 1993, all liver injuries were treated through surgery. From 1998 onwards, non-operative treatment was introduced as the standard method of treatment for liver trauma with 80% of adult liver trauma treated conservatively and 97% of children also treated non-operatively [25].

Liver injury can be mild when the trauma affects less than 25% of one lobe, moderate when the trauma affects between 25 and 50% of the lobe, and severe when the trauma affects more than 50% of the lobe.

Why liver is prone to trauma?

The liver is prone to trauma for the following reasons:

1. Fixed position of the liver: The liver is an organ which is huge and fixed at the right upper quadrant of the abdomen.

2. Liver is an organ with friable parenchyma.

3. Liver has a thin capsule.

Liver trauma can be the following:

Subcapsular haematoma, laceration, contusion, liver avulsion, bile duct injury, and gall bladder injury. Eighty percent of liver trauma involves segments 6, 7 and 8.

2. Etiology of liver trauma

The liver can be injured commonly by the following:

1. Blunt trauma commonly due to road traffic accident and can follow fall down from height. Blunt liver trauma is 10 times more fatal than penetrating trauma [7]. Blunt abdominal trauma can sustain up to 1–8% of liver injury. Hepatic trauma forms 15–20% of abdominal trauma and 80% of blunt trauma.

2. Penetrating trauma caused by a bullet or by stabbing with a sharp instrument.

3. Iatrogenic trauma is very rare during surgery or during performance of percutaneous transhepatic cholangiography (PTC). Hepatic vein injury can occur during insertion of (transjugular portosystemic shunt (TIPS).

2.1. Diagnosis of liver trauma

2.1.1. A: Clinical picture of liver trauma

1. Liver injury can be obvious.

2. Liver injury can be easily predicted.

3. Liver injury can be difficult to predict.

Obvious liver trauma:

Liver injury can be positively diagnosed where the following points are clearly established:

1. The patient is in a state of shock where he or she was involved in a road traffic accident or hit by a bullet at the right upper quadrant of the abdomen.

2. The patient is with hypotension and pain at the right upper quadrant of the abdomen after a road traffic accident.

3. Hypotensive patient shows tenderness over the right side of chest with fractured ribs after the trauma.

4. Hypotensive patient with bruises at the right upper quadrant.

Liver trauma can be easily predicted with the following points borne in mind:

1. Drop in blood pressure in a patient with road traffic accident and with guarding and tenderness at the right side of the upper abdomen.

2. Penetrating wound at the right upper quadrant of the abdomen.

Liver trauma is difficult to predict:

1. Normal blood pressure with right upper abdominal pain with guarding and tenderness at the right upper quadrant

Clinical presentation of liver trauma:

1. Pain at the right upper quadrant.

2. Fracture of right lower ribs.

3. Shock

Grading of liver trauma: **American association of trauma**

Grade I: Subcapsular haematoma less than 10% of the surface area. Laceration less than 1 cm.

Grade II: Haematoma more than 10–50% surface area. Laceration from 1 to 3 cm.

Grade III: Haematoma more than 50%. Laceration more than 3 cm.

Grade IV: Ruptured haematoma and bleeding. Laceration of the liver from 25 to 75% of the lobe.

Grade V: More than 75% of liver laceration, retrohepatic vena cava injury or hepatic vein injuries.

Grade VI: Hepatic avulsion.

2.1.2. B: Investigations

2.1.2.1. Routine investigations

Routine examination includes full blood count, electrolytes, blood sugar, urea, hemoglobin may be normal where the injury is simple, or there may be low hemoglobin indicating blood loss where the injury is severe.

Liver function tests were not done at the admission time and may not be needed if the injury is simple; it could be done if the case showed severe liver trauma. Liver function includes bilirubin, and liver enzymes include glutamic pyruvate transaminase (GPT), glutamic oxaloacetate transainase (GOT) and alkaline phosphatase (ALK) phos.

Blood group is done routinely in all patients with hepatic trauma.

2.1.2.2. Imaging investigations

Ultrasound scan for liver trauma has 99% of specificity and 88% of sensitivity [19–21]. Fast ultrasound replaced peritoneal lavage. Looking to Morrison space if there is fluid in the space indicating bleeding. The use of contrast with ultrasound scan is more beneficial in liver trauma.

CT scan: This is done on a stable patient with oral and intravenous contrast. CT scan for liver injury has more than 90% of sensitivity and specificity (**Figure 1**). Useful for diagnosis of liver injury and follow-up of liver trauma, for any hemorrhage, bile accumulation or sepsis.

X-ray: X-ray chest may show fractured ribs at the site of the liver from 7th to 9th rib but is not specific and not done to look for liver injury.

DPL Diagnostic peritoneal lavage: This is an invasive procedure done on patients with trauma when there is intraperitoneal bleeding. It is useful and produces good results when performed by expert, but nowadays, it is replaced by ultrasound scan.

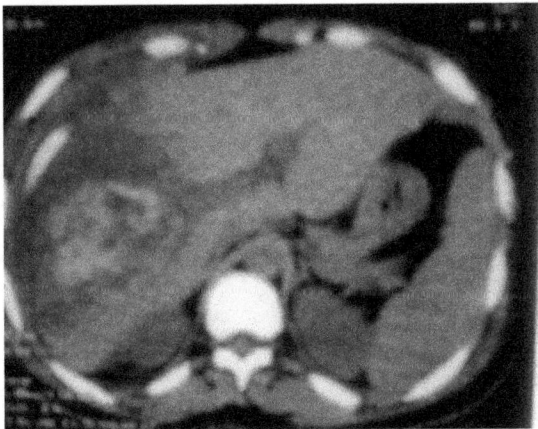

Figure 1. CT scan for a patient with massive liver trauma.

2.2. Treatment of liver trauma

Table 1 shows the number and types of liver trauma treated using different treatments in a busy general hospital.

Eighty percent of adults with liver trauma were treated conservatively, and 97% of those were children who were treated conservatively.

Healing of liver trauma: The liver has good capacity of healing once it is traumatized.

Mild liver trauma: Less than 25% of lobe damage takes 3 months to heal.

Moderate liver trauma: Between 25 and 50% takes 6 months to heal.

Severe injury: Liver injury, which encompasses more than 50% of lobe injured, takes 9 months to heal or more.

Patients with liver trauma blunt or penetrating, mild or severe once diagnosed or suspected should undergo resuscitation as usual traumatized patients, which include caring of respiration, putting good venous access for the fluids, treating emergency killing conditions like tension pneumothorax, fixing urinary catheter to know the output. After patient resuscitation, the grading of liver trauma is evaluated clinically and by imaging and the mode of treatment is planned which will include either [8–10].

1. Non-operative treatment.

2. Operative treatment.

3. Interventional radiology treatment of liver trauma.

Mode	Number of patients	Lobe	Grade	Procedure	Outcome
RTA	94	Left lobe and right lobe	Range from grade I to VI	1. Conservative treatment: 35 cases 2. Diagnostic laparoscopy: 12 suturing and insertion of drain 3. Laparotomy: 47 3-A. Repair of liver wounds: 30 3-B. Packing: 14 perihepatic packing 3-C. Resection: Three had segmental liver resection	13 died
Bullet	124	Left lobe Right lobe	Grade I and II had few patients, and most were grade III, IV	All underwent laparotomy, debridement, repair, omental packing, eight patients had perihepatic packing	18 died
Stab	13	Left lobe and right lobe	I and II	Conservative management	Nil

Table 1. Different types of hepatic trauma patients who were treated at Zliten teaching hospital.

2.2.1. Conservative treatment of liver trauma

Blunt liver trauma can be mild, moderate or severe. Mild and moderate liver trauma can be managed conservatively without surgery [3, 11, 15, 18].

Conservative treatment includes the following:

1. Full assessment of patients.
2. Full assessment of the grade of liver injury by ultrasound and CT scan.
3. Correction of blood loss by giving blood.
4. Daily monitoring of patient.
5. Discharge of patient once he is fully stable and active.
6. Post-discharge follow-up by clinical assessment and imaging.

2.2.2. Non-operative treatment of liver injury

Non operative management was firstly conducted in children than started in adult, it is not indicated in elderly patients, choosing of the patients for non-operative management (NOM) depends on clinical condition of the patients and associated injury, less on grade of the liver of injury [2, 16].

2.2.3. Advantages of NOM

1. Less hospital stay.
2. Avoidance of unnecessary laparotomy.

An unstable patient can be defined as follows:

1. Systolic blood pressure less than 90 mmhg.
2. Pulse rate more than 120 beats per minute.
3. Altered consciousness level.
4. Altered breathing.
5. Cold clammy skin.

About 80% of blunt liver trauma can be treated conservatively, provided the patient is haemo dynamically stable. It can be utilized even in grade IV.

Non-operative treatment can be performed for the following reasons:

1. Patients who are haemodynamically stable with no signs of peritonism.
2. Operative management should be available when needed.

3. Imaging facilities should be available to follow the treatments, which can lead to 100% success rate.

Liver trauma at Zliten University Hospital over a period of 9 years from 2009 to 2017 — Patients: 231, deaths: 31, patients who underwent conservative treatment: 48 (**Table 1**).

Most of our patients with liver trauma during war, the time where the weapon is scattered in many regions of the country; none of our patients with hepatic trauma having had gun shot wounds left for conservative treatment, and all patients underwent surgery. This number affected our conservative management in hepatic trauma. Our rate of conservative treatment for patients with hepatic trauma was approximately 50%.

2.2.4. Complications of NOM

Complications of NOM can be diagnosed by clinical examination including blood tests, ultrasound scan and CT scan. Complications may reach up to 7% in grade III and V.

1. Bile collection may reach up to 20% — biliary peritonitis. Haemobilia: Bile leak is treated with endoscopic retrograde cholangiopancreatography most of our patients with liver trauma were during war. If fluid collection is significant, it can be drained percutaneously, laparoscopically or open surgery. **Figure 2** shows the CT of a child with hepatic trauma managed conservatively with the development of bilioma). **Figure 3** shows bilioma collection that was treated by laparotomy.

   Nagano-classified bile leak:

   Type A: Minor bile leak, small radicle from the liver surface — resolved spontaneously.

   Type B: Bile leak from a major duct on the liver surface not tied.

   Type C: Injury of duct branch from the main duct at the hilum.

   Type D: Main bile duct transected.

2. Infection and abscess formation may reach 7% and can be treated conservatively when clinical manifestation is significant.

3. Liver necrosis can be diagnosed clinically with raised liver enzymes, coagulation abnormalities or bile leak.

4. Bleeding: Hepatic artery pseudo-aneurysm accounts to about 1–2% and can be either extrahepatic or intrahepatic — more cases of extrahepatic nature. Liver compartment syndrome due to compression of the liver by huge subcapsular haematoma may result in liver failure.

2.2.5. Surgical treatment of liver injury

1. Surgery is indicated in a patient who is unstable.

2. Surgical treatment is indicated if the patient was on conservative treatment and showed signs of deterioration, [8, 27–29].

Surgical procedures (**Figure 4** shows different repair of liver trauma).

1. Simple suturing of liver tear.

2. Debridment of unhealthy liver tissue and suturing.

3. Resection of severely damaged segment.

4. Liver lobectomy or hepatectomy for severely damaged lobe.

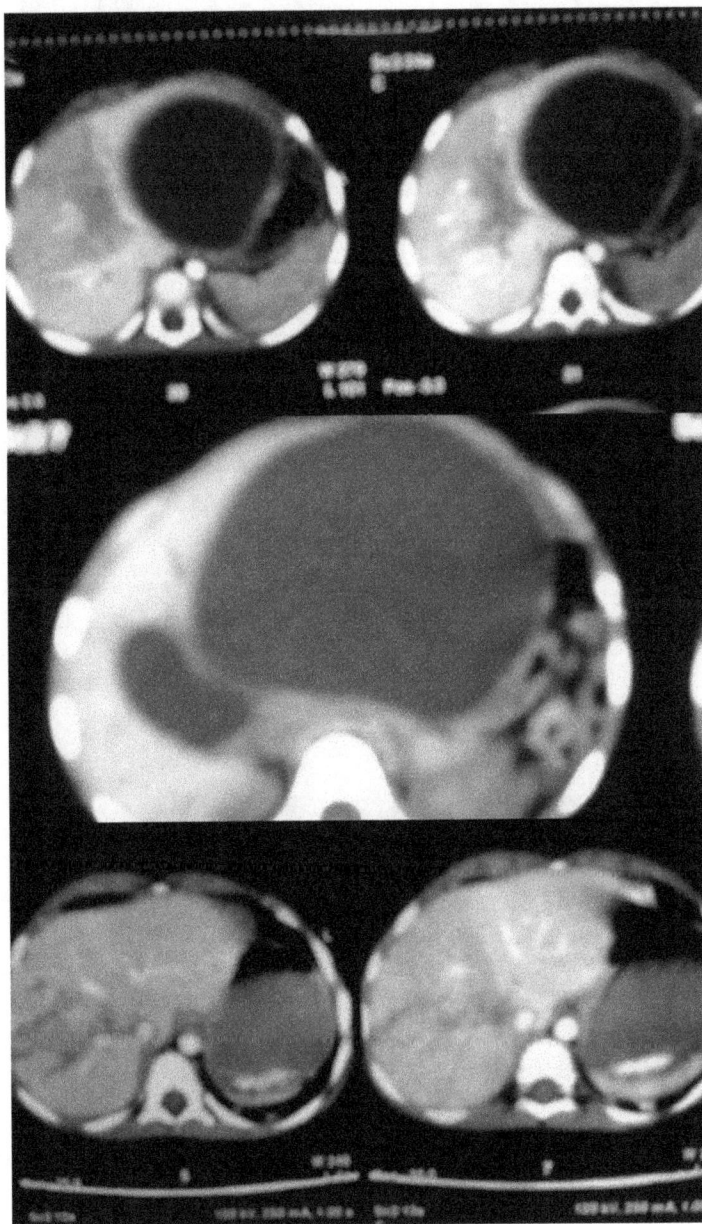

Figure 2. CT abdomen of a child who had liver trauma and was treated conservatively developed bile collection as a complication of hepatic trauma management.

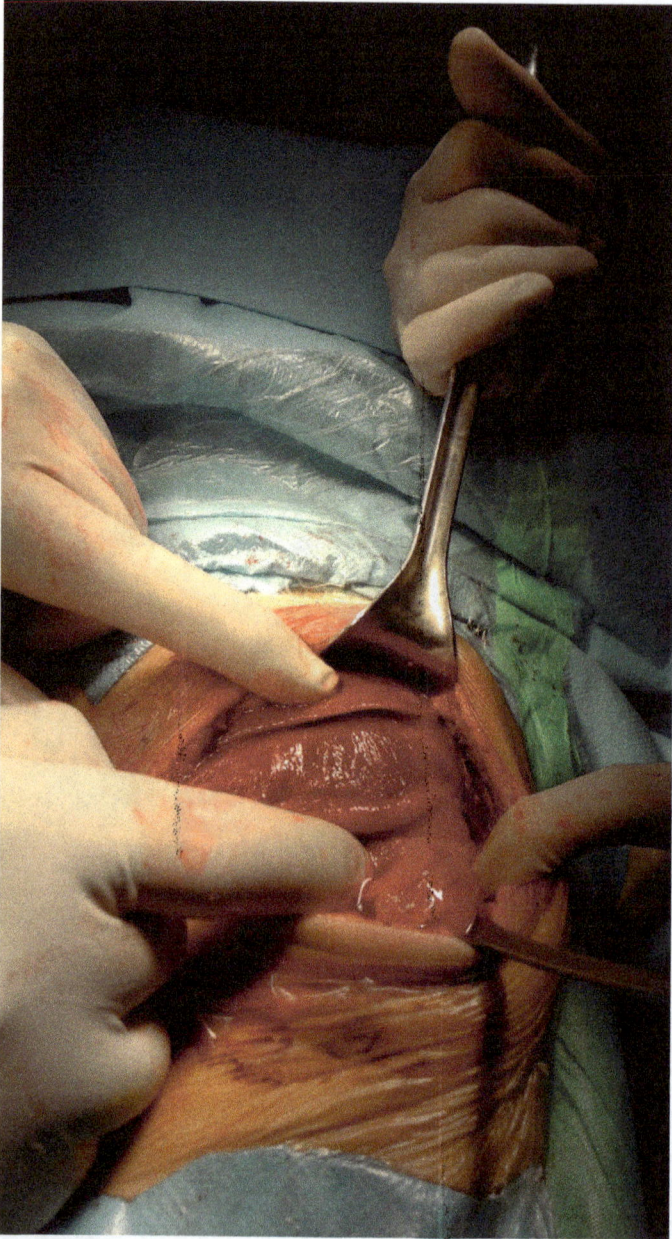

Figure 3. Child who had liver trauma managed conservatively and complicated by bile leak, presented with encysted bilioma. The child underwent laparotomy.[13].

5. Perihepatic packing for uncontrolled bleeding in unstable patients.

6. Arterial embolization which can be performed as the first option in patients who are planned for non-operative treatment or for those patient who developed bleeding after surgery [17].

Damage control in liver trauma:

Damage control is of three phases:

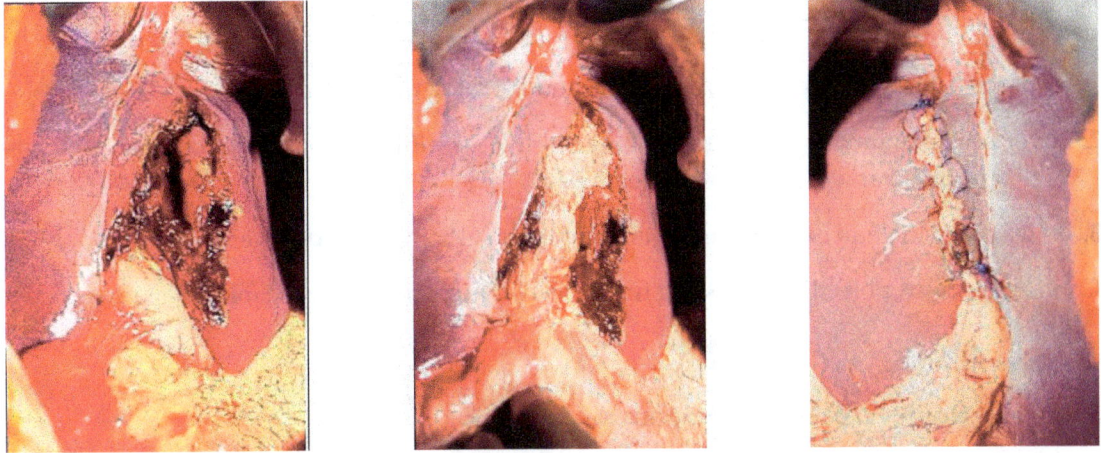

Figure 4. Liver trauma repaired and the wound packed with omentum (taken with permission from Prof. Ronald M. Stewart).

Phase I: Control of bleeding, closure of the abdomen.

Phase II: Intensive care unit resuscitation and overcome on acidosis, hypothermia, hyper-coagulability.

Phase III: Re-exploration of the abdomen.

In 1983, Stone et al. proposed damage control for trauma patient [6, 14, 22–24]. Once patient had severe liver trauma, where the condition of the patient is deteriorating during surgery and the bleeding is continuous from the damaged liver, either the damage at the posterior aspect or whole of the liver, damage control is utilized in the form of packing the liver with abdominal gauze pack which are wrapped around the liver [4–6]. This technique is useful in the management of controlling the bleeding that occurs during surgery and liver resection. Packing is also useful to avoid the three killers of the patient during surgery which includes acidosis, hypercoagulability and hypothermia, which can cause cardiac arrest. To avoid the occurrence of these bad incidents, we should change to damage control. Usually six packs are placed around the liver to stop the bleeding. The abdomen left either open or closed depending on the patient's condition with the use of Bogota bag. Packing the liver with gauze packs can be complicated when patients need to go through full resuscitation in the ICU. For the correction of the three killers including acidosis, hyperthermia, hyper-coagulability, usually it needs time for our patients 48–72 h to control sepsis with the use of antibiotics.

Complication of perihepatic packing:

The complication of perihepatic packing includes the following:

1. Compartment syndrome.

2. Respiratory embarrassment due to compression on the right dome of the diaphragm.

3. Abdominal sepsis if the packs were left longer than 3 days.

Other surgical procedure for liver trauma include

1. Laparoscopic assessment of liver trauma and suturing of liver tear [12].

2. Liver transplantation for severely damaged liver is difficult to perform because of availability of the liver and the experienced team.

3. Liver exclusion and extracorporeal circulation is seldom done for severe liver trauma.

Controlling of liver bleeding: Bleeding from the liver is controlled by the following procedures

1. Simple suturing.

2. Hepatorrhaphy and control of the arterial bleeding.

3. Use of omental pack and mattress sutures.

4. Selective hepatic artery ligation may control the bleeding.

5. Non-anatomical resection, anatomical resection, venovenous shunt, atriocaval shunts.

Mortality of blunt trauma is 27% and of penetrating trauma is 11%.

Overall, mortality of liver trauma is 10%, Grade III and IV mortality is 10% and V and VI are 75%.

There are many haemostatic materials used for liver trauma are very helpful for controlling the bleeding, which includes the following:

1. Surgical.

2. Spongostan.

3. Tacoceil.

4. Fibrin glue.

Author details

Ali Ibrahim Yahya

Address all correspondence to: aliyahyaz60@hotmail.com

Teaching Hospital, Zliten, Libya

References

[1] Koyama T, Skattum J, Engelsen P, Eken T, Gaarder C, Naess PA. Surgical intervention for paediatric liver injuries is almost history–A 12-year cohort from a major Scandinavian trauma centre. Scandinavian Journal of Trauma, Resuscitation and Emergency Medicine. 2016;**24**:139

[2] Li M, Yu WK, Wang XB, Ji W, Li JS. Non-operative management of isolated liver trauma. Hepatobiliary & Pancreatic Diseases International. 2014 Oct;13(5):545-550

[3] Letoublon C, Amariutei A, Taton N, Lacaze L, Abba J, Risse O, Arvieux C. Management of blunt hepatic trauma. Journal of Visceral Surgery. 2016 Aug;153(4 Suppl):33-43. DOI: 10.1016/j.jviscsurg.2016.07.005

[4] Ng N, McLean SF, Ghaleb MR, Tyroch A. Hepatic "BOLSA" a novel method of perihepatic wrapping for hepatic hemorrhage "BOLSA". International Journal of Surgery Case Reports. 2015;13:99-102. DOI: 10.1016/j.ijscr.2015.06.007

[5] Stassen NA, Bhullar I, Cheng JD, Crandall M, Friese R, Guillamondegui O, Jawa R, Maung A, Rohs TJ Jr, Sangosanya A, Schuster K, Seamon M, Tchorz KM, Zarzuar BL, Kerwin A. Nonoperative management of blunt hepatic injury: An Eastern Association for the Surgery of Trauma practice management guideline. Journal of Trauma and Acute Care Surgery;73(5)

[6] Lin BC, Fang JF, Chen RJ, Wong YC, Hsu YP. Surgical management and outcome of blunt major liver injuries: Experience of damage controllaparotomy with perihepatic packing in one trauma centre. Injury. 2014 Jan;45(1):122-127. DOI: 10.1016/j.injury.2013.08.022

[7] Schnüriger B, Inderbitzin D, Schafer M, Kickuth R, Exadaktylos A, Candinas D. Concomitant injuries are an important determinant of outcome of high-grade blunt hepatic trauma. The British Journal of Surgery. 2009 Jan;96(1):104-110. DOI: 10.1002/bjs.6439

[8] Girgin S, Gedik E, Taçyildiz IH. Evaluation of surgical methods in patients with blunt liver trauma. Ulusal Travma ve Acil Cerrahi Dergisi. 2006 Jan;12(1):35-42

[9] Gür S, Orsel A, Atahan K, Hökmez A, Tarcan E. Surgical treatment of liver trauma (analysis of 244 patients). Hepato-Gastroenterology. 2003 Nov-Dec;50(54):2109-2111

[10] Terrinoni V, Catroppo JF, Caramanico L, Cosimati A, Cosimati P, Bellini N, Abate O, Rengo M. The diagnostic-therapeutic picture in liver injuries: A review of the literature and clinical cases. Il Giornale di Chirurgia. 1995 Jan-Feb;16(1-2):48-54

[11] Buci S, Torba M, Gjata A, Kajo I, Bushi G, Kagjini K. The rate of success of the conservative management of liver trauma in a developing country. World Journal of Emergency Surgery. 2017;12:24

[12] Lim KH, Chung BS, Kim JY, Kim SS. Laparoscopic surgery in abdominal trauma: A single center review of a 7-year experience. World Journal of Emergency Surgery. 2015;10:16

[13] Giss SR, Dobrilovic N, Brown RL, Garcia VF. Complications of nonoperative management of pediatric blunt hepatic injury: Diagnosis, management, and outcomes. The Journal of Trauma. 2006 Aug;61(2)

[14] Kobayashi T, Kubota M, Arai Y, Ohyama T, Yokota N, Miura K, Ishikawa H, Soma D, Takizawa K, Sakata J, Nagahashi M, Kameyama H, Wakai T. Staged laparotomies based on the damage control principle to treat hemodynamically unstable grade IV blunt hepatic injury in an eight-year-old girl. Surgical Case Reports. 2016 Dec;2:134

[15] Moreno P, Von Allmen M, Haltmeier T, Candinas D, Schnüriger B. Long-term follow-up after non-operative management of blunt splenic and liver injuries: A questionnaire-based survey. World Journal of Surgery. 2017 Nov 14. DOI: 10.1007/s00268-017-4336-5

[16] Perumean JC, Martinez M, Neal R, Lee J, Olajire-Aro T, Imran JB, Williams BH, Phelan HA. Low-grade blunt hepatic injury and benefits of intensive care unit monitoring. American Journal of Surgery. 2017 Dec;**214**(6):1188-1192. DOI: 10.1016/j.amjsurg.2017.09.003

[17] Melloul E, Denys A, Demartines N. Management of severe blunt hepatic injury in the era of computed tomography and transarterial embolization: A systematic review and critical appraisal of the literature. Journal of Trauma and Acute Care Surgery. 2015 Sep;**79**(3):468-474. DOI: 10.1097/TA.0000000000000724

[18] Cirocchi R, Trastulli S, Pressi E, Farinella E, Avenia S, Morales Uribe CH, Botero AM, Barrera LM. Non-operative management versus operative management in high-grade blunt hepatic injury. Cochrane Database of Systematic Reviews. 2015 Aug 24;**8**:CD010989. DOI: 10.1002/14651858.CD010989

[19] Stengel D, Rademacher G, Ekkernkamp A, Güthoff C, Mutze S. Emergency ultrasound-based algorithms for diagnosing blunt abdominal trauma. Cochrane Database of Systematic Reviews. 2015 Sep 14;**9**:CD004446. DOI: 10.1002/14651858.CD004446.pub4

[20] Quinn AC, Sinert R. What is the utility of the Focused Assessment with Sonography in Trauma (FAST) exam in penetrating torso trauma? Injury. DOI: injury.2010.07.249

[21] Kaptanoglu L, Kurt N, Sikar HE. Current approach to liver traumas. International Journal of Surgery. 2017 Mar;**39**:255-259. DOI: 10.1016/j.ijsu.2017.02.015

[22] Recordare A, Bruno GT, Callegari P, Guarise A, Bassi N. Bleeding control by radiofre-quency in penetrating trauma of the liver. G Chir. 2011 Apr;**32**(4):203-5.25

[23] Krige JE, Bornman PC, Terblanche J. Therapeutic perihepatic packing in complex liver trauma. The British Journal of Surgery. 1992 Jan;**79**(1):43-46

[24] Reed RL 2nd, Merrell RC, Meyers WC, Fischer RP. Continuing evolution in the approach to severe liver trauma. Annals of Surgery. 1992 Nov;**216**(5):524-538

[25] van As Alastair AB, Milla JW. Management of paediatric liver trauma. Pediatric Surgery International. April 2017;**33**(4):445-453

[26] Kalil M, Amaral IM. Epidemiological evaluation of hepatic trauma victims undergoing surgery. Revista do Colégio Brasileiro de Cirurgiões. 2016 Feb;**43**(1):22-27

[27] Safi F, Weiner S, Poch B, Schwarz A, Beger HG. Surgical management of liver rupture. Der Chirurg. 1999 Mar;**70**(3):253-258

[28] John TG, Greig JD, Johnstone AJ, Garden OJ. Liver trauma: A 10-year experience. The British Journal of Surgery. 1992 Dec;**79**(12):1352-1356

[29] Vatanaprasan T. Operative Treatment of hepatic trauma in Vachira Phuket hospital. Journal of the Medical Association of Thailand. 2005 Mar;**88**(3):318-328

8

Acute Kidney Injury in Cirrhosis

Marco Antonio López Hernández

Abstract

Acute kidney injury is a very relevant feature in the liver cirrhosis. Acute renal failure is due to prerenal factors, intrinsic factors of the kidney, or postrenal. Prerenal damage is the result of renal hypoperfusion without damage to the glomeruli or renal tubules. Without treatment, prerenal acute renal failure can progress to acute tubular necrosis, a type of intrinsic renal damage. Patients with cirrhosis are prone to developing acute kidney injury. The acute decrease of the kidney function contributes to the mortality of patients with cirrhosis. The potential triggers of acute kidney injury should be recognized and removed; this includes the discontinuation of diuretics and nephrotoxic drugs, the treatment of infections and gastrointestinal bleeding, and plasma expansion in case of hypovolemia. The new International Club of Ascites-Acute Kidney Injury in cirrhosis criteria provide a simple and relevant staging system for acute kidney injury in patients with liver cirrhosis based on relative increases in serum creatinine. Vasopressors such as terlipressin and norepinephrine in combination with intravenous albumin represent the first-line therapy for hepatorenal syndrome.

Keywords: acute kidney injury, hepatorenal syndrome, cirrhosis

1. Introduction

The association of acute kidney injury (AKI) in patients with liver cirrhosis has been established in the context of the hepatorenal syndrome, but there are several etiologies besides this cause.

Acute renal failure is a therapeutic challenge in patients with liver cirrhosis. This may be related to abnormal hemodynamics with systemic arterial vasodilatation and the splanchnic bed, in addition to the vasoconstriction of extrahepatic vessels, characteristic of advanced liver cirrhosis [1]. Acute renal failure frequently occurs in the advanced stages of liver cirrhosis and entails a bad prognosis [2, 3].

Acute renal failure is due to prerenal factors, intrinsic factors of the kidney, or postrenal. Prerenal damage is the result of renal hypoperfusion without damage to the glomeruli or renal tubules. Without treatment, prerenal acute renal failure can progress to acute tubular necrosis (ATN), a type of intrinsic renal damage.

The prevalence of acute renal failure in cirrhosis has been reported from 14 to 50% in patients with cirrhosis. Its prevalence is approximately 50% in patients with cirrhosis and ascites and 20% of patients with advanced stage cirrhosis who are hospitalized [4, 5].

The definition of acute kidney injury is a reduction in the glomerular filtration rate (GFR) over a short time of period, and this is a common and severe complication in the patients with liver cirrhosis. Acute kidney failure can be triggered by a precipitating event, for example, overdose of diuretics, gastrointestinal bleeding, large-volume paracentesis without albumin replacement, bacterial infections, and so on [6]. The prevalence of acute kidney injury is approximately 20–50% among hospitalized patients with cirrhosis [6–9] and the renal failure development is more common in patients with cirrhosis compared to individuals without liver disease [10]. The presence of acute kidney failure is associated with poor prognosis in these patients and represents an important predictor for short-term mortality [11].

The criteria for acute renal failure in cirrhosis were initially proposed in 1996 [12] and redefined in subsequent years [13]. Traditionally, renal failure in cirrhosis was defined as a 50% increase in serum creatinine, with an increase greater than 1.5 mg/dL (133 μm/L) of it. The cutoff value of serum creatinine to define acute renal failure in patients with decompensated cirrhosis has changed [14, 15]. Several nephrology academic societies have proposed the use of the concept of acute renal injury to represent acute changes in kidney function. The diagnostic criteria constitute a combination of changes in the glomerular filtration rate as well as a reduction in urine output. In the past decade, the definition of acute kidney injury evolved to the classifications and diagnostic criteria known as RIFLE [16], AKIN [17], and KDIGO [18].

In 2010, the International Ascites Club (IAC) and the Acute Dialysis Quality Initiative (ADQI) decided to use the nomenclature of the Acute Kidney Injury (AKI).

In 2015, the International Ascites Club established a new definition and staging of acute renal failure for patients with liver cirrhosis [19].

2. Physiopathology of renal failure in cirrhosis

Patients with liver cirrhosis develop portal hypertension, which results in the vasodilatation of the splanchnic vascular bed, resulting in blood accumulation due to resistance in the portal venous flow. This is due to an increase in the fixed resistance of liver fibrosis, and dynamics in the splanchnic arteries is last due to

a. vasodilators such as nitric oxide, carbon monoxide, and endogenous cannabinoids [20, 21];

b. vasodilation by pro-inflammatory cytokines such as tumor necrosis factor and interleukin 6, derived from bacterial translocation of the intestine [22].

The accumulation of blood in the splanchnic bed leads to a reduction in the effective circulating volume, which leads to a compensatory increase in cardiac output through the activation of the sympathetic nervous system by the carotid baroreceptors in order to maintain adequate renal perfusion [23].

In advanced stages of cirrhosis, systemic vascular resistance is significantly reduced, and the additional increase in cardiac output cannot compensate. Thus, it is evident that cardiac output decreases as cirrhosis progresses. In advanced stages of cirrhosis, cardiac output is maintained through the activation of vasoconstrictor systems, including the sympathetic nervous system and the renin-angiotensin system, and by a non-osmotic hypersecretion of arginine-vasopressin.

These compensatory mechanisms can help to maintain effective arterial volume and of this way a relatively normal blood pressure, but this has important effects on kidney function, primarily a retention of water and sodium, which can eventually lead to the formation of ascites and edema, and renal failure conditioned by renal vasoconstriction and hypoperfusion [24, 25].

There are four factors involved in the pathogenesis of hepatorenal syndrome. These are the following:

1. Activation of the renin-angiotensin-aldosterone system and the sympathetic nervous system which causes renal vasoconstriction and a shift in the renal autoregulatory curve, which results in a renal blood flow more sensitive to changes in the arterial pressure.

2. Splanchnic vasodilatation, which causes a fall in the effective arterial blood volume and this way a decrease of the mean arterial pressure.

3. Increased synthesis of vasoactive mediators which affect renal blood flow or glomerular microcirculatory hemodynamics, such as leukotrienes, thromboxane A2, isoprostanes, and endothelin-1.

4. Impairment of cardiac function due to the development of cirrhotic cardiomyopathy, which leads to a relative impairment of the compensatory increase in cardiac output secondary to vasodilatation.

Hemodynamic disorders can have widespread impact on the body according to the severity of the cirrhosis [26]. The hemodynamic changes in cirrhosis include portal hypertension and hyperdynamic circulation which are the main cause of morbidity and mortality in patients with cirrhosis. The effective arterial blood volume and the circulating levels of RAS components and antidiuretic hormone remain normal at early stages of the disease, even with a reduced systemic vascular resistance. The elevated cardiac output and low systemic vascular resistance are characteristics of the portal hypertension and hyperdynamic circulation in cirrhosis. Arterial vasodilation in the splanchnic circulation and the resulting decrease in systemic vascular resistance are associated with portal hypertension in cirrhosis. Compensatory mechanisms following the reduction of systemic vascular resistance lead to hyperdynamic circulation. Nevertheless, hyperdynamic circulation is insufficient to correct the effective arterial hypovolemia when the disease progresses and arterial vasodilation increases, resulting in arterial hypotension and consequent activation of the circulating renin-angiotensin-aldosterone system and the sympathetic nervous system and secretion of antidiuretic hormone [27].

In the early stages of disease, the circulating RAS is not activated at early stages of the disease. The patients at the advanced stages of cirrhosis presented an activation of peripheral and splanchnic renin-aldosterone system, and a metabolic deviation toward the RAS vasodilator axis in the splanchnic circulation (**Figure 1**).

2.1. Causes of acute kidney injury in cirrhosis

The acute kidney injury has prerenal, intrarenal, or postrenal causes (**Figure 2**). The most common causes of acute kidney injury between patients with cirrhosis are the prerenal etiologies, followed by acute tubular necrosis, and the postrenal etiology is extremely rare. The prerenal and acute tubular necrosis are the etiology of 80% of cases (49% prerenal and 35% acute tubular

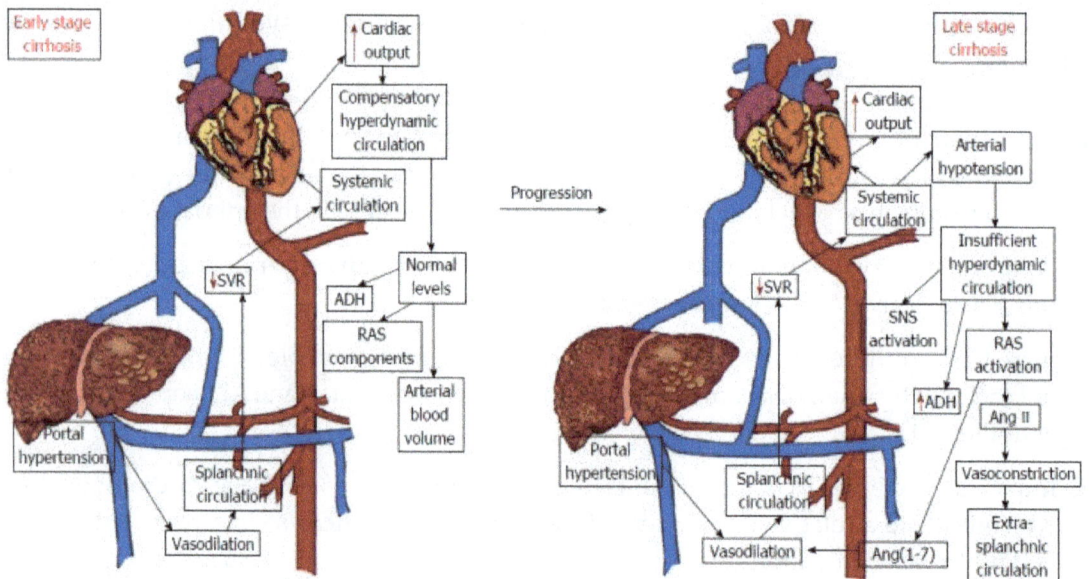

Figure 1. Hemodynamic alterations in the early and advanced stages of cirrhosis. In the early stages of cirrhosis, there is an increased cardiac output and a diminished systemic vascular resistance without changes in the circulating levels of the renin-angiotensin system components and antidiuretic hormone. In later phases of the cirrhosis, the components of the renin-angiotensin-aldosterone system are elevated, with activation of the sympathetic nervous system and secretion of the antidiuretic hormone, like a response to persistent arterial hypotension. Ang II: angiotensin II; Ang-(1–7): angiotensin (1–7); SNS: sympathetic nervous system; SVR: systemic vascular resistance.

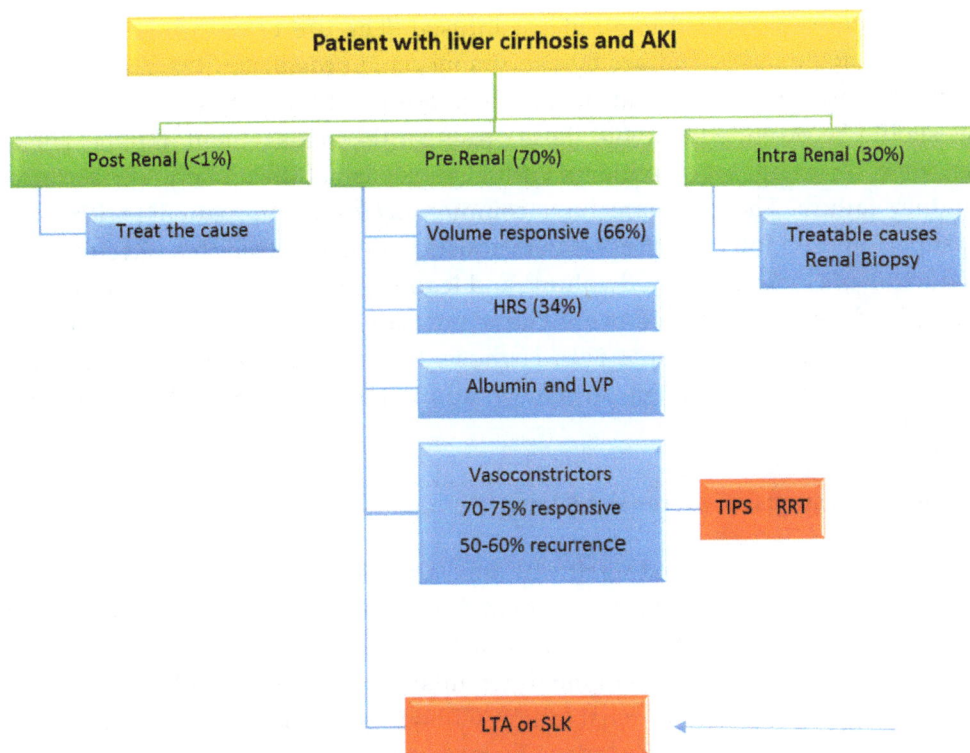

Figure 2. Management approach and algorithm for acute kidney injury in patients with cirrhosis. AKI, acute kidney injury; ESLD, end-stage liver disease; HRS, hepatorenal syndrome; LVP, large-volume paracentesis; RRT, renal replacement therapy; LTA, liver transplant alone; SLK, simultaneous liver kidney; TIPS, transjugular intrahepatic portosystemic shunt; USG, ultrasonogram.

necrosis). Postrenal injury accounted for only 0.2%. In a prospective study, among patients with cirrhosis listed for liver transplantation who had acute kidney injury, prerenal injury was the most common cause in 76% followed by intrarenal etiology in 33%, while postrenal etiology did not occur in any patient [66, 67].

3. Prerenal injury

3.1. Volume responsive prerenal AKI

The hemodynamic state in cirrhosis with vascular dilatation and reduced vascular resistance in cirrhosis is quite similar to hemodynamic state in sepsis, especially spontaneous bacterial peritonitis. Prerenal injury occurs commonly due to gastrointestinal bleeding, infections, use of diuretics, diarrhea often related to lactulose use for hepatic encephalopathy, and from large-volume paracentesis without albumin infusion. Large-volume paracentesis may be associated with intravascular volume depletion and acute kidney failure. This condition occurs in up to 70% of patients undergoing paracentesis when more than 5 L are removed and albumin is not infused. The use of any drugs like NSAIDs can precipitate acute kidney failure by decreasing renal prostaglandins and accentuating the intrarenal vasoconstriction and further decrease renal blood flow. The advice to the patients should be provided to avoid these drugs for the management of pain. The use of intravenous contrast agents in patients with cirrhosis is another potential risk factor for acute kidney failure. The infections have common occurrence in patients with cirrhosis. Hence, superimposed infections/sepsis in cirrhosis patients worsen this physiology, causing a reduction of circulating blood volume and leading to the development of AKI. Before the widespread use of antibiotic prophylaxis for acute gastrointestinal bleeding in cirrhosis, more than 20% of patients with cirrhosis hospitalized for acute gastrointestinal bleeding had a bacterial infection present on admission, with up to 50% developing an infection while hospitalized.

3.2. Volume nonresponsive prerenal AKI: hepatorenal syndrome

The volume expansion is the first treatment after acute kidney failure is diagnosed, using crystalloids or intravenous albumin and discontinuation of precipitating medications. If renal function does not normalize or improve with this intervention, it is important to consider hepatorenal syndrome (HRS) in the differential diagnosis to consider as the cause for AKI. HRS is a functional form of renal failure without any major structural or histological changes in the kidneys that is characterized by intense renal vasoconstriction. It is important to differentiate it from another intrarenal cause, because management and prognosis differ. In the absence of renal biopsy, the diagnosis of HRS remains difficult and is essentially a diagnosis of exclusion. In patients with cirrhosis, HRS develops in about 18% at 1 year and 39% at 5 years.

Approximately, 66% of all HRS cases are type 2, or HRS-AKI which are rapidly occurring with an increase in serum creatinine to over 2.5 mg/dL over 1 or 2 weeks. Type 1 HRS has high mortality with a median survival of around 50% at 2 weeks and is usually precipitated by infections. The type 2 HRS has a better outcome with a median survival of about 6 months and a slower course in the setting of refractory ascites, with slowly increasing serum creatinine to over 1.5 mg/dL. The definition of type I HRS has been recently revised and changed the value of 2.5 mg/dL serum creatinine for diagnosis, thus avoid delaying the initiation of therapy.

3.3. Volume nonresponsive intrinsic AKI: acute tubular necrosis

The most common cause for intrarenal AKI in cirrhosis is ATN. This occurs commonly either as a complication of sepsis or due to unrecognized and untreated prerenal injury. The main cause of ATN has been attributed to sepsis, followed by hypovolemia and rarely nephrotoxic drugs.

Other less common causes of intrarenal injury include tubular damage due to bile cast nephropathy from high-conjugated bilirubin excreted through the glomeruli, membranoproliferative glomerulonephritis with or without cryoglobulinemia associated with hepatitis C, and acute interstitial nephritis due to medications, such as antibiotics, NSAIDS, and proton pump inhibitors.

4. Postrenal injury

As stated earlier, postrenal injury is a rare cause of AKI in cirrhosis [66, 68]. This etiology can easily be excluded using renal ultrasound or CT scan.

4.1. Evaluation of the renal function

The glomerular filtration rate (GFR) is the universally used index to quantify kidney function. The principle of GFR determination is to determine the body clearance of a substance with the supposed exclusive renal clearance. The substance used for determinate GFR must be freely filtered and neither reabsorbed or secreted along the renal tubule. Also, no extrarenal excretion of the substance occurs, and it cannot be stored or be bound to plasma proteins: then it can be assumed that the plasmatic clearance is only due to renal clearance. Thus, the GFR can be inferred from the plasma disappearance of the substance. It is considered that the renal clearance of a marker occurs only through glomerular filtration [28].

Calculation of the eGFR requires normalization to BSA. Studies that tested the performance of this method showed a clear trend to overestimate mGFR by 4–80%. A normalization based on the assumption that the GFR is positively correlated with the basal metabolism rate of individuals which is proportional to their stature on arbitrarily fixed body surface area (BSA) set to 1.73 m^2 is commonly done [29]. This normalization has been questioned [30] and standardization on other criteria has been proposed [31]. The formula most commonly used to determine the BSA is the Dubois formula, and the adjustment on the body surface remains widely used [32].

Historically, the Cockcroft and Gault formula was the most popular before the MDRD formula was published in the early 2000s. This formula is not adjusted to the patient BSA, and the adjustment has, theoretically, to be done afterwards (even if the relevance of this adjustment remains to be assessed in cirrhotic patients). The relationship between GFR level and overestimation could be explained by the secretion of creatinine by the tubule in patients with CKD. However, the importance of this overestimation does not seem to be related to the severity of cirrhosis.

Creatinine clearance is a simple method to estimate GFR, based on the assumption that creatinine has the characteristics of a perfect renal marker. It requests the accurate recollection of urine from a 24-h period. It has several limitations: mainly, the possible inadequate urine collection by the patients, the occurrence of tubular secretion of creatinine, which leads to overestimation of the GFR, and that is on a longer or a shorter than 24-h time period.

4.2. Definition of acute kidney injury in cirrhosis

The definition of acute kidney injury in cirrhosis consists in an acute increase in serum creatinine of >0.3 mg/dL in a time lapse of 48 h or by <50% from a stable baseline serum creatinine, in the last 3 months (presumed to have developed within the past 7 days when no prior readings are available) [19, 33]. In addition, the use of urine output as part of the diagnostic criteria was eliminated, since many patients with cirrhosis and ascites maintain a preserved renal function despite being oliguric due to sodium and water retention. The main modifications over the previous, rather stringent, criteria that were based on absolute serum creatinine level, were abandoning the threshold of serum creatinine >1.5 mg/dL to diagnose acute kidney injury, because milder degrees of renal failure in cirrhotic patients had often remained underdiagnosed [34, 35].

Similar to the ICA-AKI criteria, most of these studies diagnosed AKI solely on serum creatinine. In 2013, a modified, AKIN-derived score for cirrhosis was developed, by division of AKI stage 1 into two groups depending on whether or not serum creatinine surpassed the threshold of 1.5 mg/dL and by merging AKI stages 2 and 3 into stage "C" [40]; this reclassification did not gain wide acceptance. Several clinical studies have evaluated the prognostic value of the AKIN/KDIGO criteria that constitute the basis for the International Club of Ascites (ICA)-AKI criteria in patients with cirrhosis [37–39]. The acute kidney injury can be classified into three stages according to severity. Stage 1 AKI is defined by rather small changes in serum creatinine, while stages 2 and 3 AKI are defined by a twofold and threefold increase in serum creatinine, respectively (**Table 1**) [36]. Since their publication in 2015, the newer and cirrhosis-specific ICA criteria have been assessed within one retrospective study in hospitalized patients with cirrhosis [41]. Within this study, approximately 40% of patients experienced AKI during their hospitalization with the majority of cases having been diagnosed at stage 1. Also, in patients with AKI stage 1 and a serum creatinine of <1.5 mg/dL, already a 3.5-fold increase in 30-day mortality as compared to patients without AKI was reported [41], again underlining the prognostic importance of even small increases in serum creatinine levels.

4.3. Hepatorenal syndrome type of acute kidney injury or type 1 hepatorenal syndrome

Hepatorenal syndrome (HRS) is defined as the occurrence of renal failure in a patient with advanced liver disease in the absence of an identifiable cause of renal failure [12].

The hepatorenal syndrome type I requires the fulfillment of several specific diagnostic criteria that are summarized in **Table 2**. This Acute Kidney Injury (HRS-AKI) is defined as >stage 2 ICA-AKI that is diagnosed after other causes of renal failure have been ruled out [35].

Acute kidney injury stages according to the International Club of Ascites criteria	
Stage 2	Increase in serum creatinine >0.3 mg/dl or Increase in serum creatinine by>50–100% from baseline
Stage 2	Increase in serum creatinine by100–200% from baseline
Stage 3	Increase in serum creatinine by 200% from baseline or Increase in serum creatinine to 4 mg/dL with an acute increase by 0.3 mg/dL or Need for renal replacement therapy

Table 1. Criteria of AKI of the International Club of Ascites [36].

Diagnostic criteria of hepatorenal syndrome
Presence of cirrhosis and ascites
No improvement in serum creatinine after 2 consecutive days of withdrawal of diuretics and plasma volume expansion with albumin (1 g per kg of body weight, maximum 100 g/day)
Absence of shock
Exclusion of recurrent or recent use of nephrotoxic agents (e.g.NSAIDs, aminoglycosides, contrast media)
Exclusion of parenchymal kidney disease: • **absence of proteinuria (>500 mg/day)** • **absence of microhematuria (>50 RBCs per high-power field)** • **normal renal ultrasonography**

Table 2. Diagnostic criteria for hepatorenal syndrome [12].

The Guidelines of the European Association for the Study of Liver Diseases (EASL) and the American Association for the Study of the Liver (AASLD) Clinical Practice Guidelines for ascites and hepatorenal syndrome still proclaim the threshold of 2.5 mg/dL for diagnosing HRS-AKI [42, 43]. The use of this threshold in clinical practice would mean that proper diagnosis and treatment of HRS would be withheld as long as serum creatinine does not reach this threshold. In order to prevent misclassification or even treatment delay, the newer International Club of Ascites criteria focus on the relative increase in creatinine rather than absolute values, since also smaller rises in serum creatinine have been shown to have a negative prognostic impact in patients with cirrhosis [44].

The hepatorenal syndrome is classified in two types. HRS type 1 is a quickly progressive acute renal failure. It commonly occurs in patients with end-stage cirrhosis following a septic insult such as spontaneous bacterial peritonitis or severe alcoholic hepatitis; this kind of hepatorenal syndrome frequently is developed in temporal relationship with a precipitating factor for a deterioration of liver function together with a deterioration of other organ function, although it may occur in the absence of any identifiable triggering event. Type 1 HRS is only diagnosed when the serum creatinine increases more than 100% from baseline to a final level of greater than 2.5 mg/dL.

Patients with type 2 HRS may eventually develop type 1 HRS; this can be spontaneously or following a precipitating event such as an infection [12].

HRS should be diagnosed and excludes other known causes of renal failure and by demonstrating a significant increase in serum creatinine. For practical purposes, HRS is usually diagnosed only when serum creatinine increases to >133 mol/L (1.5 mg/dL). Repeated measurement of serum creatinine over time, particularly in hospitalized patients, is helpful in the early identification of HRS.

The diverse etiologies of renal failure in cirrhosis should be excluded before to conclude the diagnosis of HRS. Parenchymal renal diseases should be suspected if there is significant proteinuria or micro-hematuria, or if renal ultrasonography demonstrates abnormalities in kidney size. The hypovolemia, shock, parenchymal renal diseases, and concomitant use of nephrotoxic drugs are common causes of acute kidney injury and must be excluded before to diagnose HRS. Renal biopsy is important in these patients to help plan the further management, including the potential need for combined liver and kidney transplantation [42].

4.3.1. Treatment

The initial management of acute kidney injury should focus on the early recognition and correction of potential trigger events and on preventing further hemodynamic deterioration [25, 33, 45]. In volume-depleted patients, diuretic therapy and/or lactulose should be withdrawn and plasma volume should be expanded with albumin, or blood transfusions in anemic patients due to gastrointestinal blood loss, is important the careful review of all medications, and consider the withdrawn of nephrotoxic agents. The use of medications that may induce or aggravate arterial should be carefully evaluated [46, 47].

Bacterial infections are a common precipitant of acute kidney injury, including the hepatorenal syndrome; in cirrhosis, these patients should be thoroughly screened for. The early initiation of empiric antibiotic treatment based on clinical suspicion and the local epidemiology and resistance patterns must be considered [48, 49].

The therapeutic response is defined as a decrease of creatinine in serum to a value within 0.3 mg/dL of baseline; in this case, the patients should be followed up closely for the early detection of recurrent episodes kidney failure. It is necessary to consider the possibility of hepatorenal syndrome In case of stage 2 or 3 or progression to a higher acute kidney injury stage, diuretics should be withdrawn immediately. The patients should receive plasma volume expansion with albumin for 2 consecutive days (1 g per kg of body weight, maximum 100 g/day). Albumin is particularly beneficial in patients with sepsis because in addition to its volume-expanding effect, it has antioxidant, scavenging, and endothelial-stabilizing functions [50]. A follow-up assessment of creatinine every 2–4 days during hospitalization and every 2–4 weeks during the first 6 months after discharge is advised [35].

In stages 2 and 3, the patients who meet diagnostic criteria of HRS-AKI should be treated with vasoconstrictors in combination with albumin [35]. The albumin initial dose is 1 g/kg body weight up to 100 g on the first day, then ongoing with 20–40 g/day, as it has been shown that the effects of intravenous albumin in the prevention and treatment of HRS are dose-dependent, with better results when higher cumulative doses were administered [51, 52]. In all large-volume paracentesis (>5 L, with 8 g/L of ascites removed), albumin should be administered since it prevents post-paracentesis circulatory dysfunction, which reduces the risk of renal dysfunction and improve survival [53, 54].

The first-line drug therapy of type 1 hepatorenal syndrome is the use of terlipressin (1 mg/4–6 h intravenous bolus) in combination with albumin. The therapeutic target improves renal function enough to decrease serum creatinine to less than 133 mol/L (1.5 mg/dL); this is considered a complete response. If serum creatinine does not decrease at least 25% after 3 days, the dose of terlipressin should be increased in a stepwise manner up to a maximum of 2 mg/4 h. For patients with partial response (serum creatinine does not decrease <133 mol/L) or in those patients without reduction of serum creatinine, treatment should be discontinued within 14 days.

The terlipressin is the most intensively studied vasoconstrictor for the treatment of HRS-AKI. A bolus of terlipressin induces a significant reduction in the portal pressure for over a 3- to 4-h period and also increases the mean arterial pressure [55]. Hyponatremia must be considered, and this commonly occurs in less advanced liver disease and normal baseline serum sodium levels [56, 57]. Considering the pharmacodynamic profile and the costs of terlipressin, continuous infusion might be preferred over bolus administration. Although terlipressin has been consistently shown to improve renal function, its impact on survival is less clear [58]. Terlipressin is particularly beneficial in patients with sepsis and might also prevent variceal bleeding during the period of discontinuation of nonselective beta blockers [59].

Norepinephrine is an alternative to the use of terlipressin with an initial dose: 0.5 mg/h, and a max. Dose studied in randomized controlled trials of 3 mg/h, norepinephrine is equally effective and inexpensive. A meta-analysis of four randomized-controlled trials demonstrated similar efficacy for HRS, when compared to terlipressin [60]. The therapy recommended for type 2 hepatorenal syndrome is similar [61, 62]; however, HRS type 2 commonly recurs after termination of treatment with vasoconstrictors [63].

Complete response is defined by a decrease in serum creatinine to a value within 0.3 mg/dL of baseline, while a regression of at least one AKI stage is considered as partial response [35]. If there is no response after 3 days of treatment, the vasoconstrictor dose should be increased. In nonresponders, treatment should be discontinued after 14 days. In responders, longer treatment durations can be used as a bridging therapy to liver transplantation.

Potential alternative therapies to terlipressin include norepinephrine or midodrine plus octreotide, both in association with albumin, but there is very limited information with respect to the use of these drugs in patients with type 1 HRS. Treatment with terlipressin should be repeated and is frequently successful. The recurrence of type 1 HRS after discontinuation of terlipressin therapy is relatively uncommon.

Cardiovascular ischemic disease is a contraindication to terlipressin therapy. Patients on terlipressin should be carefully monitored for signs of splanchnic or digital ischemia, the development of cardiac arrhythmias and fluid overload, and treatment modified or stopped accordingly.

The use of TIPS may improve renal function in some patients; there are insufficient data in patients with type 1 HRS to support the use of TIPS as a treatment. The renal replacement therapy may be useful when the patients do not respond to vasoconstrictor therapy. There are limited data on the use of artificial liver support systems, and further studies are required for its use [43].

4.4. Hepatitis C and acute kidney injury

Hepatitis C (HCV) infection can induce kidney injury, mainly due to the formation of immune complexes and cryoglobulins, and possibly to a direct cytopathic effect. HCV is responsible for membranous glomerulonephritis or mesangiocapillary and accelerates the progression of chronic kidney disease due to other causes. It may cause acute kidney injury as a part of systemic vasculitis and augments the risk of AKI due to other etiologies. HCV-infected patients are at an increased risk of acute posttransplant complications. HCV infection increases cardiovascular and liver-related mortality in patients on regular dialysis. Long-term graft survival is compromised by chronic transplant glomerulopathy or recurrent or de novo glomerulonephritis. The increased incidence of diabetes, sepsis, posttransplant lymphoproliferative disease, and liver failure compromises the patient survival. Directly acting antiviral agents (DAAs) are currently available for treatment at different stages of kidney disease. It is concluded that the thoughtful use of DAAs will result in a significant change in the epidemiology and clinical profiles of kidney disease, as well as improvement of dialysis and transplant outcomes, in endemic areas [64].

The acute kidney failure induced by HCV is a systemic disease reported in <5% of HCV-infected (HCV+ve) patients. It is characterized by multiorgan involvement, mainly affecting the lungs and kidneys, skin, musculoskeletal system, and peripheral nerves. The fundamental lesion is endothelial injury, perivascular inflammation with lymphocytic and neutrophilic infiltration, small vessel necrosis, and luminal occlusion by cryoglobulins and fibrin thrombi.

4.5. Cryoglobulinemic vasculitis

In the kidneys, this leads to focal fibrinoid necrosis of the glomerular tufts, often with crescent formation (**Figure 3**). The renal tubules are affected by ischemic and inflammatory lesions and contain hyaline and blood casts. The ureteric and bladder mucosa may display vasculitic purpuric lesions. The interstitium is infiltrated with inflammatory cells and found edematous.

The mechanism of vascular injury is typically attributed to component C1q of the complement, complement activation generates chemotactic factors, C3a and C5a, which recruit and activate pro-inflammatory leucocytes. It also leads to the formation of C5–9, the membrane attack complex that may have an important role in endothelial damage, the active complement component incorporated within the cryoglobulin complex. This leads to endothelial injury by dual effects, namely the activation of the complement cascade via the classical pathway and binding to endothelial complement receptors, thereby localizing the injury in target capillary beds.

The clinical presentation has a wide range from isolated hematuria to acute kidney injury, sometimes associated with thrombotic microangiopathy (**Figure 4**). If left untreated, the

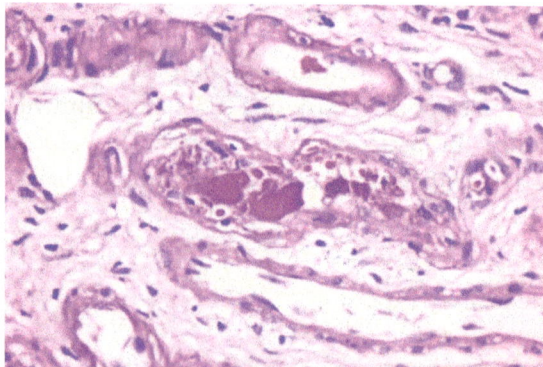

Figure 3. Cryoglobulinemic renal vasculitis. Renal arteriole showing endothelialitis and cryoglobulin deposits in a patient with AKI due to HCV-associated cryoglobulinemia. Hematoxylin and eosin stain. Reproduced with permission from Ref. [64].

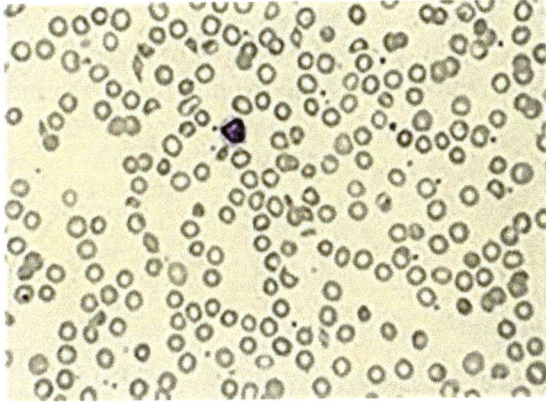

Figure 4. Blood smear in a patient with cryoglobulinemic vasculitis and thrombotic microangiopathy. Note the red cell fragmentation with microcytes and schistocytes.

prognosis becomes bad for the renal function, as well as patient survival. The successful treatment may lead to complete or partial recovery, unless the damage has already been extensive, leading to healing with focal or global sclerosis.

4.6. Non-cryoglobulinemic AKI

HCV-infected patient, compared to the general population are at many-fold risk of developing acute kidney injury of diverse etiology. The most frequent cause of kidney injury is hypovolemia associated with excessive vomiting or diarrhea. The second common cause was bacterial infection in the lungs, urinary, or gastrointestinal tract; 7.3% of patients had advanced cirrhosis and developed AKI following an episode of hematemesis, presumably due to ischemic acute tubular necrosis, and 6.5% were associated with hepatic encephalopathy including the hepatorenal syndrome. Decompensated liver disease, diabetes mellitus, history of intravenous drug abuse, and high baseline serum creatinine were independent predictors of developing AKI. End-stage kidney disease eventually developed in 17.5% of patients who developed AKI, compared to 1% of those who did not. Risk factors for end-stage renal kidney disease were preexisting hypertension, diabetes, or chronic kidney disease [65].

5. Summary

Patients with cirrhosis are prone to developing acute kidney failure. The acute decrease of the kidney function contributes to the mortality of patients with cirrhosis. The criteria of the International Club of Ascites for acute kidney injury provide a simple and relevant staging system for acute kidney injury in patients with liver cirrhosis based on relative increases in serum creatinine. It is very important to consider the potential triggers of renal failure, and this should be recognized early and removed; this includes discontinuation of nephrotoxic drugs and diuretics, treatment of infections and gastrointestinal bleeding, and plasma expansion in case of hypovolemia.

Cardiovascular ischemic disease is a contraindication to terlipressin therapy. Patients on terlipressin should be carefully monitored for signs of splanchnic or digital ischemia, the development of cardiac arrhythmias and fluid overload, and treatment modified or stopped accordingly.

Author details

Marco Antonio López Hernández

Address all correspondence to: niklaus2003@yahoo.com.mx

Internal Medicine Department, Tacuba General Hospital, Mexico City, Mexico

References

[1] Wong F. Recent advances in our understanding of hepatorenal syndrome. Nature Reviews. Gastroenterology & Hepatology. 2012;9:382-391

[2] D'Amico G, Garcia-Tsao G, Pagliaro L. Natural history and prognostic indicators of survival in cirrhosis: A systematic review of 118 studies. Journal of Hepatology. 2006; 44:217-231

[3] du Cheyron D, Bouchet B, Parienti JJ, Ramakers M, Charbonneau P. The attributable mortality of acute renal failure in critically ill patients with liver cirrhosis. Intensive Care Medicine. 2005;31:1693-1699

[4] Montoliu S, Ballesté B, Planas R, Alvarez MA, Rivera M, Miquel M, et al. Incidence and prognosis of different types of functional renal failure in cirrhotic patients with ascites. Clinical Gastroenterology and Hepatology. 2010;8:616-622

[5] Wu CC, Yeung LK, Tsai WS, Tseng CF, Chu P, Huang TY, et al. Incidence and factors predictive of acute renal failure in patients with advanced liver cirrhosis. Clinical Nephrology. 2006;65:28-33

[6] Gerbes AL. Liver cirrhosis and kidney. Digestive Diseases. 2016;34:387-390

[7] Piano S, Rosi S, Maresio G, et al. Evaluation of the Acute Kidney Injury Network criteria in hospitalized patients with cirrhosis and ascites. Journal of Hepatology. 2013;59:482-489

[8] Follo A, Llovet J, Navasa M, et al. Renal impairment after spontaneous bacterial peritonitis in cirrhosis: Incidence, clinical course, predictive factors and prognosis. Hepatology. 1994;20:1495-1501

[9] Hampel H, Bynum GD, Zamora E, El-Serag HB. Risk factors for the development of renal dysfunction in hospitalized patients with cirrhosis. The American Journal of Gastroenterology. 2001;96:2206-2210

[10] Garcia-Tsao G, Parikh CR, Viola A. Acute kidney injury in cirrhosis. Hepatology. 2008; **48**:2064-2077

[11] Cardenas A, Gines P, Uriz J, et al. Renal failure after upper gastrointestinal bleeding in cirrhosis: Incidence, clinical course, predictive factors, and short-term prognosis. Hepatology. 2001;**34**:671-676

[12] Arroyo V, Gines P, Gerbes AL, et al. Definition and diagnostic criteria of refractory ascites and hepatorenal syndrome in cirrhosis. Hepatology. 1996;**23**:164-176

[13] Salerno F, Gerbes A, Gines P, et al. Diagnosis, prevention and treatment of the hepatorenal syndrome in cirrhosis a consensus workshop of the International Ascites Club. Gut. 2007;**56**:1310-1318

[14] Wong F, Nadim MK, Kellum JA, et al. Working Party proposal for a revised classification system of renal dysfunction in patients with cirrhosis. Gut. 2011;**60**:702-709

[15] Angeli P, Sanyal A, Moller S, et al. Current limits and future challenges in the management of renal dysfunction in patients with cirrhosis: Report from the International Club of Ascites. Liver International. 2013;**33**:16-23

[16] Bellomo R, Ronco C, Kellum JA, Mehta RL, Palevsky P; Acute Dialysis Quality Initiative workgroup. Acute renal failure–Definition, outcome measures, animal models, fluid therapy and information technology needs: The Second International Consensus Conference of the Acute Dialysis Quality Initiative (ADQI) Group. Critical Care 2004;**8**:R204-R212

[17] Mehta RL, Kellum JA, Shah SV, Molitoris BA, Ronco C, Warnock DG, et al. Acute Kidney Injury Network: Report of an initiative to improve outcomes in acute kidney injury. Critical Care. 2007;**11**:R31

[18] Kidney Disease: Improving Global Outcomes (KDIGO) Acute Kidney Injury Work Group. KDIGO clinical practice guideline for acute kidney injury. Kidney International. 2012;**2**(Suppl 1):1-138

[19] Angeli P, Gines P, Wong F, Bernardi M, Boyer TD, Gerbes A, et al. Diagnosis and management of acute kidney injury in patients with cirrhosis: Revised consensus recommendations of the International Club of Ascites. Gut. 2015;**64**:531-537

[20] Martin PY, Ginès P, Schrier RW. Nitric oxide as a mediator of hemodynamic abnormalities and sodium and water retention in cirrhosis. The New England Journal of Medicine. 1998;**339**:533 541

[21] Ros J, Clària J, To-Figueras J, Planagumà A, Cejudo-Martín P, Fernández-Varo G, et al. Endogenous cannabinoids: A new system involved in the homeostasis of arterial pressure in experimental cirrhosis in the rat. Gastroenterology. 2002;**122**:85-93

[22] Navasa M, Follo A, Filella X, Jiménez W, Francitorra A, Planas R, et al. Tumor necrosis factor and interleukin-6 in spontaneous bacterial peritonitis in cirrhosis: Relationship with the development of renal impairment and mortality. Hepatology. 1998;**27**:1227-1232

[23] Ginès P, Schrier RW. Renal failure in cirrhosis. The New England Journal of Medicine. 2009;**361**:1279-1290

[24] Schrier RW, Arroyo V, Bernardi M, Epstein M, Henriksen JH, Rodés J. Peripheral arterial vasodilatation hypothesis: A proposal for the initiation of renal sodium and water retention in cirrhosis. Hepatology. 1988;**8**:1151-1157

[25] Arroyo V, Ginès P, Gerbes AL, et al. Definition and diagnostic criteria of refractory ascites and hepatorenal syndrome in cirrhosis. Hepatology. 1996;**23**:164-176

[26] Kim MY, Baik SK, Lee SS. Hemodynamic alterations in cirrhosis and portal hypertension. The Korean Journal of Hepatology. 2010;**16**:347-352

[27] Vilas-Boas WW, Ribeiro-Oliveira A, Pereira RM, Ribeiro Rda C, Almeida J, Nadu AP, Simões e Silva AC, dos Santos RA. Relationship between angiotensin-(1-7) and angiotensin II correlates with hemodynamic changes in human liver cirrhosis. World Journal of Gastroenterology. 2009;**15**:2512-2519

[28] Israni AK, Kasiske BL. Laboratory assessment of kidney disease: Clearance, urinalysis and kidney biopsy. In: Brenner and Rector's The Kidney. 8th ed. Philadelphia: Saunders Elsevier; 2008. pp. 724-750

[29] Mccance RA, Widdowson EM. The correct physiological basis on which to compare infant and adult renal function. Lancet. 1952;**2**:860-862

[30] Delanaye P, Krzesinski JM. Indexing of renal function parameters by body surface area: Intelligence or folly? Nephron. Clinical Practice. 2011;**119**:c289-c292

[31] Eriksen BO, Melsom T, Mathisen UD, Jenssen TG, Solbu MD, Toft I. GFR normalized to total body water allows comparisons across genders and body sizes. Journal of the American Society of Nephrology. 2011;**22**:1517-1525

[32] Du Bois D, Du Bois EF. A formula to estimate the approximate surface area if height and weight be known. Nutrition. 1989;**5**:303-311

[33] Garcia-Tsao G, Parikh CR, Viola A. Acute kidney injury in cirrhosis. Hepatology. 2008; **48**:2064-2077

[34] Wong F, O'Leary JG, Reddy KR, et al. New consensus definition of acute kidney injury accurately predicts 30-day mortality in patients with cirrhosis with infection. Gastroenterology. 2013;**145**:1280-1288

[35] Angeli P, Wong P. Hepatology snapshot: New diagnostic criteria and management of Acute Kidney Injury Hepatology Snapshot. Journal of Hepatology. 2016;**xx**:1-2

[36] Angeli P, Gine's P, Wong F, et al. Diagnosis and management of acute kidney injury in patients with cirrhosis: Revised consensus recommendations of the International Club of Ascites. Journal of Hepatology. 2015;**62**:986-974

[37] Angeli P, Rodrıguez E, Piano S, et al. Acute kidney injury and acute-on-chronic liver failure classifications in prognosis assessment of patients with acute decompensation of cirrhosis. Gut. 2015;**64**:1616-1622

[38] Bucsics T, Mandorfer M, Schwabl P, et al. Impact of acute kidney injury on prognosis of patients with liver cirrhosis and ascites: A retrospective cohort study. Journal of Gastroenterology and Hepatology. 2015;**30**:1567-1565

[39] Elia C, Graupera I, Barreto R, et al. Severe acute kidney injury associated with non-steroidal antiinflammatory drugs in cirrhosis: A case-control study. Journal of Hepatology. 2015;**63**:593-600

[40] Fagundes C, Barreto R, Guevara M, et al. A modified acute kidney injury classification for diagnosis and risk stratification of impairment of kidney function in cirrhosis. Journal of Hepatology. 2013;**59**:474-481

[41] Tandon P, James MT, Abraldes JG, Karvellas CJ. Relevance of new definitions to incidence and prognosis of acute kidney injury in hospitalized patients with cirrhosis: A retrospective population-based cohort study. PLoS. 2016;**11**:1-15

[42] Runyon BA. AASLD practice guideline: Management of adult patients with ascites due to cirrhosis: Update 2012. AASLD Practice Guidelines. 2012. pp. 1-96

[43] European Association for the Study of the Liver. EASL clinical practice guidelines on the management of ascites, spontaneous bacterial peritonitis, and hepatorenal syndrome in cirrhosis. European Journal of Hepatology. 2010;**53**:397-417

[44] Wong F, O'Leary JG, Reddy KR, et al. New consensus definition of acute kidney injury accurately predicts 30-day mortality in patients with cirrhosis with infection. Gastroenterology. 2013;**145**:1280-1288

[45] Wong F. Diagnosing and treating renal disease in cirrhotic patients. Minerva Gastroenterologica e Dietologica. 2016;**62**:253-266

[46] Mandorfer M, Bota S, Schwabl P, et al. Nonselective b blockers increase risk for hepatorenal syndrome and death in patients with cirrhosis and spontaneous bacterial peritonitis. Gastroenterology. 2014;**146**:1680-1690

[47] Mandorfer M, Reiberger T. Beta blockers and cirrhosis, 2016. Digestive and Liver Disease. 2017;**49**:3-10

[48] Arabi YM, Dara SI, Memish Z, et al. Antimicrobial therapeutic determinants of outcomes from septic shock among patients with cirrhosis. Hepatology. 2012;**56**:2305-2315

[49] Jalan R, Fernandez J, Wiest R, et al. Bacterial infections in cirrhosis: A position statement based on the EASL Special Conference 2013. Journal of Hepatology. 2014;**60**: 1310-1324

[50] Bernardi M, Ricci CS, Zaccherini G. Role of human albumin in the management of complications of liver cirrhosis. Journal of Clinical and Experimental Hepatology. 2014; **4**:302-311

[51] Afinogenova Y, Tapper EB. The efficacy and safety profile of albumin administration for patients with cirrhosis at high risk of hepatorenal syndrome is dose dependent. Gastroenterology Report (Oxf). 2015;**3**:216-221

[52] Salerno F. Albumin treatment regimen for type 1 hepatorenal syndrome: A dose–response meta-analysis. BMC Gastroenterology. 2015;15:1-11

[53] Bernardi M, Caraceni P, Navickis RJ, Wilkes MM. Albumin infusion in patients undergoing large-volume paracentesis: A meta-analysis of randomized trials. Hepatology. 2012;55:1172-1181

[54] Gine's P, Tilo L, Arroyo V, et al. Randomized comparative study of therapeutic paracentesis with and without intravenous albumin in cirrhosis. Gastroenterology. 1988; 94:1493-1502

[55] Escorsell A, Bandi JC, Moitinho E, et al. Time profile of the haemodynamic effects of terlipressin in portal hypertension. Journal of Hepatology. 1997;26:621-627

[56] Sola E, Lens S, Guevara M, et al. Hyponatremia in patients treated with terlipressin for severe gastrointestinal bleeding due to portal hypertension. Hepatology. 2010;52: 1783-1790

[57] Cavallin M, Piano S, Romano A, et al. Terlipressin given by continuous intravenous infusion versus intravenous boluses in the treatment of hepatorenal syndrome: A randomized controlled study. Hepatology. 2016;63:983-992

[58] Boyer TD, Sanyal AJ, Wong F, et al. Terlipressin plus albumin is more effective than albumin alone in improving renal function in patients with cirrhosis and hepatorenal syndrome type 1. Gastroenterology. 2016;150:1579-1589

[59] Choudhury A, Kedarisetty CK, Vashishtha C, et al. A randomized trial comparing terlipressin and noradrenaline in patients with cirrhosis and septic shock. Liver Int. 2017 Apr;37(4):552-561

[60] De Mattos ÂZ, De Mattos AA, Ribeiro RA. Terlipressin versus noradrenaline in the treatment of hepatorenal syndrome: Systematic review with meta-analysis and full economic evaluation. European Journal of Gastroenterology & Hepatology. 2016;28:345-351

[61] Alessandria C, Venon WD, Marzano A, Barletti C, Fadda M, Rizzetto M. Renal failure in cirrhotic patients: Role of terlipressin in clinical approach to hepatorenal syndrome type 2. European Journal of Gastroenterology & Hepatology. 2002;14:1363-1368

[62] Piano S, Tonon M, Cavallin M, et al. Reply to: 'A cut-off serum creatinine value of 1.5 mg/dl for AKI—to be or not to be'. Journal of Hepatology. 2015;62:744-746

[63] Rodriguez E, Pereira GH, Solá E, et al. Treatment of type 2 hepatorenal syndrome in patients awaiting transplantation: Effects on kidney function and transplantation outcomes. Liver Transplantation. 2015;21:1347-1354

[64] Rashad S, Emad AW, Soha SK. Hepatitis C and kidney disease: A narrative review. Journal of Advanced Research. 2017 Mar;8(2):113-130

[65] Satapathy SK, Lingisetty CS, Williams SE. Acute kidney dysfunction in patients with chronic hepatitis C virus infection: Analysis of viral and non-viral factors. Journal of Clinical and Experimental Hepatology. 2014;4(1):8-13

[66] Moreau R, Durand F, Poynard T, Duhamel C, Cervoni JP, Ichaï P, et al. Terlipressin in patients with cirrhosis and type 1 hepatorenal syndrome: A retrospective multicenter study. Gastroenterology. 2002;**122**:923-930

[67] Russ KB, Kuo YF, Singal AK. Renal function and acute kidney injury among cirhosis patients listed for liver transplantation: A prospective study. The American Journal of Gastroenterology. 2014;**109**:S173

[68] Kirk BR, Todd MS, Singhal AK. Acute kidney injury in patients with cirrhosis. Journal of Clinical and Translational Hepatology. 2015;**3**:195-204

9

Management of Nonalcoholic Fatty Liver Disease (NAFLD)

Monjur Ahmed

Abstract

Although there is an epidemic of NAFLD throughout the world, the management of NAFLD is not very satisfactory at the present time. Lifestyle modification is the main mode of therapy. Other modalities like pharmacotherapy and bariatric endoscopy or surgery should be individualized. Various pharmacological agents are being investigated to optimize the treatment of NAFLD.

Keywords: nonalcoholic fatty liver disease, fatty liver, hepatic steatosis, nonalcoholic steatohepatitis, NASH, treatment of NAFLD

1. Introduction

When we consider the management of Nonalcoholic Fatty Liver Disease (NAFLD), two aspects should be considered. One is that it can be a part of the metabolic syndrome [1]. About 80% of patients with metabolic syndrome have NAFLD [2]. Although the prevalence of NAFLD is 20–40% in the general population, about 70% of type 2 diabetes mellitus [3] and 85% of patients with morbid obesity (BMI ≥ 40) have NAFLD [4]. In the general population, 80% of patients with NAFLD are overweight and 20% of NAFLD patients have normal weight as per ultrasonography [5]. Another aspect is that it covers a spectrum of hepatic involvement as it progresses slowly from one stage to another. Initially, it starts as simple steatosis or benign fatty liver disease or nonalcoholic fatty liver (NAFL), where there is only macrovesicular hepatic steatosis (>5% of hepatocytes are affected) without any inflammation, hepatocellular injury or fibrosis [6]. The second phase is nonalcoholic steatohepatitis (NASH) where there is not only hepatic steatosis but also ballooning degeneration of hepatocytes and mixed inflammatory cells (lymphocytes, plasma cells, monocytes, neutrophils and eosinophils) infiltrates mainly involving the hepatic acini [7]. The third phase is hepatic fibrosis which generally starts from zone 3 and progresses to bridging fibrosis, cirrhosis of liver and hepatocellular cancer. Prognosis depends on the degree of liver fibrosis [8].

2. Purpose

The main purpose of management of NAFLD is to halt the process as soon as it is diagnosed. The three main modalities of therapy include lifestyle modification, pharmacotherapy and bariatric surgery. Lifestyle modification is applicable to all stages of NAFLD, whereas pharmacotherapy and bariatric surgery should not be considered for patients with simple steatosis. Pharmacotherapy should be considered only for patients with biopsy-proven NASH and hepatic fibrosis as per the guideline of American Association for the Study of Liver Diseases (AASLD).

3. Lifestyle modification

As NAFLD is related to insulin resistance, gradual weight loss is extremely important in overweight and obese individuals [9]. Rapid weight loss can cause portal inflammation and fibrosis [10]. About 7–10% of weight loss over one year by lifestyle changes has been associated with histological improvement in simple steatosis and NASH [11]. Another study showed vigorous and moderate exercises were equally effective in reducing hepatic triglyceride content largely through weight loss [12]. Diet and moderate aerobic exercise are the first line measures to reduce weight and improve insulin resistance [13]. Dietary counseling should be highly encouraged. Consumption of high fructose containing food is the main cause of epidemic of obesity [14]. Patient should avoid high fructose containing foods like sweet, soda, desserts, breakfast cereals, granola bars and cakes. One study showed that in patients with NAFLD, fructokinase and fatty acid synthase activity are increased [15]. NAFLD may occur when there is a combination of genetic predisposition, sedentary life style and consumption of high-calorie foods [16]. One meta-analysis suggested that Omega-3 fatty acid supplementation in diet was beneficial in patients with NAFLD/NASH [17]. Patients should be encouraged to eat food rich in Omega-3 fatty acid (fish, canola, olive, perilla and chia). Food with high glycemic effects and saturated fat should be avoided [18].

In summary, lifestyle modification is the first line intervention in the management of NAFLD. This includes [1] weight loss of about 7–10% of body weight by a combination of diet and exercise [2], low-calorie diet [3], diet with high fructose and saturated fat should be avoided [4], diet with Omega-3 fatty acid supplement should be encouraged.

4. Pharmacotherapy

There are various pharmacological agents available for the management of NAFLD. Many of them have been found to be ineffective and some of them have high risk-benefit ratio [19]. There are various clinical trials ongoing. Here, we discuss the common agents available and the agents recommended by the American Association for the Study of Liver Diseases (ASSLD).

4.1. Antioxidants

Progression of simple steatosis to steatohepatitis is related to oxidative stress and free radical formation. Vitamin E has been studied in different clinical trials. One study showed that patients with vitamin E deficiency and NAFLD did not respond to the classical diet for NAFLD [20]. In PIVENS trial, vitamin E 800 units per day was associated with improvement of serum transaminases and liver histology in nondiabetic NAFLD patients [21]. Fibrosis scores were not improved in this trial [22]. In SELECT trial, vitamin E supplementation 400 units per day in healthy individuals was associated with significant increase in prostate cancer [23].

Currently, vitamin E 800 units per day is recommended in nondiabetic individuals with biopsy-proven NASH [19].

4.2. Insulin sensitizing agents

4.2.1. Thioglitazones (TZD)

They are agonists/selective ligands of nuclear transcription factor PPAR-ɣ (peroxisome proliferator-activated receptor-gamma) which is present in pancreatic β-cells, adipocytes, skeletal muscles, endothelial cells and macrophages. They increase insulin sensitivity in NAFLD and thus, promote fatty acid transportation from liver and skeletal muscles into adipose tissue, decrease serum-free fatty acid concentration and increase fatty acid oxidation in the liver [24]. Pioglitazone 30 mg/day improved hepatic steatosis, steatohepatitis and transaminitis in nondiabetic patients with NASH in the PIVENS trial but histological response did not reach statistical significance [22]. Another study showed that in prediabetic and diabetic patients, long-term treatment with pioglitazone 45 mg/day improved not only steatotic and inflammatory activity but also hepatic fibrosis [25]. There are few concerns about the side effects of TZD and these include weight gain [26], bone loss [27] and congestive heart failure [28].

As pioglitazone improves histology of NASH in both diabetic and nondiabetic individuals, it can be used in biopsy-proven NASH. Patients should be informed about the efficacy and side effects of this medication.

4.2.2. Incretin-based therapy

Glucagon-like peptide 1 (GLP-1) receptor agonists (liraglutide and exenatide) not only improves insulin sensitivity but also causes weight loss by suppressing appetite and inhibiting gastric emptying [29]. They are primarily used to control diabetes mellitus at this time. There are case reports of improvement of hepatic steatosis by GLP-1 receptor agonists [30]. Another study found that liraglutide given daily improved steatohepatitis and decreased progression of fibrosis [31].

Although incretin mimetics have been found to be helpful in diabetic patients with NAFLD, they are currently not recommended solely to treat NASH or NAFLD [19].

4.2.3. Bariatric surgery

As sustained weight loss is achievable by bariatric surgery, all the features of metabolic syndrome improve and there is reduction in mortality [32]. In a prospective study, NASH disappeared in 70% (severe NASH) to 94% (mild NASH) of patients 1 year after bariatric surgery [33]. There are various bariatric surgical and endoscopic procedures available and approved for morbid obesity at the present time. Laparoscopic sleeve gastrectomy is most commonly done in the United States [34]. Other surgical procedures include gastric bypass, biliointestinal bypass, biliopancreatic diversion with duodenal switch, vertical band gastroplasty and gastric banding. Various endoscopic procedures include intragastric balloon placement, endoscopic sleeve gastroplasty [35] and duodenal mucosal resurfacing [36]. Bariatric endoscopy is successful in reducing more weight than pharmacological agents but less effective than bariatric surgery but has less complications than bariatric surgery. Bower et al. found in a systematic review of studies that bariatric surgery improved steatosis, steatohepatitis and fibrosis in NAFLD [37]. Patients with cirrhosis of liver due to NAFLD are at a higher risk for bariatric surgery [38]. Another study showed that perioperative mortality was higher in patients with NAFLD with cirrhosis than in patients with NAFLD without cirrhosis [39].

Nowadays, bariatric surgery is not recommended as a primary treatment of NAFLD but it can be considered in obese individuals with noncirrhotic NAFLD [19].

4.2.4. Ursodeoxycholic acid (UDCA)

UDCA has cytoprotective effect and can improve serum transaminases in NAFLD but cannot alter liver histology [40].

UDCA is not recommended for the treatment of NAFLD or NASH [19].

4.2.5. Omega-3 fatty acids

Although in animal models, omega-3 fatty acid treatment improved hepatic steatosis [41, 42], recent studies did not show any significant effect on serum transaminases or liver histology [43]. Omega-3 fatty acid is not recommended for the treatment of NAFLD or NASH.

4.2.6. Obeticholic acid (OCA)

OCA is a ligand of farnesoid X receptor (FXR) which is a nuclear receptor present in liver, kidneys, intestine and adipose tissue. FXR controls target genes involved in bile acid synthesis and transport as well as lipid and carbohydrate metabolism. In the farnesoid X receptor ligand obeticholic acid in NASH treatment (FLINT) trial, OCA induced weight loss and improved hepatic fibrosis but resolution of NASH was not statistically more than placebo. OCA decreased serum transaminases but increased serum alkaline phosphatase, LDL and blood glucose levels [44].

Currently, OCA is not recommended in the routine management of NAFLD awaiting the completion of phase 3 trial (REGENERATE) of OCA for the treatment of NASH patients with liver fibrosis [45].

5. Elafibranor

Elafibranor is an agonist of PPAR-α and δ receptor. It has anti-inflammatory activity and can improve insulin sensitivity and lipid metabolism. It was evaluated in a phase II international study for the treatment of NASH [46]. In the post hoc analysis, elafibranor (120 mg/day for 1 year) group showed resolution of NASH without progression of fibrosis more than placebo (19% vs. 12%).

As the improvement was marginal, further studies are needed before using this agent in the treatment of NAFLD.

5.1. Statins

Hyperlipidemia is frequently seen in patients with NAFLD as part of the metabolic syndrome. Statins are commonly used for the treatment of hyperlipidemia, and low-to-moderate dose of statins have been found to be safe with low hepatic toxicity [47]. Statins decrease hepatic transaminases and hepatic fat but have no effect on hepatic fibrosis [48, 49].

Statins are not currently recommended solely for the treatment of NAFLD unless the patient has concomitant hyperlipidemia.

5.2. Orlistat

Orlistat is used as a weight reducing agent as it induces fat malabsorption by inhibiting enteric and pancreatic lipase [50]. A randomized controlled trial showed that orlistat improved transaminitis and hepatitis steatosis in obese individuals with NAFLD [51]. Subsequent study suggested that orlistat did not have any direct effect on NAFLD, overweight subjects improved their hepatic histology if they achieved ≥5% weight loss irrespective of taking orlistat [52].

Currently, orlistat cannot be recommended primarily for NAFLD.

5.3. NAFLD and cirrhosis

Patients should be managed the same way as in other cirrhosis. Patients with NAFLD-cirrhosis have 2.6% annual cumulative risk of developing hepatocellular cancer [53]. For every 6 months, abdominal ultrasound is recommended for screening of hepatocellular carcinoma. In obese individuals, if ultrasound is technically difficult, CT or MRI should be considered. As obesity and hyperinsulinemia are risk factors for malignancy, liver cancer can occur even in noncirrhotic NAFLD [54]. Screening for esophageal and gastric varices should be done at base-line of diagnosis of cirrhosis and at regular intervals—no varices: every 2–3 years, small varices—every 1–2 years and decompensated cirrhosis—yearly once [55].

With the epidemic of NAFLD, NASH-cirrhosis and hepatocellular carcinoma will be the leading indication of liver transplantation in future. As patients with NAFLD have multiple metabolic and cardiovascular comorbidities, they should be managed posttransplant appropriately. Management of NAFLD involves multiple specialties which include primary care physicians, gastroenterologists, hepatologists, endocrinologists, bariatric surgeons, transplant surgeons, dietitians and nutritionists.

6. Future therapy

As hepatic inflammation, fibrosis, cirrhosis and subsequent malignancy are the main concerns of NAFLD, plenty of research and studies on anti-inflammatory and anti-fibrotic agents are on-going.

7. Summary

The management of NAFLD patients should be individualized (**Table 1**).

- Lifestyle change is the first line therapy: healthy food habit, increased physical activity, exercise and weight loss of 7–10%.

- Pharmacotherapy is to be considered when lifestyle changes fail to achieve the goal: vitamin E in nondiabetic biopsy-proven NASH, pioglitazone in both diabetic and nondiabetic biopsy-proven NASH, incretin mimetics in diabetes mellitus and NAFLD, statins in hyperlipidemia and NAFLD, orlistat in NAFLD and obesity when life-style changes fail to reduce weight loss.

- Bariatric surgery should be considered in obese individuals and noncirrhotic NAFLD.

Lifestyle changes	First line therapy of NAFLD
Vitamin E	Nondiabetic biopsy-proven NASH
Pioglitazone	Both diabetic and nondiabetic biopsy-proven NASH
Incretin mimetics	Diabetes mellitus and NAFLD
Statins	Hyperlipidemia and NAFLD
Orlistat	NAFLD and obesity when lifestyle changes fail
Bariatric surgery	Morbid obesity and noncirrhotic NAFLD

Table 1. Summary of management of NAFLD.

Author details

Monjur Ahmed

Address all correspondence to: monjur.ahmed@jefferson.edu

Thomas Jefferson University, Philadelphia, PA, USA

References

[1] Lonardo A, Ballestri S, Marchesini G, Angulo P, Loria P. Nonalcoholic fatty liver disease: A precursor of the metabolic syndrome. Digestive and Liver Disease. 2015;**47**(3):181-190. DOI: 10.1016/j.dld.2014.09.020 Epub 2014 Nov 18

[2]   Antunes C, Bhimji S. Fatty Liver. StatPearls [Internet]. Treasure Island (FL): StatPearls Publishing; 2017. PMID: 28723021

[3]   Leite NC, Salles GF, Araujo AL, Villela-Nogueira CA, Cardoso CR. Prevalence and associ-ated factors of non-alcoholic fatty liver disease in patients with type-2 diabetes mellitus. Liver International. 2009;**29**(1):113-119. DOI: 10.1111/j.1478-3231.2008.01718.x Epub 2008 Apr 1

[4]   Fabbrini E, Sullivan S, Klein S. Obesity and Nonalcoholic Fatty Liver Disease: Biochemical, Metabolic and Clinical Implications. Hepatology. 2010;**51**(2):679-689. DOI: 10.1002/hep.23280

[5]   Bellentani S, Tiribelli C. The spectrum of liver disease in the general population: Lesson from the Dionysos study. Journal of Hepatology. 2001;**35**(4):531-537 PMID: 11682041

[6]   Contos MJ, Sanyal AJ. The clinicopathologic spectrum and management of nonalcoholic fatty liver disease. Advances in Anatomic Pathology. 2002;**9**(1):37-51 PMID: 11756758

[7]   Harmon RC, Tiniakos DG, Argo CK. Inflammation in nonalcoholic steatohepatitis. Expert Review of Gastroenterology and Hepatology. 2011;**5**(2):189-200. DOI: 10.1586/egh.11.21

[8]   Angulo P, Machado MV, Diehl AM. Fibrosis in nonalcoholic Fatty liver disease: Mecha-nisms and clinical implications. Seminars in Liver Disease. 2015;**35**(2):132-145. DOI: 10.1055/ s-0035-1550065 Epub 2015 May 14

[9]   Harrison SA, Day CP. Benefits of lifestyle modification in NAFLD. Gut. 2007;**56**(12):1760-1769. DOI: 10.1136/gut.2006.112094 PMCID: PMC2095707

[10] Andersen T, Gluud C, Franzmann MB, Christoffersen P. Hepatic effects of dietary weight loss in morbidly obese subjects. Journal of Hepatology. 1991;**12**(2):224-229 PMID: 2051001

[11] Tilg H, Moschen A. Weight loss: Cornerstone in the treatment of non-alcoholic fatty liver disease. Minerva Gastroenterologica e Dietologica. 2010;**56**(2):159-167

[12] Zhang HJ, He J, Pan LL, Ma ZM, Han CK, Chen CS, Chen Z, Han HW, Chen S, Sun Q, Zhang JF, Li ZB, Yang SY, Li XJ, Li XY. Effects of moderate and vigorous exercise on nonalcoholic fatty liver disease: A randomized clinical trial. JAMA Internal Medicine. 2016;**176**(8):1074-1082. DOI: 10.1001/jamainternmed.2016.3202

[13] Wilkins T, Tadkod A, Hepburn I, Schade RR. Nonalcoholic fatty liver disease: Diagnosis and management. American Family Physician. 2013;**88**(1):35-42

[14] Bray GA, Nielson SJ, Popkin BM. Consumption of high-fructose corn syrup in beverages may play a role in the epidemic of obesity. American Journal of Clinical Nutrition. 2004;**79**(4):537-543

[15] Ouyang X, Cirillo P, Sautin Y, McCall S, Bruchette JL, Diehl AM, Johnson RJ, Abdelmalek MF. Fructose consumption as a risk factor for non-alcoholic fatty liver disease. Journal of Hepatology. 2008;**48**(6):993-999. DOI: 10.1016/j.jhep.2008.02.011 Epub 2008 Mar 10

[16] Dongiovanni P, Romeo S, Valenti L. Genetic factors in the pathogenesis of nonalcoholic fatty liver and steatohepatitis. Biomed Research International. 2015;**2015**:460190. DOI: 10.1155/2015/460190 Epub 2015 Jul 27. PMID: 26273621. PMCID: PMC4530215

[17] Lu W, Li S, Li J, Wang J, Zhang R, Zhou Y, Yin Q, Zheng Y, Wang F, Xia Y, Chen K, Liu T, Lu J, Zhou Y, Guo C. Effects of omega-3 fatty acid in nonalcoholic fatty liver disease: A meta-analysis. Gastroenterology Research and Practice. 2016;**2016**:1459790. DOI: 10.1155/2016/1459790 PMCID: PMC5019889

[18] Ferolla SM, Silva LC, Ferrari MDLA, Cunha ASD, Martins FDS, Couto CA, Ferrari TCA. Dietary approach in the treatment of nonalcoholic fatty liver disease. World Journal of Hepatology. 2015;**7**(24):2522-2534. DOI: 10.4254/wjh.v7.i24.2522 PMCID: PMC4621466

[19] Chalasani N, Younossi Z, Lavine JE, Charlton M, Cusi K, Rinella M, Harrison SA, Brunt EM, Sanyal AJ. The diagnosis and management of nonalcoholic fatty liver disease: Practice guidance from the American Association for the Study of Liver Diseases. Hepatology. 2017. DOI: 10.1002/hep.29367 [Epub ahead of print]. PMID: 28714183

[20] Cankurtaran M, Kav T, Yavuz B, Shorbagi A, Halil M, Coskun T, Arslan S. Serum vitamin-E levels and its relation to clinical features in nonalcoholic fatty liver disease with elevated ALT levels. Acta Gastro-enterologica Belgica. 2006;**69**(1):5-11

[21] Chalasani NP, Sanyal AJ, Kowdley KV, Robuck PR, Hoofnagle J, Kleiner DE, Unalp A, Tonascia J, NASH CRN Research Group. Pioglitazone versus vitamin E versus placebo for the treatment of non-diabetic patients with non-alcoholic steatohepatitis: PIVENS trial design. Contemporary Clinical Trials. 2009;**30**(1):88-96. DOI: 10.1016/j.cct. 2008.09.003 Epub 2008 Sep 10

[22] Sanyal AJ, Chalasani N, Kowdley KV, McCullough A, Diehl AM, Bass NM, Neuschwander-Tetri BA, Lavine JE, Tonascia J, Unalp A, Van Natta M, Clark J, Brunt EM, Kleiner DE, Hoofnagle JH, Robuck PR, NASH CRN. Pioglitazone, vitamin E, or placebo for nonalcoholic steatohepatitis. New England Journal of Medicine. 2010;**362**(18):1675-1685. DOI: 10.1056/NEJMoa0907929 Epub 2010 Apr 28

[23] Klein EA, Thompson IM Jr, Tangen CM, Crowley JJ, Lucia MS, Goodman PJ, Minasian LM, Ford LG, Parnes HL, Gaziano JM, Karp DD, Lieber MM, Walther PJ, Klotz L, Parsons JK, Chin JL, Darke AK, Lippman SM, Goodman GE, Meyskens FL Jr, Baker LH. Vitamin E and the risk of prostate cancer: The Selenium and Vitamin E Cancer Prevention Trial (SELECT). Journal of the American Medical Association. 2011;**306**(14):1549-1556. DOI: 10.1001/jama.2011.1437

[24] Mehta SR. Advances in the treatment of nonalcoholic fatty liver disease. Therapeutic Advances in Endocrinology and Metabolism. 2010;**1**(3):101-115. DOI: 10.1177/204201 8810379587 PMCID: PMC3475281

[25] Cusi K, Orsak B, Bril F, Lomonaco R, Hecht J, Ortiz-Lopez C, Tio F, Hardies J, Darland C, Musi N, Webb A, Portillo-Sanchez P. Long-term pioglitazone treatment for patients with nonalcoholic steatohepatitis and prediabetes or type 2 diabetes mellitus: A randomized trial. Annals of Internal Medicine. 2016;**165**(5):305-315. DOI: 10.7326/M15-1774 Epub 2016 Jun 21. PMID: 27322798

[26] Aghamohammadzadeh N, Niafar M, Dalir Abdolahinia E, et al. The effect of pioglitazone on weight, lipid profile and liver enzymes in type 2 diabetic patients. Therapeutic Advances in Endocrinology and Metabolism. 2015;**6**(2):56-60. DOI: 10.1177/204201881 5574229

[27] Lecka-Czernik B. Bone loss in diabetes: Use of antidiabetic thiazolidinediones and secondary osteoporosis. Current Osteoporosis Reports. 2010;8(4):178-184. DOI: 10.1007/s11914-010-0027 PMID: 20809203

[28] Jearath V, Vashisht R, Rustagi V, Raina S, Sharma R. Pioglitazone-induced congestive heart failure and pulmonary edema in a patient with preserved ejection fraction. Journal of Pharmacology & Pharmacotherapeutics. 2016;7(1):41-43. DOI: 10.4103/0976-500X.179363

[29] Prasad-Reddy L, Isaacs D. A clinical review of GLP-1 receptor agonists: Efficacy and safety in diabetes and beyond. Drugs Context. 2015;4:212283. DOI: 10.7573/dic.212283 PMCID: PMC4509428

[30] Tushuizen ME, Bunck MC, Pouwels PJ, van Waesberghe JH, Diamant M, Heine RJ. Incretin mimetics as a novel therapeutic option for hepatic steatosis. Liver International. 2006;26(8):1015-1017. DOI: 10.1111/j.1478-3231.2006.01315.x 16953843

[31] Armstrong MJ, Gaunt P, Aithal GP, Barton D, Hull D, Parker R, Hazlehurst JM, Guo K, LEAN trial team, Abouda G, Aldersley MA, Stocken D, Gough SC, Tomlinson JW, Brown RM, Hübscher SG, Newsome PN. Liraglutide safety and efficacy in patients with non-alcoholicsteatohepatitis (LEAN): A multicentre, double-blind, randomised, placebo-controlled phase 2 study. Lancet. 2016;387(10019):679-690. DOI: 10.1016/S0140-6736(15)00803-X Epub 2015 Nov 20

[32] Adams TD, Gress RE, Smith SC, Halverson RC, Simper SC, Rosamond WD, Lamonte MJ, Stroup AM, Hunt SC. Long-term mortality after gastric bypass surgery. New England Journal of Medicine. 2007;357(8):753-761 PMID: 17715409

[33] Lassailly G, Caiazzo R, Buob D, Pigeyre M, Verkindt H, Labreuche J, Raverdy V, Leteurtre E, Dharancy S, Louvet A, Romon M, Duhamel A, Pattou F, Mathurin P. Bariatric surgery reduces features of nonalcoholic steatohepatitis in morbidly obese patients. Gastroenterology. 2015;149(2):379-388; quiz e15-6. DOI: 10.1053/j.gastro.2015.04.014 Epub 2015 Apr 25

[34] Donatelli G, Dumont JL, Cereatti F, Ferretti S, Vergeau BM, Tuszynski T, Pourcher G, Tranchart H, Mariani P, Meduri A, Catheline JM, Dagher I, Fiocca F, Marmuse JP, Meduri B. Treatment of leaks following sleeve gastrectomy by endoscopic internal drainage (EID). Obesity Surgery. 2015;25(7):1293-1301. DOI: 10.1007/s11695-015-1675-x PMID: 25913755

[35] Choi HS, Chun HJ. Recent trends in endoscopic bariatric therapies. Clinical Endoscopy. 2017;50(1):11-16. DOI: 10.5946/ce.2017.007

[36] Cherrington AD, Rajagopalan H, Maggs D, Devière J. Hydrothermal duodenal mucosal resurfacing: Role in the treatment of metabolic disease. Gastrointestinal Endoscopy Clinic of North America. 2017;27(2):299-311. DOI: 10.1016/j.giec.2016.12.002

[37] Bower G, Toma T, Harling L, Jiao LR, Efthimiou E, Darzi A, Athanasiou T, Ashrafian H. Bariatric surgery and non-alcoholic fatty liver disease: A systematic review of liver biochemistry and histology. Obesity Surgery. 2015;25(12):2280-2289. DOI: 10.1007/s11695-015-1691-x

[38] Grimm IS, Schindler W, Haluszka O. Steatohepatitis and fatal hepatic failure after bilio-pancreatic diversion. American Journal of Gastroenterology. 1992;**87**(6):775-779 PMID: 1590319

[39] Mosko JD, Nguyen GC. Increased perioperative mortality following bariatric surgery among patients with cirrhosis. Clinical Gastroenterology and Hepatology. 2011;**9**(10):897-901. DOI: 10.1016/j.cgh.2011.07.007 Epub 2011 Jul 23

[40] Lindor KD, Kowdley KV, Heathcote EJ, Harrison ME, Jorgensen R, Angulo P, Lymp JF, Burgart L, Colin P. Ursodeoxycholic acid for treatment of nonalcoholic steatohepatitis: Results of a randomized trial. Hepatology. 2004;**39**(3):770-778. DOI: 10.1002/hep.20092 PMID: 14999696

[41] Di Minno MND, Russolillo A, Lupoli R, Ambrosino P, Di Minno A, Tarantino G. Omega-3 fatty acids for the treatment of non-alcoholic fatty liver disease. World Journal of Gastroenterology: WJG. 2012;**18**(41):5839-5847. DOI: 10.3748/wjg.v18.i41.5839

[42] Scorletti E, Bhatia L, McCormick KG, Clough GF, Nash K, Hodson L, Moyses HE, Calder PC, Byrne CD, WELCOME Study. Effects of purified eicosapentaenoic and docosahexaenoic acids in nonalcoholic fatty liver disease: Results from the Welcome* study. Hepatology. 2014;**60**(4):1211-1221. DOI: 10.1002/hep.27289 PMID: 25043514

[43] Sanyal AJ, Abdelmalek MF, Suzuki A, Cummings OW, Chojkier M, EPE-A Study Group. No significant effects of ethyl-eicosapentanoic acid on histologic features of nonalcoholic steatohepatitis in a phase 2 trial. Gastroenterology. 2014;**147**(2):377-84.e1. DOI: 10.1053/j.gastro.2014.04.046 Epub 2014 May 9

[44] Makri E, Cholongitas E, Tziomalos K. Emerging role of obeticholic acid in the management of nonalcoholic fatty liver disease. World Journal of Gastroenterology. 2016;**22**(41):9039-9043. DOI: 10.3748/wjg.v22.i41.9039

[45] Randomized Global Phase 3 Study to Evaluate the Impact on NASH With Fibrosis of Obeticholic Acid Treatment (REGENERATE). https://clinicaltrials.gov/ct2/show/NCT02548351

[46] Ratziu V, Harrison SA, Francque S, Bedossa P, Lehert P, Serfaty L, Romero-Gomez M, Boursier J, Abdelmalek M, Caldwell S, Drenth J, Anstee QM, Hum D, Hanf R, Roudot A, Megnien S, Staels B, Sanyal A, GOLDEN-505 Investigator Study Group. Elafibranor, an agonist of the peroxisome proliferator-activated receptor-α and δ, induces resolution of nonalcoholic steatohepatitis without fibrosis worsening. Gastroenterology. 2016;**150**(5):1147-1159.e5. DOI: 10.1053/j.gastro.2016.01.038 Epub 2016 Feb 11

[47] Athyros VG, Mikhailidis DP, Didangelos TP, Giouleme OI, Liberopoulos EN, Karagiannis A, Kakafika AI, Tziomalos K, Burroughs AK, Elisaf MS. Effect of multifactorial treatment on non-alcoholic fatty liver disease in metabolic syndrome: A randomised study. Current Medical Research and Opinion. 2006;**22**(5):873-883

[48] Lowyck I, Fevery J. Statins in hepatobiliary diseases: Effects, indications and risks. Acta Gastro-enterologica Belgica. 2007;**70**(4):381-388 18330098

[49] Eslami L, Merat S, Malekzadeh R, Nasseri-Moghaddam S, Aramin H. Statins for non-alcoholic fatty liver disease and non-alcoholic steatohepatitis. Cochrane Database of Systematic Reviews. 2013;**12**:CD008623. DOI: 10.1002/14651858.CD008623.pub2

[50] Guerciolini R. International Journal of Obesity and Related Metabolic Disorders: Journal of the International Association for the Study of Obesity. 1997;**21**(Supplement 3):S12-S23

[51] Zelber-Sagi S, Kessler A, Brazowsky E, Webb M, Lurie Y, Santo M, Leshno M, Blendis L, Halpern Z, Oren R. A double-blind randomized placebo-controlled trial of orlistat for the treatment of nonalcoholic fatty liver disease. Clinical Gastroenterology and Hepatology. 2006;**4**(5):639-644 Epub 2006 Apr 17

[52] Harrison SA, Fecht W, Brunt EM, Neuschwander-Tetri BA. Orlistat for overweight subjects with nonalcoholic steatohepatitis: A randomized, prospective trial. Hepatology. 2009;**49**(1):80-86. DOI: 10.1002/hep.22575

[53] Ascha MS, Hanouneh IA, Lopez R, Tamimi TA, Feldstein AF, Zein NN. The incidence and risk factors of hepatocellular carcinoma in patients with nonalcoholic steatohepatitis. Hepatology. 2010;**51**(6):1972-1978. DOI: 10.1002/hep.23527

[54] Kawada N, Imanaka K, Kawaguchi T, Tamai C, Ishihara R, Matsunaga T, Gotoh K, Yamada T, Tomita Y. Hepatocellular carcinoma arising from non-cirrhotic nonalcoholic steatohepatitis. Journal of Gastroenterology. 2009;**44**(12):1190-1194. DOI: 10.1007/s00535-009-0112-0

[55] Garcia-Tsao G, Sanyal AJ, Grace ND, Carey W. Practice Guidelines Committee of the American Association for the Study of Liver Diseases; Practice Parameters Committee of the American College of Gastroenterology. Prevention and management of gastroesophageal varices and variceal hemorrhage in cirrhosis. Hepatology. 2007;**46**(3):922-938. DOI: 10.1002/hep.21907 PMID: 17879356

10

Intraoperative Ultrasound of the Liver: Actual Status and Indications

Adrian Bartoş, Ioana Iancu, Caius Breazu and
Dana Bartoş

Abstract

Intraoperative liver ultrasound represents an essential component in the hepatobiliary surgery arsenal, having an essential role in describing liver lesions, their topography, and loco-regional extension. It also has an important role in establishing surgical strategy, in modulating the surgeon decisions, and thus in preventing postoperative complications. This chapter tries to make a synthetic review of principal indications for using ultrasound in liver surgical treatment, underlining the liver's lesions characteristics and advantages brought by this method. Also, we wanted to underline the importance that ultrasound has for guiding the surgeon in interventional intraoperative techniques or in any anatomical liver resection. The role of enhanced contrast intraoperative ultrasound is put in front by the better diagnostic results obtained for both primary and metastatic tumors of the liver.

Keywords: intraoperative ultrasound, liver tumors, contrast enhanced ultrasound

1. Introduction: brief history

The main advantage of the ultrasound imaging method is the real-time visualization of the anatomy and structure of the liver lesions, allowing for the adaptation of the therapeutic decision during surgery.

The concept of intraoperative ultrasound (IOUS) was first introduced in the 60s and was used to evaluate renal lithiasis when doing nephrolithotomy. Due to the limitations of A-mode ultrasonography (difficulty in interpreting images), IOUS began to be more applicable in the surgical sphere later, in the early 80s [1], when high-frequency real-time B mode-ultrasound was introduced [2]. The use of IOUS in hepato-bilio-pancreatic surgery was emphasized for the first time in the literature in the mid-80s [3]; later, it became an exploratory technique routinely performed in specialized centers for staging liver disease and guiding surgical procedures on patients diagnosed with hepatocarcinoma on cirrhotic liver [4–7]. Studies in the 90s showed that the information provided by IOUS may modify the initial therapeutic plan in up to 53% of cases [8, 9].

Although first reports related to laparoscopic transducers used in A-mode date back to early 1964, the laparoscopic IOUS technique has been developed relatively recent [10].

2. General aspects

Currently, there is a wide range of equipment for IOUS, probes of different types and shapes, adapted according to the type and localization of the lesion. Standard transductors for trans-abdominal ultrasound can also be used, but there may be some limitations on image resolution and on the large size of the transducer that do not offer optimal maneuverability [1]. Conventional transducers can be used at the beginning of the liver examination to obtain an overview of the organ anatomy [1, 11]. The transducers used in IOUS usually operate at high frequency: 7.5–10 MHz [12]. There are different shapes: linear T-shaped probes, interdigital probes, microconvex probes and more recently, T-shaped probes with trapezoidal scanning window [13]. In case of liver surgery, the ideal transducer should be a small one that can be easily manipulated in narrow spaces, with a special design to allow the probe to be held in the palm between two fingers, thus allowing the operator to have permanent contact with the surface of the liver, without omitting to scan some areas [11, 14] (**Figure 1**).

When necessary, IOUS can also be used in laparoscopic surgery, with special transducers suitable for this type of approach. Transducers used during laparoscopic surgery are either linear or curved, mounted at the end of a long, thin articulated arm, with a design that allows insertion and manipulation inside the trocar (**Figure 2**) [15].

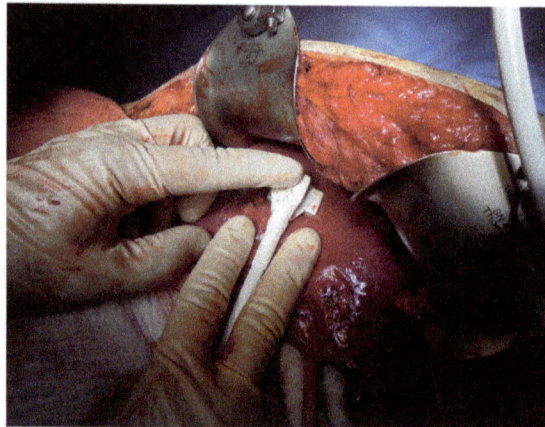

Figure 1. Scanning the liver surface with a intraoperative mini-convex probe, 1–13 MHz, 65°, Hitachi Aloka Medical, Ltd., Japan (intraoperative aspect, from the personal archive of the authors).

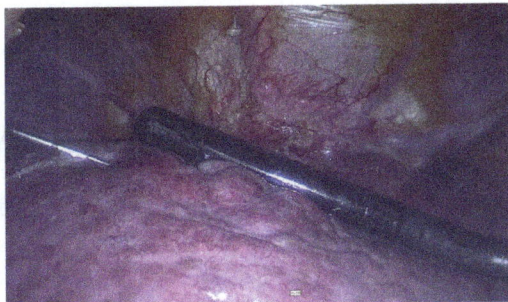

Figure 2. Intraoperative laparoscopic ultrasound of the liver. HCC on cirrhotic liver. L44LA intraoperative probe, 13–2 MHz, 36 mm, Hitachi Aloka Medical, Ltd., Japan (intraoperative aspect, from the personal archive of the authors).

The possibility of performing intra-operative contrast ultrasound (CE-IOUS) is an important factor in choosing the ultrasound equipment. Nowadays, the most commonly used contrast agents are SonoVue (Gaseous sulfur hexafluoride, Bracco, Milan Italy) and Sonazoid (Gaseous perflutane, GE Healthcare, Norway/DaiichiSankyo, Japan) [11, 16–19].

In order to ensure a good examination, the ultrasound machine should be positioned in front of the main operator, the patient (the organ to be examined) being located between the surgeon and the monitor (a collinearity between operator, organ and monitor) in order to view simultaneously the ultrasound monitor and the surgical field. The ultrasound monitor should have size and resolution large enough to allow optimal remote viewing. Examination must always begin with the inspection and palpation of the liver and of the entire peritoneal cavity. These steps should not be avoided in favor of IOUS [20]. Mobilization of the liver begins with the sectioning of suspensory ligaments, thus creating enough space to manipulate the ultrasound transducer. Worth mentioning some of the artifacts that may appear on the examination of the VIIIth and IVa liver segments after the sectioning of the cavo-hepatic adhesions. Therefore, in the case of suspected lesions located in these areas (adjacent to the cavo-hepatic region), dissection at this level should be performed only after ultrasound exploration.

3. IOUS of the liver: benign tumors

Benign tumors can develop on a normal or steatotic liver, may be solitary or multiple, with increased echogenity (hemangiomas, focal nodular hyperplasia) or anechogenic, with posterior acoustic strengthening (serous cysts) and distinct contours (hydatid cysts), with no vascularization or characteristic circulatory pattern; may have a mass effect on liver structures or even adjacent organs. A characteristic for benign tumors is the fact that they have elastic consistency and do not invade vascular elements [20, 21].

Hemangiomas are benign tumors, mostly asymptomatic, incidentally discovered. These tumors can present themselves under various echographic aspects; most commonly, are well-defined, round, hyperecogenic, homogeneous, usually small (<3 cm), and may present the posterior acoustic strengthening effect [22]. As hemangiomas grow in size, they can change their echogenicity, from homogeneous to heterogeneous, with their edges becoming irregular. These features make them more difficult to differentiate from malignant tumor formations. When surgery is indicated, IOUS has the role to localize and visualize the relationships of the hemangioma with the intrahepatic structures. The surgeon can trace the hepatic resection line outside the hemangioma, minimizing hemorrhagic risk, and preserving the healthy hepatic parenchyma to its full potential. The CE-IOUS can be useful, capturing the contrast agent by the hemangioma being most of the time characteristic. Differentiation from malignant tumor formation becomes difficult for arterial hemangiomas or for those with arterio-venous shunts [21].

For *focal nodular hyperplasia*, the central location of a fibrous scar is characteristic. This tumor appears as a well-defined lesions with variable size, usually unique, of solid consistency and inhomogeneous structure. Rarely, the central scar can be distinguished when using simple ultrasound, without contrast agent. When using CE-IOUS, in the arterial phase, there is a central filling followed by a complete capture in the venous phase. At this stage, the center of the tumor becomes hypoechoic. In the late phase, the tumor remains isogenic together with the hepatic parenchyma, which strengthens the diagnosis of benign lesion [21].

Hepatic adenoma appears ecographically as a well-defined solid tumor lesion; it may have an inhomogeneous structure in the presence of intratumoral hemorrhage. Doppler ultrasound does not detect a vascular signal. When using CE-IOUS, in the arterial phase, there is a centripetal and inconsistent capture; in the venous phase, a moderate washout may be noted. In the late phase, the appearance is isoechoic or hyperechoic [21].

Differentiation between focal nodular hyperplasia and hepatic adenoma is important for establishing the therapeutic indication, surgery being indicated for large adenomas, due to the risk of rupture and hemorrhage as well as due to its malignant potential.

Because sometimes it is difficult to make a benign-malignant US differentiation, intraoperatory, when the situation imposes, might by necessary to make a bioptic puncture for establishing a correct diagnosis [20]. IOUS has an important guiding role, especially in the case of lesions located in the depth of the liver parenchyma, hard to reach when palpating.

Simple hepatic cysts (biliary cysts) are benign tumors with no malignant potential, usually asymptomatic, that can be easily diagnosed with ultrasound imaging. They are described by ultrasound as well-defined lesions with very thin walls, no Doppler signal, anechoic, with transonic content due to the liquid composition. Simple hepatic cysts have therapeutic indications only when they become symptomatic, often due to symptoms related to the mass effect they have on neighboring structures.

Percutaneous ultrasound guided treatment with cyst evacuation is often possible, but is followed by an increased risk of relapse, with the rebound of collection. In this idea, the laparoscopic surgical resection of the cystic dome is indicated. This technique is easy if the lesions are located superficially, in segments II, III, IVB, V, VI (after Couinaud) [23]. The lesions localized intraparenchymatous can be approached safely only when using IOUS [24].

Depending on the evolutionary stage, *hydatid cysts* may appear as single or multiple lesions, anechoic, with membranes and sediment inside, with thin or calcified walls. They may be multilocular or may contain multiple fluid compartments (daughter vesicles). IOUS helps the surgeon in finding the cysts and in some situations it can detect bile duct communication. These lesions can compress the intrahepatic vessels with mass effect, signs of invasion, or embedding of these structures being absent [21]. IOUS has the same indications as in the case of simple cysts, being a real help for the surgeon, for establishing surgical tactics and for checking the radicality of the treatment (the content of the remaining cavity, residual content, multilocular abscesses, etc.) [25].

4. IOUS of the liver: malignant tumor

IOUS finds its usefulness in liver surgery for both primary and secondary malignant lesions facilitating the detection, characterization of lesions and guiding the surgical procedure [26, 27]. Most studies have evaluated the role of IOUS for treatment of hepatocarcinomas and hepatic metastases due to colorectal cancer, these pathologies being considered the most common liver malignant lesions. Intraoperative detection and local treatment of these lesions may have a major impact in choosing surgical strategy [28, 29].

4.1. Hepatocarcinoma (HCC)

HCC is the most common primary malignancy in the liver, and is frequently associated with cirrhosis [30, 31].

Ecographically, this tumor has the appearance of a solid tumor with irregular contours, heterogeneous, uni-, or multilocular ("encephaloid form"). Typically, it invades the liver vessels, primarily the portal branches, but also the suprahepatic veins. Doppler screening usually highlights a high-speed arterial flow. Vessel distribution is irregular, disordered. CE-US shows hypercaptation in the arterial phase with a specific "washout" of contrast substance in the venous phase. In the late phase, the tumor appears as hypoechoic. This behavior is usually described in tumor nodules larger than 2 cm [21].

In the case of HCC, IOUS is superior in detecting lesions measuring less than 1 cm, preoperative MRI having a lower sensitivity and specificity for these lesions [11, 32]. It has also been shown in several studies that CE-IOUS can modify in 19–29% of the cases the initial treatment plan [33, 34]. CE-IOUS finds its usefulness especially in cirrhotic patients when it comes to differential diagnosis between malignant lesions and regenerative nodules [29, 35]. It has been demonstrated that neoangiogenesis of tumor nodules is a specific criteria for distinguishing hepatocarcinomas from dysplastic or regenerative nodules [35].

CE-IOUS has a sensitivity of 100%, a specificity between 69 and 100% and can modify the surgical strategy in up to 79% of patients [36–38], most frequently by detecting new lesions. The literature emphasizes that the filling pattern of the contrast agent in nodules found by IOUS can guide surgical resection [36]. It has also been shown that the vascular pattern of HCC visualized by using CE-IOUS has been associated with the expression of some genetic profiles, suggesting that CE-IOUS images can be used as an indicator for predicting prognosis of patients [39].

During hepatic resection, which is the standard treatment for HCC, particular attention should be paid in preserving as much hepatic parenchyma as we can, the remaining hepatic volume being an important prognostic factor for the short outcome [37, 39, 40]. Thus, local resection of the tumor formation or its ablation under IOUS guidance may be chosen to minimize the

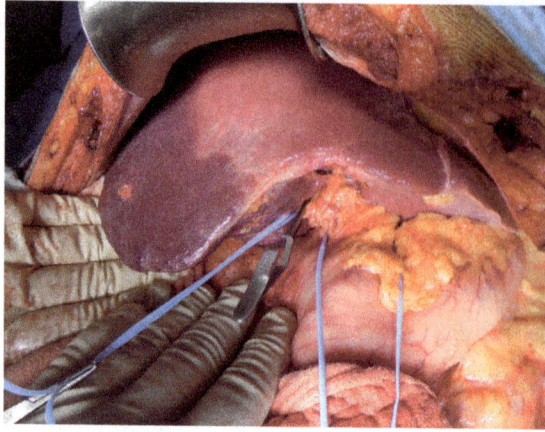

Figure 3. Anatomical resection: ischemic delimitation of sixth and seventh liver segments (intraoperative aspect, from the personal archive of the authors).

volume of resected liver parenchyma, respecting the oncological resection margin. Also, in order to minimize the risk of postoperative complications (hemorrhage, necrosis of the liver parenchyma) and remote relapse (by satellite micrometastases, specific for HCC), the use of IOUS is vital in guiding anatomical resections. These involve the ultrasound identification of vascular pedicles corresponding to the affected hepatic segments and through various associated maneuvers (digital compression, injection of contrast agents) an exact delimitation of the targeted resection area can be obtained (**Figure 3**). More details will be given in the following rows, in the sub-section dedicated to the role of IOUS in guiding hepatic resections.

4.2. Hepatic metastases

Despite significant advances in preoperative staging diagnostic procedures (conventional CE-US, multi-sliced CT, CE-MRI, and PET-CT), studies have shown that 10–30% of the patients with colo-rectal cancer remain with undiagnosed hepatic metastases during primary tumor surgery [41–46].

In this respect, IOUS and CE-IOUS have a special role in completing the diagnosis, in addition to the liver's palpation technique. IOUS is considered the "gold standard" in open surgery for colorectal cancer since 1980, being able to detect liver metastases that cannot be palpated intra-operatively and that have not been visualized with preoperative imaging techniques [8, 47–50].

Liver metastases have a non-characteristic echographic appearance, being circumscribed lesions with imprecise or halo delineation, with a homogeneous or heterogeneous pattern. They may be solitary (usually liver metastases from colonic neoplasms) or multiple. Their echogenicity is variable. When they are large, they can compress the bile ducts (which may appear to be dilated) and the liver vessels. As for their vascularization, they may be hypo-vascular (in gastric, colon, pancreatic, or ovarian cancers) with hypoechoic pattern in arterial phase and similar in the venous and late phases or hypervascular (neuroendocrine tumors, malignant melanomas, sarcomas, renal tumors, breast, or thyroids), with a hyperechoic appearance during the arterial phase, with wash out during the venous phase and hypoechoic pattern at about 30 s after the injection of the contrast substance [51].

Several studies in the literature have shown that after the surgical treatment of the primary tumor, the ultrasound of metastasis after colorectal cancer can be correlated with prognosis. Thus, Gruenberger et al. [52] demonstrated that in patients with hyperechoic ultrasound liver metastases, survival is longer than in those with the hypoechoic aspect of the lesions. This suggests that the role of IOUS is more than a diagnostic one and can be useful in establishing prognosis [53].

The CE-IOUS applied for colorectal liver metastases has an 96% accuracy, in contrast to 74 and 79%, percentages associated with pre-operative CT and MRI [34, 54]. The fact that undetected preoperative liver metastases represent the main cause of recurrent neoplasia [55] highlights the important role that IOUS has in the management of patients diagnosed with colorectal cancer. This is why routine IOUS is recommended in these patients [56].

Chemotherapy is an important, standardized element in regard with the adjuvant and neo-adjuvant therapy in colorectal cancer patients. [57, 58] Regarding hepatic metastases, good results of cytostatic treatment mean either stagnation or regression of these lesions [59, 60]. A particular situation is when liver metastases are no longer visible in CT and/or MRI performed after chemotherapy. Literature indicates that the complete, real response is found in up to 66% of cases [61, 62]. For the rest of the cases (34%), chemotherapy can affect the echogenity of the metastases making them difficult to be identified with preoperative imaging (CT, MRI, even IOUS) [13, 33]. In these situations, CE-IOUS allows the surgeon to check areas where hepatic lesions have been described before chemotherapy [11]. The role of this technique is highlighted in many studies that have shown that only be confirmation given by the CE-IOUS in regard with the lack of lesions can be associated with a complete therapeutic response [59, 62].

Resection or ablation of all lesions is the gold standard in the treatment of colorectal liver metastases [63]. Even in patients with unresectable metastases, local ablation or combination between ablation and surgical resection of the lesions has been shown to be able to locally control the disease [64]. It is obvious that IOUS plays a major role in liver surgery for the detection and localization of metastatic lesions [28].

5. The role of laparoscopic approach

The laparoscopic approach and minimally invasive surgery have more and more indications and thus the role of IOUS in laparoscopic surgery has become increasingly important. Of course, laparoscopic surgery has some disadvantages in assessing the liver because the surgeon loses the advantage of palpating the structures and lesions. IOUS manages to compensate for most of these laparoscopic minuses by providing intraoperative high utility imaging with greater sensitivity in detecting liver lesions than most preoperative imaging techniques [65–69]. Intraoperative laparoscopic ultrasound (LIOUS) has a sensitivity and specificity similar to that in open surgery [69]. Several authors have suggested routine use of LIOUS in laparoscopic colorectal surgery [70] and prior to planned laparotomies for liver resections [71]. In cases where hepatic disease is known, with the help of LIOUS data, around 64% of cases could be exempted from laparotomy [71, 72].

The success of the laparoscopic approach depends primarily on the location of the lesions [73, 74]. Guiding surgical maneuvers by the use of LIOUS is possible especially in superficial tumors on the left lobe or on the anterior segments of the right lobe (hepatic segments II, III,

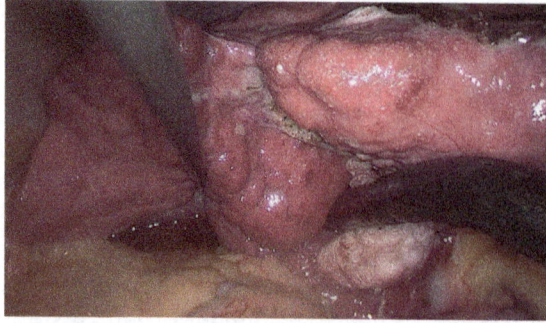

Figure 4. Laparoscopic ultrasound guided radiofrequency ablation of HCC on cirrhotic liver (intraoperative aspect, from the personal archive of the authors).

IVb, V, and VI). Direct visualization and LIOUS should be used to compensate for the impossibility of liver palpation in laparoscopic surgery [75, 76]. In the case of laparoscopically treated malignant lesions, it is important to mark by IOUS imaging the oncological resection margins, this way ensuring their tracing by minimally invasive approach. Furthermore, the completion of the treatment is possible using ablative techniques (radiofrequency, microwave). The laparoscopic approach finds its indications especially for higher-risk cirrhotic patients (altered hepatic markers, clotting disorders) with subcapsular neoplastic lesions (**Figure 4**).

With the evolution of technology and the experience of surgical teams, laparoscopic approaches to hepatectomies have become more and more used in centers of excellence. Several studies have shown that laparoscopic hepatectomy is a safe procedure and could have advantages over open surgery, translated by reduced blood loss and a shorter hospitalization stays [77, 78]. As for LIOUS, it should guarantee the same performance as the ultrasound used in conventional liver surgery. Although, LIOUS has been introduced since 1981, few studies have addressed this subject. Although reported to be a safe and accurate method [79], it is currently not routinely used in laparoscopic surgery [80], although the reliability of LIOUS in the staging of liver disease has been demonstrated to be similar to conventional IOUS [81]. Moreover, although many articles mention LIOUS as an important technique, few scientific papers described this technique [82–85].

6. Ultrasound-guided techniques

It has been demonstrated that making biopsies under IOUS guidance, laparoscopic or "classic," have a high diagnostic accuracy and are considered safe procedures with possible impact on surgical management [86, 87]. For example, liver metastases detected intra-operatively and confirmed by histopathological examination as having pancreatic origin could be a contraindication for pancreatic radical surgery [58].

In terms of non-excisional treatment of hepatic tumor formations, this can also be achieved by ablative techniques, such as ethanol injection [88], RFA (coagulation necrosis induced by high-frequency alternating currents-thermal energy) [89] and MWA (same as RFA, although

MWA uses different parts of the electromagnetic spectrum) [90]. Although the elective treatment is by percutaneous approach, there are situations when both classical or laparoscopic method are indicated.

Laparoscopic approach is particularly preferred on patients who are on the waiting list for liver transplantation or for those who cannot benefit from liver resection due to comorbidities, liver cirrhosis, or hepatic dysfunction due to chemotherapy, especially when percutaneous procedures are not possible [91–93]. Indications are subcapsular lesions located in the immediate vicinity of important structures (diaphragm, stomach, and gallbladder) or difficult to approach (caudal lobe). [84, 94–96]. Moreover, these ablation techniques can be combined with hepatic resections or can be performed serially after surgical resections, improving the oncological outcome and prognosis [97–99]. In the majority of cases treated by these procedures, IOUS is used as a guidance tool and for evaluation the efficacy of the treatment and appearance of complications [94].

Multiple studies have demonstrated that IOUS-guided ablations are a safe and an effective treatment option that provides excellent local control of both primary and secondary hepatic tumor lesions [64, 94, 100–102]. Recent studies have also reported that intraoperative RFA has a local recurrence rate equivalent to that obtained from low-grade HCC surgery [11, 96] and colorectal hepatic metastases [64, 100].

7. Guiding liver resections

Localization of liver lesions is related to portal branches and suprahepatic veins, which are used to define segmental boundaries. Without the use of IOUS, it would probably be impossible to define correctly, anatomically, the hepatic segments and often the limits of the tumors, especially due to the existence of multiple anatomical variants [13].

Hepatic resections are known to be the standard treatment for malignant liver tumor formations, being the only procedure that provides oncological radicality [58]. Preservation of hepatic parenchyma should be a goal of the surgical team, especially in patients with cirrhotic liver, whose liver function and prognostic could be influenced by extensive resection. In these situations, IOUS plays an essential role because it allows the evaluation of the intrahepatic tumors, facilitating a limited but oncological liver resection. Thus, in modern hepatic surgery, whether HCC or colorectal liver metastases, the use of IOUS allows the realization of the so-called "radical but conservative surgery." Thus, obtaining continuous information on the relationship between liver lesions and intrahepatic bilio-vascular structures, the surgeon can guide his resection line, respecting the Glisson pedicles, and suprahepatic veins, with the ultimate goal of preserving as much functional hepatic parenchyma as possible [11, 12, 103, 104].

IOUS is also a real help for anatomical resections. This technique involves the compression of segmental portal branches between the transducer and the operator's fingers, resulting in a transient ischemia of the target parenchyma. This area can be marked with the electrocautery, and then the resection is made along the demarcation line [105–110].

Starting from the use of IOUS, Torzilli introduces new types of resection, such as mini-meso-hepatectomy, for tumor formations located at the confluence of the cave vein with superhepatic veins [11, 12, 111]. These resections are based on the ultrasound study of the relationship between the tumor and the suprahepatic veins and the analysis of the blood flow at this level after clamping the proposed vein for resection. Evidence of an inverse flow in the peripheral portion of the compressed vein or of a collateral shunt between the clamped vein and the other superhepatic vein or cava vein will allow the ligation and segregation of the tumor-affected suprahepatic vein and the achievement of a limited resection, while maintaining the principles of oncological radicality [11, 12].

Summarizing, the use of IOUS allows the extension of surgical indications for certain liver lesions that were either considered unresectable or required major surgery [104].

8. Future perspectives

IOUS is still characterized by several drawbacks: it cannot detect lesions smaller than 3 mm, its accuracy is dependent on the surgeon's skill and experience, the images are 2D and there is a "blind area "of about 1 cm below the surface of the liver, which is particularly problematic in the case of small hepatic metastases due to colorectal cancer that are mainly located on the surface of the liver. Of course, associating contrast agents has greatly improved IOUS accuracy; however, the disadvantage of visualization of the lesions for a too short period of time makes this technique to be of limited applicability in guiding hepatic resections that may last between 2 and 6 h [112].

Recently, a new fluorescent approach, using indocyanine green (ICG), has been proposed to improve the intraoperative detection of neoplastic lesions [113, 114]. ICG is a non-specific molecule that allows detection of tumor tissue, but with limited specificity. The main advantage of its use is its safety and its commercial availability as a contrast substance. The imaging technique of intraoperative fluorescence using ICG was initially used for the detection of sentinel lymph nodes in patients with gastric, colon, and breast cancer [115, 116]. Several studies have shown that malign liver tumors show strong fluorescence when preoperative ICG administration is made [117, 118]. This technique is based on the fact that ICG binds to plasma proteins and together emit light with a peak wavelength of approximately 830 nm when illuminated with infrared light [119].

Initially, ICG-fluorescence imaging was limited to open surgery alone. After year 2010, as laparoscopic and robotic imaging systems with fluorescence have developed, ICG-fluorescence imaging has been extended to minimally invasive abdominal surgery, especially for the visualization of extrahepatic biliary tract anatomy (during laparoscopic/robotic cholecystectomies) [120], an approach known as fluorescence cholangiography [121]. In 2014, the use of ICG-fluorescence imaging was reported for the identification of subcapsular hepatic tumors before liver transection [122]. A new laparoscopic imaging system is starting to be used, this system overlapping pseudo-color fluorescence images with white color-light images in real-time (fusion ICG-fluorescence imaging) with the proposal to identify segmental hepatic margins and localization of liver tumors [123]. Thus, ICG has the ability to "label" bile ducts

[121, 124–126], hepatic tumors [118, 127–130], edges of liver segments [117, 131–133], this being due both to ICG fluorescence [134], and to its property to be excreted into the bile [135]. Due to the property of being eliminated for more than 6 h after intravenous injection [126, 135], ICG-fluorescence imaging can also be used to identify small biliary fistulas after hepatectomy [136].

As for ICG-fluorescence imaging sensitivity in detecting liver metastases, it varies between 69 and 100%. However, sensitivity is limited because the examination does not have the ability to detect hepatic lesions at a depth greater than 8 mm in the hepatic parenchyma. It has also been shown that this method can detect new metastatic lesions in up to 43% of cases [137]. In fact, it has been reported that ICG-fluorescence imaging can detect superficial lesions of up to 2 mm in both HCC and metastases liver disease due to colorectal cancers [127, 129].

Currently, a combination of a fluorophore, such as ICG, with an anti-tumor antibody is evaluated in preclinical studies. These new molecules could present a major advantage in the future for clinical applications that would allow the detection of tumor lesions with a higher TBR (tumor-to-background ratio between the intensity of fluorescence in tumor tissue and normal surrounding tissue). Recently, Harlaar et al. reported the first clinical trial using IRD-800CW-labeled bevacizumab for the detection of peritoneal metastases of colorectal origin [138].

9. Key points

- The IOUS has applications in both open or laparoscopic abdominal surgery.

- For benign hepatic tumors, IOUS has the role to localize and to visualize the relationships with the intrahepatic structures.

- For intraoperative interventional maneuvers (biopsies, ablative techniques), IOUS guidance is mandatory.

- In the case of HCC, IOUS is superior in detecting lesions measuring less than 1 cm.

- In the case of HCC, CE-IOUS finds its usefulness especially in cirrhotic patients for the differential diagnosis between malignant lesions and regenerative nodules.

- IOUS is considered the "gold standard" in open surgery for colorectal cancer.

- CE-IOUS allows the surgeon to check areas where hepatic metastasis have been described before chemotherapy.

- IOUS is mandatory for anatomic resections and for limited but radical hepatectomy.

Acknowledgements

Bartoș Adrian is the coordinator of this chapter.

Conflict of interest

The authors have no conflict of interest.

Author details

Adrian Bartoş[1]*, Ioana Iancu[1,2], Caius Breazu[3] and Dana Bartoş[1,2]

*Address all correspondence to: bartos.adi@gmail.com

1 Regional Institute of Gastroenterology and Hepatology, Surgery Department, Cluj-Napoca, Romania

2 Anatomy and Embryology Department, UMF, Cluj-Napoca, Romania

3 Regional Institute of Gastroenterology and Hepatology, ICU Department, Cluj-Napoca, Romania

References

[1] Kruskal JB, Kane RA. Intraoperative ultrasonography of the liver. Critical Reviews in Diagnostic Imaging. 1995;**36**:175-226

[2] Makuuchi M, Torzilli G, Machi J. History of intraoperative ultrasound. Ultrasound in Medicine & Biology. 1998;**24**:1229-1242

[3] Staren ED, Gambla M, Deziel DJ, et al. Intraoperative ultrasound in the management of liver neoplasms. The American Surgeon. 1997;**63**:591-596

[4] Adam R, Majno P, Castaing D, et al. Treatment of irresectable liver tumors by percutaneous cryosurgery. The British Journal of Surgery. 1998;**85**:1493-1494

[5] Livraghi T, Giorgio A, Marin G, et al. Hepatocellular carcinoma and cirrhosis in 746 patients: Long-term results of percutaneous ethanol injection. Radiology. 1995;**197**:101-108

[6] Makuuchi M, Yamazaki S, Hasegawa H, et al. Ultrasonically guided liver surgery. Japanese Journal of Medical Ultrasound Technology. 1980;**7**:45-49

[7] Solbiati L, Livraghi T, Goldberg SN, et al. Percutaneous radiofrequency ablation of hepatic metastases from colorectal cancer in 117 patients. Radiology. 2001;**221**:159-166

[8] Luck AJ, Maddern GJ. Intraoperative abdominal ultrasonography. The British Journal of Surgery. 1999;**86**:5-16

[9] Solomon MJ, Stephen MS, Gallinger S, et al. Does intraoperative hepatic ultrasonography change surgical decision making during liver resection? American Journal of Surgery. 1994;**168**:307-310

[10] Yamakawa K, Yoshioka A, Shimizu K, et al. Laparoechography: An ultrasonic diagnosis under laparoscopic observation. Japanese Journal of Medical Ultrasound Technology. 1964;**2**:26

[11] Donadon M, Costa G, Torzilli G. State of the art of intraoperative ultrasound in liver surgery: Current use for staging and resection guidance. Ultraschall in der Medizin. 2014;**35**:500-511

[12] Torzilli G, Procopio F, Fabbro D. Technological requirements for ultrasound-guided liver surgery. In: Torzilli G, editor. Ultrasound-Guided Liver Surgery. Italia: Springer; 2014. pp. 3-14

[13] Donadon M, Torzilli G. Intraoperative ultrasound in patients with hepatocellular carcinoma: From daily practice to future trends. Liver Cancer. 2013;**2**:16-24

[14] Patel N, Roh M. Utility of intraoperative liver ultrasound. Surgical Clinics of North America. 2004;**84**:513-524

[15] Horwhat JD, Gress F. Defining the diagnostic algorithm in pancreatic cancer. Journal of the Pancreas. 2004;**5**:289-303

[16] von Herbay A, Westendorff J, Gregor M. Contrastenhanced ultrasound with SonoVue: Differentiation between benign and malignant focal liver lesions in 317 patients. Journal of Clinical Ultrasound. 2010;**38**:1-9

[17] Trillaud H, Bruel JM, Valette PJ, Vilgrain V, Schmutz G, et al. Characterization of focal liver lesions with SonoVueÂ®-enhanced sonography: International multicenter-study in comparison to CT and MRI. World Journal of Gastroenterology. 2009;**15**:3748-3756

[18] Luo W, Numata K, Kondo M, Morimoto M, Sugimori K. Sonazoid-enhanced ultrasonography for evaluation of the enhancement patterns of focal liver tumors in the late phase by intermittent imaging with a high mechanical index. Journal of Ultrasound in Medicine. 2009;**28**:439-448

[19] Imazu H, Uchiyama Y, Matsunaga K, Ikeda K, Kakutani H, et al. Contrast-enhanced harmonic EUS with novel ultrasonographic contrast (Sonazoid) in the preoperative T-staging for pancreaticobiliary malignancies. Scandinavian Journal of Gastroenterology. 2010;**45**:732-738

[20] Machi J, Staren E. Intraoperative ultrasound of the liver. In: Machi J, editor. Ultrasound for Surgeons. Vol. 15. Philadelphia: Lippincott Williams & Wilkins; 2005. pp. 341-343

[21] Badea R, Ioanitescu S. Ultrasound imaging of liver tumors—Current clinical applications. In: Liver Tumors. Vol. 5. Croatia: InTech; 2012. pp. 75-102

[22] Kim KW, Kim TK, Han JK, et al. Hepatic hemangiomas: Spectrum of US appearances on gray-scale, power Doppler, and contrast-enhanced US. Korean Journal of Radiology. 2000;**1**:191-197

[23] Couinaud C. Surgical anatomy of the liver. Several new aspects. Chirurgie. 1986;**112**:337-342

[24]   Mulholland M, Hussain H, Fritze D. Hepatic Cyst Disease. In: Yeo C, McFadden D, editors. Shackelford's Surgery of the Alimentary Tract. Philadelphia: Elsevier; 2013. pp. 1453-1462

[25]   Bartos A, Betea I, Bartos D. Intraoperative ultrasound: Applications in digestive surgery. Sonography. 2016;1:3-16

[26]   Nanashima A, Tobinaga S, Abo T, Kunizaki M, Takeshita H, Hidaka S, et al. Usefulness of sonazoid-ultrasonography during hepatectomy in patients with liver tumors: A preliminary study. Journal of Surgical Oncology. 2011;103:152-157

[27]   Zacherl J, Scheuba C, Imhof M, Zacherl M, Langle F, Pokieser P, et al. Current value of intraoperative sonography during surgery for hepatic neoplasms. World Journal of Surgery. 2002;26:550-554

[28]   Schulz A, Dormagen JB, Drolsum A, Bjornbeth BA, Labori KJ, Klow NE. Impact of contrast-enhanced intraoperative ultrasound on operation strategy in case of colorectal liver metastasis. Acta Radiologica. 2012;53:1081-1087

[29]   Torzilli G, Olivari N, Moroni E, Del Fabbro D, Gambetti A, Leoni P, et al. Contrast-enhanced intraoperative ultrasonography in surgery for hepatocellular carcinoma in cirrhosis. Liver Transplantation. 2004;10(2 Suppl 1):S34-S38

[30]   Yuen MF, Hou JL, Chutaputti A, Asia Pacific Working Party on Prevention of Hepatocellular Carcinoma. Hepatocellular carcinoma in the Asia Pacific region. Journal of Gastroenterology and Hepatology. 2009;24:346-353

[31]   Nagaoki Y, Hyogo H, Aikata H, Tanaka M, Naeshiro N, Nakahara T, et al. Recent trend of clinical features in patients with hepatocellular carcinoma. Hepatology Research. 2012;42:368-375

[32]   Hammerstingl R, Huppertz A, Breuer J, Balzer T, Blakeborough A. Diagnostic efficacy of gadoxetic acid (Primovist)-enhanced MRI and spiral CT for a therapeutic strategy: Comparison with intraoperative and histopathologic findings in focal liver lesions. European Radiology. 2008;18:457-467

[33]   Leen E, Ceccotti P, Moug SJ, Glen P, MacQuarrie J. Potential value of contrast-enhanced intraoperative ultrasonography during partial hepatectomy for metastases: An essential investigation before resection? Annals of Surgery. 2006;243:236-240

[34]   Bartos A, Iancu C. Tratamentul chirurgical al cancerului colo-rectal cu metastaze hepatice rezecabile. In: Grigorescu M, Irimie A, Beuran M, editors. Tratat de Oncologie Digestiv Äf. III. Bucuresti: Editura Academiei RomÃ¢ne. 2015:425-433

[35]   Roncalli M, Roz E, Coggi G, Di Rocco MG, Bossi P, et al. The vascular profile of regenerative and dysplastic nodules of the cirrhotic liver: Implications for diagnosis and classification. Hepatology. 1999;30:1174-1178

[36]   Torzilli G, Palmisano A, Del Fabbro D, Marconi M, Donadon M, Spinelli A, Bianchi PP, Montorsi M. Contrast-enhanced intraoperative ultrasonography durino surgery for hepatocellular carcinoma in liver cirrhosis: Is it useful or useless? A prospective cohort study of our experience. Annals of Surgical Oncology. 2007;14:1347-1355

[37] Lu Q, Luo Y, Yuan CX, Zeng Y, Wu H, Lei Z, Zhong Y, Fan YT, Wang HH, Luo Y. Value of contrast-enhanced intraoperative ultrasound for cirrhotic patients with hepatocellular carcinoma: A report of 20 cases. World Journal of Gastroenterology. 2008;14:4005-4010

[38] Wu H, Lu Q, Luo HXL, Zeng Y. Application of contrast-enhanced intraoperative ultrasonography in the decision-making about hepatocellular carcinoma operation. World Journal of Gastroenterology. 2010;16:508-512

[39] Kaibori M, Matsui Y, Kitade H, Kwon AH, Kamiyama Y. Hepatic resection for hepatocellular carcinoma in severely cirrhotic livers. Hepato-Gastroenterology. 2003;50:491-496

[40] Ezaki T, Yamamoto K, Yamaguchi H, Sasaki Y, Ishida T, Mori M, et al. Hepatic resection for hepatocellular carcinoma existing with liver cirrhosis. Hepato-Gastroenterology. 2002;49:1363-1368

[41] van de Velde CJ, Boelens PG, Borras JM, Coebergh JW, Cervantes A, Blomqvist L, et al. EURECCA colorectal: Multidisciplinary management: European consensus conference colon & rectum. European Journal of Cancer. 2014;50:e1-e34

[42] De Greef K, Rolfo C, Russo A, Chapelle T, Bronto G, Passiglia F, et al. Multisciplinary management of patients with lives metastasis from colorectal cancer. World Journal of Gastroentrology. 2016;22:7215-7225

[43] GI Cancer [Internet]. 2013. Available from: www.GICancer.dk/klinische retningslinier for kolorectal lever metastaser [Accessed: June 01, 2016]

[44] Finlay IG, McArdle CS. Occult hepatic metastases in colorectal carcinoma. The British Journal of Surgery. 1986;73:732-735

[45] Bonanni L, De'liguori Carino N, Deshpande R, Ammori BJ, Sherlock DJ, Valle JW, et al. A comparison of diagnostic imaging modalities for colorectal liver metastases. European Journal of Surgical Oncology: The Journal of the European Society of Surgical Oncology and the British Association of Surgical Oncology. 2014;40:545-550

[46] Takeuchi N, Ramirez JM, Mortensen NJ, Cobb R, Whittlestone T. Intraoperative ultrasonography in the diagnosis of hepatic metastases during surgery for colorectal cancer. International Journal of Colorectal Disease. 1996;11:92-95

[47] Machi J, Sigel B. Operative ultrasound in general surgery. American Journal of Surgery. 1996;172:15-20

[48] Cervone A, Sardi A, Conaway GL. Intraoperative ultrasound (IOUS) is essential in the management of metastatic colorectal liver lesions. The American Surgeon. 2000;66:611-615

[49] Elias D, Sideris L, Pocard M, de Baere T, Dromain C, Lassau N, et al. Incidence of unsuspected and treatable metastatic disease associated with operable colorectal liver metastases discovered only at laparotomy (and not treated when performing percutaneous radiofrequency ablation). Annals of Surgical Oncology. 2005;12:298-302

[50] Larsen LP, Rosenkilde M, Christensen H, Bang N, Bolvig L, Christiansen T, et al. The value of contrast enhanced ultrasonography in detection of liver metastases from colorectal cancer: A prospective double-blindedstudy. European Journal of Radiology. 2007;62:302-307

[51] Larsen LPS. Role of contrast enhanced ultrasonography in the assessment of hepatic metastases: A review. World Journal of Hepatology. 2010;2(1):8-15

[52] Gruenberger T, Jourdan JL, Zhao J, et al. Echogenicity of liver metastases is an independent prognostic factor after potentially curative treatment. Archives of Surgery. 2000;135:1285-1290

[53] Seifert J, Morris D. Pretreatment echogenicity of colorectal liver metastases predicts survival after hepatic cryotherapy. Diseases of the Colon and Rectum. 1999;42:43-49

[54] Winter J, Auer AC. Metastatic malignant liver tumors: Colorectal cancer. In: Jarnagin WR, editor. Blumgart's Surgery of the Liver, Biliary Tract and Pancreas. 5th ed. Vol. 2. Philadelphia: Elsevier Saunders; 2012. pp. 1290-1304

[55] Yoshidome H, Kimura F, Shimizu H, Ohtsuka M, Kato A, et al. Interval period tumor progression: does delayed hepatectomy detect occult metastases in synchronous colorectal liver metastases? Journal of Gastrointestinal Surgery: Official Journal of the Society for Surgery of the Alimentary Tract. 2008;12:1391-1398

[56] Claudon M, Dietrich CF, Choi BI, Cosgrove DO, Kudo M, et al. Guidelines and good clinical practice recommendations for contrast enhanced ultrasound (CEUS) in the liver—Update 2012: A WFUMB-EFSUMB initiative in cooperation with representatives of AFSUMB, AIUM, ASUM, FLAUS and ICUS. Ultrasound in Medicine & Biology. 2013;39:187-210

[57] National Comprehensive Cancer Network Guidelines version 2. 2016. Rectal Cancer; 2016. www.ncc.org [Accessed: 2017]

[58] National Comprehensive Cancer Network Guidelines version 1. 2016. Pancreatic Adenocarcinoma; 2016. www.ncc.org [Accessed: 2017]

[59] Joo I. The role of intraoperative ultrasonography in the diagnosis and management of focal hepatic lesions. Ultrasonography. 2015;34:246-257

[60] Garden OJ, Rees M, Poston GJ, Mirza D, Saunders M. Guidelines for resection of colorectal cancer liver metastases. Gut. 2006;55(iii):1-8

[61] Auer RC, White RR, Kemeny NE, Schwartz LH, Shia J. Predictors of a true complete response among disappearing liver metastases from colorectal cancer after chemotherapy. Cancer. 2010;116:1502-1509

[62] Ferrero A, Langella S, Russolillo N, Vigano L, Lo Tesoriere R, et al. Intraoperative detection of disappearing colorectal liver metastases as a predictor of residual disease. Journal of Gastrointestinal Surgery: Official Journal of the Society for Surgery of the Alimentary Tract. 2012;16:806-814

[63] Penna C, Nordlinger B. Surgery of liver metastases from colorectal cancer: New promises. British Medical Bulletin. 2002;64:127-140

[64] Mulier S, Ni Y, Jamart J, Michel L, Marchal G, Ruers T. Radiofrequency ablation versus resection for resectable colorectal liver metastases: Time for a randomized trial? Annals of Surgical Oncology. 2008;15:144-157

[65] Cuschieri A. Laparoscopic management of cancer patients. Journal of the Royal College of Surgeons of Edinburgh. 1995;**40**:1-9

[66] Hunderbein M, Rau B, Schlag PM. Laparoscopy and laparoscopic ultrasound for staging of upper gastrointestinal tumors. European Journal of Surgical Oncology. 1995;**21**:50-55

[67] Gouma DJ, De Wit LT, Nieveen van Dijkum E, et al. Laparoscopic ultrasonography for staging of gastrointestinal malignancy. Scandinavian Journal of Gastroenterology. Supplement. 1996;**218**:43-49

[68] Goletti O, Buccianti P, Chiarugi M, et al. Laparoscopic sonography in screening metastases from gastrointestinal cancer: Comparative accuracy with traditional procedures. Surgical Laparoscopy & Endoscopy. 1995;**5**:176-182

[69] Tandan VR, Asch M, Margolis M, et al. Laparoscopic vs. open intraoperative ultrasound examination of the liver: A controlled study. Journal of Gastrointestinal Surgery. 1997;**1**:146-151

[70] Hartley JE, Kumar H, Drew PJ, et al. Laparoscopic ultrasound for the detection of hepatic metastases during laparoscopic colorectal cancer surgery. Diseases of the Colon and Rectum. 2000;**43**:320-324

[71] Barbot DJ, Marks JH, Feld RI, et al. Improved staging of liver tumors using laparoscopic intraoperative ultrasound. Journal of Surgical Oncology. 1997;**64**:63-67

[72] John TG, Greig JD, Crosbie JL, et al. Superior staging of liver tumors with laparoscopy and laparoscopic ultrasound. Annals of Surgery. 1994;**220**:711-719

[73] Biertho L, Waage A, Gagner M. Hepatectomies sous laparoscopie. Annales de Chirurgie. 2002;**127**:164-170

[74] Cherqui D, Husson E, Hammoud R, Malassagne B, Ste'phan F, Bensaid S, Rotman N, Fagniez PL. Laparoscopic liver resections: A feasibility study in 30 patients. Annals of Surgery. 2000;**232**:753-762

[75] Gigot JF, Glineur D, et al. Laparoscopic liver resection for malignant liver tumors: Preliminary results of a multicenter European study. Annals of Surgery. 2003;**236**:90-97

[76] Berends FJ, Meijer S, Prevoo W, Bonjer HJ, Cuesta MA. Technical considerations in laparoscopic liver surgery: A solid organ easily forgotten? Surgical Endoscopy. 2000;**15**:794-798

[77] Nguyen KT, Laurent A, Dagher I, Geller DA, Steel J, Thomas MT, Marvin M, Ravindra KV, Mejia A, Lainas P, Franco D, Cherqui D, Buell JF, Gamblin TC. Minimally invasive liver resection for metastatic colorectal cancer: A multi-institutional, international report of safety, feasibility, and early outcomes. Annals of Surgery. 2009;**250**:842-848

[78] Croome KP, Yamashita MH. Laparoscopic vs open hepatic resection for benign and malignant tumors: An updated metaanalysis. Archives of Surgery. 2010;**145**:1109-1118

[79] Machi J, Johnson JO, Deziel DJ, Soper NJ, Berber E, Siperstein A, Hata M, Patel A, Singh K, Arregui ME. The routine use of laparoscopic ultrasound decreases bile duct injury: A multicenter study. Surgical Endoscopy. 2009;**23**:384-388

[80] Vapenstad C, Rethy A, Langø T, Selbekk T, Ystgaard B, Hernes TA, Marvik R. Laparoscopic ultrasound: A survey of its current and future use, requirements, and integration with navigation technology. Surgical Endoscopy. 2010;**24**:2944-2953

[81] Vigano` L, Ferrero A, Amisano M, Russolillo N, Capussotti L. Comparison of laparoscopic and open intraoperative ultrasonography for staging liver tumours. The British Journal of Surgery. 2013;**100**:535-542

[82] Araki K, Conrad C, Ogiso S, Kuwano H, Gayet B. Intraoperative ultrasonography of laparoscopic hepatectomy: Key technique for safe liver transection. Journal of the American College of Surgeons. 2014;**218**:e37-e41

[83] Silas AM, Kruskal JB, Kane RA. Intraoperative ultrasound. Radiologic Clinics of North America. 2001;**39**:429-448

[84] Kim HO, Kim SK, Son BH, Yoo CH, Hong HP, Cho YK, et al. Intraoperative radiofrequency ablation with or without tumorectomy for hepatocellular carcinoma in locations difficult for a percutaneous approach. Hepatobiliary & Pancreatic Diseases International. 2009;**8**:591-596

[85] Crucitti A, Danza FM, Antinori A, Vincenzo A, Pirulli PG, Bock E, et al. Radiofrequency thermal ablation (RFA) of liver tumors: Percutaneous and open surgical approaches. Journal of Experimental & Clinical Cancer Research. 2003;**22**(4 Suppl):191-195

[86] Charnley RM, Sheffield JP, Hardcastle JD. Evaluation of a biopsy gun for guided biopsy of impalpable liver lesions using intraoperative ultrasound. HPB Surgery. 1990;**2**:265-267

[87] Mortensen MB, Fristrup C, Ainsworth A, Pless T, Larsen M, Nielsen H, et al. Laparoscopic ultrasound-guided biopsy in uppergastrointestinal tract cancer patients. Surgical Endoscopy. 2009;**23**:2738-2742

[88] Koda M, Murawaki Y, Mitsuda A, Oyama K, Okamoto K, Idobe Y, et al. Combination therapy with transcatheter arterial chemoembolization and percutaneous ethanol injection compared with percutaneous ethanol injection alone for patients with small hepatocellular carcinoma: A randomized control study. Cancer. 2001;**92**:1516-1524

[89] Kim YS, Rhim H, Lim HK, Choi D, Lee MW, Park MJ. Coagulation necrosis induced by radiofrequency ablation in the liver: Histopathologic and radiologic review of usual to extremely rare changes. Radiographics. 2011;**31**:377-390

[90] Iannitti DA, Martin RC, Simon CJ, Hope WW, Newcomb WL, McMasters KM, et al. Hepatic tumor ablation with clustered microwave antennae: The US Phase II trial. HPB: The Official Journal of the International Hepato Pancreato Biliary Association. 2007;**9**:120-124

[91] Howard JH, Tzeng CW, Smith JK, Eckhoff DE, Bynon JS. Radiofrequency ablation for unresectable tumors of the liver. The American Surgeon. 2008;**74**:594-600

[92] Seidenfeld J, Korn A, Aronson N. Radiofrequency ablation of unresectable liver metastases. Journal of the American College of Surgeons. 2002;**195**:378-386

[93] Curley SA, Marra P, Beaty K, Ellis LM, Vauthey JN. Early and late complications after radiofrequency ablation of malignant liver tumors in 608 patients. Annals of Surgery. 2004;**239**:450-458

[94] Machi J, Uchida S, Sumida K, Limm WM, Hundahl SA, Oishi AJ, et al. Ultrasound-guided radiofrequency thermal ablation of liver tumors: Percutaneous, laparoscopic, and open surgical approaches. Journal of Gastrointestinal Surgery. 2001;**5**:477-489

[95] Ishiko T, Beppu T, Sugiyama S, Masuda T, Takahashi M, Komori H, et al. Radiofrequency ablation with hand-assisted laparoscopic surgery for the treatment of hepatocellular carcinoma in the caudate lobe. Surgical Laparoscopy, Endoscopy & Percutaneous Techniques. 2008;**18**:272-276

[96] El-Gendi A, El-Shafei M, Abdel-Aziz F, Bedewy E. Intraoperative ablation for small HCC not amenable for percutaneous radiofrequency ablation in Child A cirrhotic patients. Journal of Gastrointestinal Surgery. 2013;**17**:712-718

[97] Razafindratsira T, Isambert M, Evrard S. Complications of intraoperative radiofrequency ablation of liver metastases. HPB: The Official Journal of the International Hepato Pancreato Biliary Association. 2011;**13**:15-23

[98] Park IJ, Kim HC, Yu CS, Kim PN, Won HJ, Kim JC. Radiofrequency ablation for metachronous liver metastasis from colorectal cancer after curative surgery. Annals of Surgical Oncology. 2008;**15**:227-232

[99] Cheung TT, Ng KK, Chok KS, Chan SC, Poon RT, Lo CM, et al. Combined resection and radiofrequency ablation for multifocal hepatocellular carcinoma: Prognosis and outcomes. World Journal of Gastroenterology. 2010;**16**:3056-3062

[100] Leblanc F, Fonck M, Brunet R, Becouarn Y, Mathoulin-Pelissier S, Evrard S. Comparison of hepatic recurrences after resection or intraoperative radiofrequency ablation indicated by size and topographical characteristics of the metastases. European Journal of Surgical Oncology. 2008;**34**:185-190

[101] Eng OS, Tsang AT, Moore D, Chen C, Narayanan S, Gannon CJ, et al. Outcomes of microwave ablation for colorectal cancer liver metastases: A single center experience. Journal of Surgical Oncology. 2015;**111**:410-413

[102] Stattner S, Jones RP, Yip VS, Buchanan K, Poston GJ, Malik HZ, et al. Microwave ablation with or without resection for colorectal liver metastases. European Journal of Surgical Oncology. 2013;**39**:844-849

[103] Donadon M, Procopio F, Torzilli G. Tailoring the area of hepatic resection using inflow and outflow modulation. World Journal of Gastroenterology. 2013;**19**:1049-1055

[104] Torzilli G, Procopio F. State of the art of intraoperative ultrasound in liver surgery: Current use for resection-guidance. Chirurgia. 2017;**112**:320-325

[105] Torzilli G, Procopio F, Costa G. Resection guidance. In: Torzilli G, editor. Ultrasound-Guided Liver Surgery. Italia: Springer; 2014. pp. 117-168

[106] Xiang C, Liu Z, Dong J, Sano K, Makuuchi M. Precise anatomical resection of the ventral part of Segment VIII. International Journal of Surgery Case Reports. 2014;**5**:924-926

[107] Torzilli G, Procopio F, Palmisano A, Donadon M, Del Fabbro D. Total or partial anatomical resection of segment 8 using the ultrasound-guided finger compression technique. HPB: The Official Journal of the International Hepato Pancreato Biliary Association. 2011;**13**:586-591

[108] Torzilli G, Procopio F, Palmisano A, Cimino M, Del Fabbro D. New technique for defining the right anterior section intraoperatively using ultrasound-guided finger counter-compression. Journal of the American College of Surgeons. 2009;**209**:e8-11

[109] Torzilli G, Makuuchi M. Ultrasound-guided finger compression in liver subsegmentectomy for hepatocellular carcinoma. Surgical Endoscopy. 2004;**18**:136-139

[110] Torzilli G, Donadon M, Cimino M, Del Fabbro D, Procopio F. Systematic subsegmentectomy by ultrasound-guided finger compression for hepatocellular carcinoma in cirrhosis. Annals of Surgical Oncology. 2009;**16**:1843

[111] Torzilli G, Donadon M, Palmisano A, Del Fabbro D, Spinelli A. Back-flow bleeding control during resection of right-sided liver tumors by means of ultrasound-guided finger compression of the right hepatic vein at its caval confluence. Hepato-Gastroenterology. 2007;**54**:1364-1367

[112] Peloso A, Franchi E, et al. Combined use of intraoperative ultrasound and indocyanine green fluorescence imaging to detect liver metastases from colorectal cancer. HPB. 2013;**15**:928-934

[113] Uchiyama K, Ueno M, Ozawa S, Kiriyama S, Shigekawa Y, Yamaue H. Combined use of contrast-enhanced intraoperative ultrasonography and a fluorescence navigation system for identifying hepatic metastases. World Journal of Surgery. 2010;**34**:2953-2959

[114] Frangioni JV. In vivo near-infrared fluorescence imaging. Current Opinion in Chemical Biology. 2003;**7**:626-634

[115] Noura S, Ohue M, Seki Y, et al. Feasibility of a lateral region sentinel node biopsy of lower rectal cancer guided by indocyanine green using a near-infrared camera system. Annals of Surgical Oncology. 2010;**17**:144-151

[116] Murawa D, Hirche C, Dresel S, et al. Sentinel lymph node biopsy in breast cancer guided by indocyanine green fluorescence. The British Journal of Surgery. 2009;**96**:1289-1294

[117] Aoki T, Yasuda D, Shimizu Y, et al. Image-guided liver mapping using fluorescence navigation system with indocyanine green for anatomical hepatic resection. World Journal of Surgery. 2008;**32**:1763-1767

[118] Gotoh K, Yamada T, Ishikawa O, et al. A novel imageguided surgery of hepatocellular carcinoma by indocyanine green fluorescence imaging navigation. Journal of Surgical Oncology. 2009;**100**:75-79

[119] Kikuchi M, Hosokawa K. Near-infrared fluorescence venography: A navigation system for varicose surgery. Dermatologic Surgery. 2009;**35**:1495-1498

[120] Spinoglio G, Priora F, Bianchi PP, Lucido FS, Licciardello A, Maglione V, Grosso F, Quarati R, Ravazzoni F, Lenti LM. Real-time near-infrared (NIR) fluorescent cholangiography in single-site robotic cholecystectomy (SSRC): A single-institutional prospective study. Surgical Endoscopy. 2013;**27**:2156-2162

[121] Ishizawa T, Bandai Y, Kokudo N. Fluorescent cholangiography using indocyanine green for laparoscopic cholecystectomy: An initial experience. Archives of Surgery. 2009;**144**:381-382

[122] Kudo H, Ishizawa T, Tani K, Harada N, Ichida A, Shimizu A, Kaneko J, Aoki T, Sakamoto Y, Sugawara Y, Hasegawa K, Kokudo N. Visualization of subcapsular hepatic malignancy by indocyanine-green fluorescence imaging during laparoscopic hepatectomy. Surgical Endoscopy. 2014;**28**:2504-2508

[123] Terasawa M, Ishizawa T, et al. Applications of fusion-fluorescence imaging using indocyanine green in laparoscopic hepatectomy. Surgical Endoscopy. 2017;**31**(12):5111-5118. DOI: 10.1007/s00464-017-5576-z

[124] Ishizawa T, Tamura S, Masuda K, Aoki T, Hasegawa K, Imamura H, Beck Y, Kokudo N. Intraoperative fluorescent cholangiography using indocyanine green: A biliary road map for safe surgery. Journal of the American College of Surgeons. 2008;**208**:e1-e4

[125] Mitsuhashi N, Kimura F, Shimizu H, Imamaki M, Yoshidome H, Ohtsuka M, Kato A, Yoshitomi H, Nozawa S, Furukawa K, Takeuchi D, Takayashiki T, Suda K, Igarashi T, Miyazaki M. Usefulness of intraoperative fluorescence imaging to evaluate local anatomy in hepatobiliary surgery. Journal of Hepato-Biliary-Pancreatic Surgery. 2008;**15**:508-514

[126] Ishizawa T, Bandai Y, Ijichi M, Kokudo N. Fluorescent cholangiography illuminating the biliary tree during laparoscopic cholecystectomy. The British Journal of Surgery. 2010;**97**:1369-1377

[127] Ishizawa T, Fukushima N, Shibahara J, Masuda K, Tamura S, Aoki T, Hasegawa K, Beck Y, Fukayama M, Kokudo N. Real-time identification of liver cancers by using indocyanine green fluorescent imaging. Cancer. 2009;**115**:2491-2504

[128] Yokoyama N, Otani T, Hashidate H, Maeda C, Katada T, Sudo N, Manabe S, Ikeno Y, Toyoda A, Katayanagi N. Real-time detection of hepatic micrometastases from pancreatic cancer by intraoperative fluorescence imaging: Preliminary results of a prospective study. Cancer. 2012;**118**:2813-2819

[129] van der Vorst JR, Schaafsma BE, Hutteman M, Verbeek FP, Liefers GJ, Hartgrink HH, Smit VT, CW Löwik, van de Velde CJ, Frangioni JV, Vahrmeijer AL. Near-infrared fluorescence-guided resection of colorectal liver metastases. Cancer. 2013;**119**(18):3411-3418

[130] Ishizawa T, Masuda K, Urano Y, Kawaguchi Y, Satou S, Kaneko J, Hasegawa K, Shibahara J, Fukayama M, Tsuji S, Midorikawa Y, Aburatani H, Kokudo N. Mechanistic background and clinical applications of indocyanine green-fluorescence imaging of hepatocellular carcinoma. Annals of Surgical Oncology. 2014;21:440-448

[131] Ishizawa T, Zuker NB, Kokudo N, Gayet B. Positive and negative staining of hepatic segments by use of fluorescent imaging techniques during laparoscopic hepatectomy. Archives of Surgery. 2012;147:393-394

[132] Inoue Y, Arita J, Sakamoto T, Ono Y, Takahashi M, Takahashi Y, Kokudo N, Saiura A. Anatomical liver resections guided by 3-dimensional parenchymal staining using fusion indocyanine green fluorescence imaging. Annals of Surgery. 2015;262(1):105-111

[133] Miyata A, Ishizawa T, Tani K, Shimizu A, Kaneko J, Aoki T, Sakamoto Y, Sugawara Y, Hasegawa K, Kokudo N. Reappraisal of a dye-staining technique for anatomic hepatectomy by the concomitant use of indocyanine green fluorescence imaging. Journal of the American College of Surgeons. 2015;221:e27-e36

[134] Landsman ML, Kwant G, Mook GA, Zijlstra WG. Lightabsorbing properties, stability, and spectral stabilization of indocyanine green. Journal of Applied Physiology. 1976;40:575-583

[135] Cherrick GR, Stein SW, Leevy CM, Davidson C. Indocyanine green: Observations on its physical properties, plasma decay, and hepatic extraction. The Journal of Clinical Investigation. 1960;39:592-600

[136] Kaibori M, Ishizaki M, Matsui K, Kwon AH. Intraoperative indocyanine green fluorescent imaging for prevention of bile leakage after hepatic resection. Surgery. 2011;150(1):91-98

[137] Liberale G, Bourgeois P. Indocyanine green fluoresce-guided surgery after IV injection in metastatic colorectal cancer: A systematic review. European Journal of Surgical Oncology. 2017;43:1656-1667

[138] Harlaar NJ, Koller M, de Jongh SJ, et al. Molecular fluorescenceguided surgery of peritoneal carcinomatosis of colorcetal origin: A single-centre feasibility study. The Lancet Gastroenterology & Hepatology. 2016;1:283-290

11

Psychosocial Aspects of Liver Transplantation and Liver Donation

Margörit Rita Krespi

Abstract

The construct of adjustment may help to understand the demands of end-stage liver failure (ESLF) and liver transplantation. Adjustment can be operationally defined on the basis of whether or not recipients and donors suffer from psychological problems and the ways in which they perceive their quality of life. For recipients of a transplant, evidence suggests that ESLF is related to the experience of psychological problems and poor quality of life, whereas transplantation is associated with less psychological problems and improvement in quality of life. Among donors, there is some evidence to suggest that organ donation surgery is associated with deterioration in quality of life and high levels of psychological problems. However, findings have been contradictory regarding the extent of these difficulties. Attempts to predict these outcomes are limited. More research is therefore needed. The construct of beliefs in general and the self-regulatory model of illness and qualitative research in particular could guide future attempts to explain these outcomes. Qualitative findings suggest that recipients and their donors experience ESLF and/or transplantation surgery or organ donation surgery in ways that are not identified by quantitative research. These findings can be used not only to develop ESLF-specific quality of life or emotional well-being questionnaires but also patient- or donor-derived interventions to improve poor outcomes.

Keywords: liver transplantation, liver donation, adjustment, quality of life, mood and anxiety disorders

1. Introduction

Two concepts including disease and illness can be differentiated. The concept of disease refers to changes that occur in the structure or functions of bodily systems, whereas the concept of illness refers to patients' perception of their symptoms and their own and their significant others' reactions to these symptoms [1].

In medicine, the concept of 'chronic patient' is a relatively recent concept [2]. Approximately, in the last 3 decades, a considerable amount of attention is given to chronic physical illnesses for two main reasons. First, medicine can effectively control infectious diseases [2]. Second, the number of patients with a chronic physical illness is increasing. A chronic physical illness refers to a long-lasting and incurable physical illness, although patients may not experience the symptoms all the time [2]. Currently, in developed countries, common causes of death are chronic physical illnesses [3]. Healthcare professionals dealing with patients with a chronic physical illness need to pay attention to both concepts of disease and illness if the aim is to provide a high quality of care which is responsive to all the needs of the patients and their significant others.

The treatment of chronic physical illnesses aims to slow down their course as well as to reduce distress resulting from associated physical symptoms. In many cases, medicine is uncertain about the mechanisms of cause and cure of these illnesses [2]; as a result the growing number of patients with a chronic physical illness presents themselves as a big challenge to healthcare professionals. In general, treatment involves changes in lifestyle (such as dietary restrictions), dependence on medical technology such as the use of medication and artificial means to replace bodily functions.

The main characteristic of the ESLF is the liver failing to execute its main functions of digesting, metabolizing and storing the essential nutrients [4]. ESLF occurs due to a number of causes. Hepatitis, liver diseases, metabolic conditions and cancer of the liver constitute some causes of ESLF [5]. Cadaveric and living donor transplantations are the main choices of treatment. Transplantation not only aims to achieve maximal quality and quantity of life but also to minimize the effects of illness and its costs [6].

Cadaveric transplantation is preferred over living donor transplantation, but the former has a number of disadvantages including long waiting time and low chance of survival [7]. In addition, cadaveric liver transplantation generally requires inpatient treatment and care which may also decrease the chances for survival [7]. The waiting time of the cadaveric liver transplantation is generally long, but available cadaveric donors are scarce [7–10].

In living donor transplantation, a healthy individual related by blood or an individual who is considered by the ethical committee as suitable to donate, although not related by blood, provides a transplant. This form of transplantation has the advantage of decreasing the time that candidates wait for a transplant and increasing the survival rate [11]. However, adult-to-adult transplantation is a complicated procedure because approximately 60% of the liver of the donor, in other words the entire right lobe, is used [12].

Due to advances in liver transplant procedures and immunosuppressive medications, the prognosis following transplantation is good, and the survival rate after 1 year and 8 years of transplantation is approximately 85–90 and 61%, respectively [6, 13]. Some donors are likely to develop complications after organ donation surgery such as biliary problems, reoperation and persistent physical symptoms [9, 14–16]. Donor mortality ranges from 0.1 to 0.3% [17].

This means that transplantation has the possibility of endangering the health of donors. Therefore, in order to maintain their health, they are asked to go through an interdisciplinary preoperative evaluation involving a series of medical as well as psychosocial assessments. This evaluation aims to ensure that they made autonomous and voluntary decisions to donate, and they can cope with the requirements and/or outcomes of organ donation surgery [18–20]. In general, medical inclusion criteria for liver donation include being between the age of 21 and 55, being within the normal weight range, the absence of any liver disease or any other significant disease such as cardiovascular diseases or diabetes and being free of any viral infection such as viral hepatitis or HIV [21, 22].

Recipients of a liver transplant and their donors are required to change their behavior or lifestyle to meet the demands brought by ESLF and transplantation or surgery for liver donation. Therefore, they both tend to face adaptational difficulties. The construct of adjustment may help to understand these difficulties. Adjustment can be defined in different ways depending on different assumptions. One way of defining adjustment involves whether or not the recipients or donors experience psychological problems (such as depression, anxiety or distress) or difficulties in overall functioning. Another way of defining adjustment is to do it in global terms by, for example, in terms of overall quality of life.

The impact of chronic illness in general and ESLF in particular goes beyond the patient himself or herself to all individuals who the patient is interacting with [1]. In general, a chronic illness can potentially influence various dimensions of life including interpersonal relationships, economic conditions and daily as well as social functioning [1]. Therefore, it is essential to understand the ways in which transplantation or surgery for liver donation influences both recipients and donors in order to formulate appropriate criteria for selecting suitable donors and promote donors and recipients' adjustment.

While reviewing the adaptational difficulties of recipients and their donors, it is important to review the difficulties experienced at pre-transplant and the ways in which these difficulties change across different time points following transplantation or organ donation surgery. Moreover, the adaptational difficulties will be reviewed on the basis of the construct of adjustment. For the purpose of this chapter, the construct of adjustment will be operationally defined on the basis of whether or not recipients and donors suffer from psychological problems and the ways in which they perceive their quality of life.

To that effect the search strategy aimed to identify all studies relevant to the experience of adaptational difficulties by recipients of a liver transplant and their donors. A number of databases were searched from 1985 to 2017. These databases included Medline, Embase, Psychinfo, PsycArticles and the Cochrane Library. A number of keywords were used. These keywords included chronic liver disease, ESLF, adjustment, quality of life, anxiety, depression, emotional well-being, mood disorders, psychological distress, psychological problems and psychiatric problems.

2. Recipients' experience

Both quantitative and qualitative studies have aimed to understand the adaptational difficulties experienced by the recipients.

2.1. Quantitative research

2.1.1. Psychological problems

Among candidates of liver transplant, reviews [23] have shown that the most common psychological problems at pre-transplant period include delirium, alcohol and substance misuse, anxiety and depressive disorders. In particular, the rates of depression, anxiety and delirium have varied from 4.5–64%, 20–50% and 50–56%, respectively [24–32].

Suitability of candidates with major mental illnesses for liver transplantation is subject to controversy. It has been argued that the presence of a major mental illness should not be an automatic exclusion criterion. Indeed evidence suggests that candidates with schizophrenia can be successfully transplanted [33]. It has been found that 27% of the sample had a severe personality disorder and 40% of this subsample were put on the transplantation list [34]. Therefore, specific exclusion criteria for those who suffer from a major mental illness may include poor compliance with medical and psychiatric follow-up appointments and poor quality of social support [33].

At post-transplantation, psychological problems experienced by the recipients include delirium, anxiety, depression, dysthymia, adjustment disorder, psychosis, post-traumatic stress disorder (PTSD) and substance related disorder [35–38]. Eighteen to twenty-seven percent of recipients report at least one disorder [38–40]. For example, it was reported that 23% of recipients experienced symptoms of PTSD, and among these recipients, 50% also experienced major depression [38]. However, the rate of depression has ranged from 5–46% across different studies [38, 41]. Nevertheless, the rate of psychological problems was the same as the general population [38].

Some studies have examined whether or not at post-transplant, the rate of psychological problems changes compared to that of pre-transplant. For example, while within 3 months post-transplant, the rate of these problems has been estimated to be 54% [36] at 1- and 3-year follow-up this rate has been estimated to be 7 and 2%, respectively [42]. Research has also shown that levels of different mood problems such as depression and anxiety have got reduced after transplantation [43]. In contrast another study found that there was no difference in terms of depressive symptoms prior and following transplantation [44].

Recipients also tend to experience different psychological problems at different time periods following transplantation. For example, it was found that recipients experienced depressive symptoms more commonly while they were in the intensive care unit, whereas they experienced anxiety symptoms more commonly after discharge from hospital [45].

2.1.2. Quality of life

Reviews [46] have shown that quality of life of candidates is poor at pre-transplantation. Indeed, the extent of impairment is greater than that of hospitalized patients with pneumonia, outpatients with rheumatoid arthritis, patients with minor nonacute conditions and the general population but similar to those of patients with peripheral vascular illness and osteoarthritis [47, 48].

After transplantation, systematic reviews and individual studies [44, 49–52] have shown that recipients have better quality of life. Studies indicate improvement in many areas including emotional, cognitive, social, behavioral, vocational, domestic and sexual areas [53]. A review showed that transplantation improved many dimensions of quality of life. These dimensions included physical health, sexual and social functioning, daily activities as well as overall quality of life [46]. Most positive changes were reported in physical, sexual and daily functioning and overall quality of life, whereas less positive changes were reported in psychological and social areas.

Prospective studies have also shown similar findings. One such study showed that recipients' general well-being was improved and the experience of physical symptoms (including tiredness, exhaustion and weakness) got reduced 1 year post-transplantation [54]. Similarly another prospective study reported improvements in cognitive areas and overall quality of life [55].

In contrast, evidence also suggests that observed positive changes in quality of life disappear when this is adjusted for those who died and that at a follow-up of 10 years, recipients' cognitive functioning and quality of life are poor [56, 57].

In addition, some systematic reviews and individual studies [51, 52] have shown that recipients have poorer quality of life in most dimensions of quality of life than healthy controls. In contrast, other studies have shown that quality of life of recipients is not different from or is higher than those of general population and patients with chronic liver disease at 1 year post-transplantation [58, 59].

Other studies have shown that high levels of psychological difficulties such as anxiety and depression reduce quality of life directly or as a mediator. For example, it was found that at pre-transplant, 31.1 and 25.8% of recipients were clinically significant for anxiety and depression, respectively, as compared to the rates observed in the general population (12.6 and 3.6% for anxiety and depression, respectively [59]). Those recipients with anxiety and depression within clinically significant levels also reported worse quality of life at post-transplantation. Similarly, following transplantation quality of life gets improved, and improvement in mood following transplantation is also related to improvement in quality of life [4, 43, 46, 54, 60, 61]. For example, one of these studies found that recipients without anxiety or depression symptoms at pre-transplant reported quality of life within the normal range at post-transplantation [60].

2.2. Qualitative research

Studies have shown that patients with ESLF experience their illness by going through two stages including 'becoming ill' and 'not living' [62]. Accordingly, the stage of 'becoming ill' includes interpreting the illness as an illness which develops insidiously, doubting the illness in the absence of experiencing its signs and managing the illness (such as by being positive, independent and supported by the family and friends) and managing its physical symptoms (such as tiredness). The stage of 'not living' includes losing independence due to deterioration in physical functioning, becoming disabled and wishing to return to a normal life by regaining independence. Other studies have provided specific information on the ways in which recipients of a transplant progress from physical, social and psychological dependence to independence [63]. The same study also showed that at pre-transplant period, recipients recounted that their quality of life was poor and their physical problems prevented their inde-pendence, their social activity, the fulfillment of personal goals and management of psycho-logical issues. At post-transplant period, recipients recounted that they wished to socially integrate and achieve control but significant others limited their independence by overpro-tecting them. A principled personality, optimistic outlook, incentives and professional sup-port helped toward independence.

Candidates or recipients of liver transplant reported that they not only experienced nega-tive emotions (such as fear, guilt, anxiety, frustration, embarrassment and uncertainty), mood fluctuations, lack of activity and energy and physical symptoms (such as pain and discomfort) but also negative social changes such as isolation, stigma, dependence on carers, carers' over-protection and restrictions in lifestyle [64–69].

Only one study examined the views of donors on the ways in which recipients evaluated their life as a result of the diagnosis of ESLF and transplantation [70]. Accordingly, donors felt that prior to transplantation in addition to experiencing social limitations, recipients experienced others both negatively (such as being frightened of getting infected by ESLF and others being insensitive) and positively (such as being supported by others). The experience of negative (such as feeling down, hopeless, like a loser) and positive feelings (such as feeling happy and relaxed) as well as improvement in life characterized recipients' experience according to donors. Improvement in life included not only physical and social improvements but also altering life perspective (such as appreciating that ESLF is serious and holding onto life).

3. Donors' experience

Both quantitative and qualitative studies have aimed to understand the adaptational difficul-ties experienced by donors.

3.1. Quantitative research

3.1.1. Becoming a donor

The experience of becoming a donor was characterized with ambivalence. There are two dif-ferent types of ambivalence [71]. Residual ambivalence comprised uncertainty feelings and hesitation about the process of donation (such as being frightened of going through with donation) that continue to be present after medical assessments. Acute ambivalence refers to feelings of indecision present during the psychosocial assessment which prevent the prospec-tive donor to give informed consent [18]. Acute ambivalence is uncommon (less than 2%) [72–74], whereas residual ambivalence is common (75%) [75–79].

Studies suggest that donors tend to make decisions that are not informed. A systematic review showed that a high percentage (89–95%) of donors felt they comprehended medical information provided by healthcare professionals regarding drawbacks and benefits of dona-tion, although they reported that their needs for information and knowledge regarding the risks and possible complications were not met [80].

Although a small minority of donors (less than 5%) report to regret their decision to donate [81–84], the majority (80–100%) of donors report to be willing to donate again [77, 84–87]. Those donors who are hesitant or regret donating explain this on the basis of the specific characteristics of their situation (such as risky behaviors of the recipient) rather than the characteristics of the donation process (such as medical risks). Relatedly, donors who believe that the recipient is healthy are willing to donate again, whereas donors who believe that recipients risk their transplant are not willing to donate again.

3.1.2. Psychological problems

Compared to studies which examined the extent of psychological problems among candidates or recipients of liver transplant, not many studies have examined the extent of these problems among donors.

At pre- and/or post-donation periods, psychological problems that are experienced include low self-esteem, stress and low confidence [88, 89] and mood and anxiety disorders [37, 38, 90–92].

Although some studies suggest that donors' mental health gets improved at post-donation period [88, 93–95], other studies report that the extent of psychological distress is one in every four donors [85, 95, 96].

3.1.3. Quality of life

As in the case of candidates or recipients of liver transplant, the findings regarding to quality of life of donors have been mixed both at pre-donation and post-donation.

Before liver donation, evidence has suggested that quality of life of donors is low [97]. Yet many studies have suggested that the levels are better than that of general population [87, 92, 98, 99], whereas other studies have shown that donors report poorer quality of life based on mental dimensions [100] as compared to healthy controls.

After donation quality of life has been found to be high among donors [15, 94], and physical and mental aspects of quality of life are equivalent to and even higher than that of general population [81, 84, 86, 87, 90, 100–102]. Recent systematic reviews [103] have shown similar findings.

Evidence suggests that prior to organ donation, quality of life of donors is good, but following donation quality of life gets reduced particularly with regard to physical aspects and activities of daily living [99]. Compared to general population, evidence suggests that prior to donation, quality of life of donors is equal to and in some cases higher but following donation the physical but not mental dimensions of quality of life deteriorate, and this level returns to starting levels at 6-month to 1-year follow-up [87, 100]. More specifically, in one of these studies, donors returned to work at 1 year post-donation, but their levels of physical functioning contrasted with those of mental functioning [87]. With regard to social aspects, most donors do not report any changes in their relationship with recipients or report that their relationship gets improved post-donation [84, 87]. However, closer relationships including relationship with the spouse get worsened [81, 101, 104].

Relatedly, studies show that donors rate their physical health as fair to poor or worse following donation [77, 95, 101, 105]. More specifically, it was shown that quality of life was worse at 2-year than 5-year follow-up [106]. Donors also suffer from debilitating symptoms including pain around the scar, fatigue and poor body image [84, 87–89, 94–96, 105, 107]. In particular, difficulties in quality of life are related to financial difficulties, negative changes in employment status or social relationships as indicated by reviews [15].

As in the case with recipients of transplant, reviews [15] show that donors who report poor quality of life also report psychological problems.

3.2. Qualitative research

More qualitative research has been undertaken to examine the experience of donors than that of recipients.

A number of qualitative studies have explored the donors' views on becoming a donor. Accordingly, donors perceive the process of becoming a donor as an automatic response and as an opportunity to help the loved one [67, 108, 109]. The donors felt that they had no choice and decided to be a donor by prioritizing the recipient's life, viewing transplantation as the last chance for the recipient and her family and feeling obligated to save the recipient [110]. More specifically, this study showed that donors decided on becoming a donor by going through five stages [110]. The first stage, recognition, involves learning of liver transplantation from recipients, family, doctors or media; the second stage, digestion, involves realizing the seriousness of liver transplantation and wanting to save recipients from suffering and avoiding the guilt; the third stage consists of making a decision; the fourth stage, reinforcement, involves the donors reinforcing themselves psychologically; the final stage, resolution, involves preparedness and acceptance of donation. Relatedly, it was also reported that donors give three types of consent [111]. 'Unconditional consent' is a voluntary consent to save family members' life; 'pressured consent' is a consent whereby the donor feels pressurized to become a donor but he/she feels frightened. 'Ulterior-motivated consent' refers to the situation when the donor has a hidden motive.

Relatedly, other studies have shown that donors consider donation to cope with guilt regarding their own health and to reduce the responsibility for the ESLF of the recipient [112]. In the same study, donors recounted that they would only donate to certain family members or close friends [88]. By contrast, in another study donors recounted that they would donate to people who were related by blood as well as to anybody whom they felt close to regardless of whether or not they were related by blood [113].

Only one study explored donors' beliefs of the ESLF of the recipients, their transplantation and their own organ donation surgery [113]. This study found that donors' beliefs could be viewed in a number of groups including beliefs about recipients ESLF, beliefs about being a donor, beliefs about surgery for organ donation and beliefs about organ donation. Beliefs about recipients' ESLF included diverse explanations for ESLF (such as spontaneous failure of the liver, worry, stress, senseless drug use, blaming oneself and physicians) and physical symptoms (such as cramps, itching, weakness, developmental slowing down). Beliefs about being a donor consisted of reasons for donating (such as being related by blood, saving a life, doing the right thing, being healed), barriers to being a donor (such as pregnancy, obesity, other people being senseless and selfish), ways of managing these barriers (such as getting significant others' consent and acting on one's gut feeling) and factors helping toward donation (such as the feeling that one does not have any responsibility). Beliefs about organ donation surgery included physical effects (such as pain, opening of stiches, putting on weight). The views that it is necessary to encourage organ donation and to raise people's awareness made up beliefs about organ donation.

In other qualitative studies, donors reported various feelings related to being a donor including not only negative emotions but also positive emotions. The former included feeling frightened, sad, anxious, angry and disappointed as well as feeling of being a failure, whereas positive emotions included feeling motivated and certain [109, 114, 115]. There was also the feelings of disappointment and anger toward medical system and insurance and the views that donation was not valued, that one is not supported and is not taken seriously by the medical staff [115]. Another study found that when the transplant did not fail, donors felt happy for having saved life. When the transplant failed, donors comforted themselves by the fact that they did everything they could [108].

On the other hand, a recent study found that donors experienced not only emotional changes but also changes in character. The former consisted of both negative (such as feeling angry, hopeless, down and helpless) and positive emotions (such as feeling appreciated, reputable, conscientiously comfortable). Changes in character were characterized by both worsening of (such as changing into an aggressive person) and positive changes in character (such as turning into a believer and stronger) [116].

The relationship of the donor with the recipient has been idealized [109], and difficulties about accepting recipients' ESLF have been experienced [114]. Research has also shown that there is a special bond between the recipient and the donor [116], in that the donor and the recipient become closer and donation is considered as a "proof of love" and the scar as a symbol of a special experience shared by the recipient and the donor only [117]. Moreover, the latter study also found that donation enhanced the positive or conflicting characteristics of the donor recipient relationship and there was not any deterioration in this relationship. Donors sometimes minimized the negative characteristics of this relationship and emphasized the improvements [117]. Similarly, another study reported that the extent of marital breakdown was lower than the general population. In the case of no marital breakdown, marital relationship has become stronger because of donation. In the case of marital breakdown, causes were independent of transplantation or donation process [108]. By contrast, another study reported that donors recounted mixed relationships. These included not only a continuum of feeling supported by significant others/doctors and not feeling supported by mothers or spouses but also formation of a special bond and worsening of close relationships [116]. Relatedly, it was reported that donors tend to postpone their personal needs such as emotional needs associated with rehabilitating oneself [108].

4. Correlates

A small number of quantitative studies have examined the effect, of a number of factors on outcomes among recipients of a liver transplant and their donors. For example, it was found that that 51–58% of the variance in quality of life was explained by a number of factors [60]. After transplantation among recipients, employment, age, and depression predicted physical aspects, whereas anxiety and depression predicted mental dimensions of quality of life. Transplant-related factors such as rejection of the transplant, the number and length of hospital stays, effectiveness of the medication and complications did not predict anxiety symptoms. However, more patients suffering from anxiety and/or depression went through re-transplantation.

Studies have shown that the experience of feelings including ambivalence about donation, hesitation and uncertainty are important predictors of poor adjustment and quality of life at post-donation period among donors [76, 86]. Moreover, it was also shown that donors who were concerned about their own health, finances and close relationships at pre-donation period had a history of psychiatric illness or present psychiatric illness and held a graduate degree reported poorer quality of life, although donors' medical complications were unre-lated to their quality of life [86].

5. Conclusion

To date, there are numerous studies among candidates or recipients of a liver transplant and their donors on their adjustment. Evidence suggests that ESLF is associated with adjustment difficulties including experience of psychological problems and poor quality of life among candidates or recipients of a liver transplant. However, findings have been contradictory regarding the extent of these difficulties partly due to different approaches that studies have taken to defining and measuring psychological problems and quality of life. Transplantation is associated with less psychological problems and improvement in quality of life, with more improvements in physical functioning and less improvements in psychosocial areas. However, although it can be argued that quality of life improves after transplantation, the ways in which this improvement continues over time are not clear. Some studies show that quality of life remains similar during follow-up, whereas other studies show subsequent deterioration. In studies which examine quality of life across different time points following transplantation, recipients with high mortality rates need to be accounted for to avoid bias.

There is also some evidence to suggest that contrary to recipients of a transplant, organ dona-tion surgery is associated with deterioration in quality of life, particularly in physical func-tioning among donors and experience of psychological problems and poor quality of life among donors. However, findings have also been contradictory regarding the extent of these difficulties partly due to different approaches that studies have taken to defining and measur-ing psychological problems and quality of life.

As mentioned above, contradictory or inconsistent findings may be due to methodological problems. More specifically, studies have mainly used generic measures of quality of life [81, 85, 101]. Such measures may not be specific and sensitive enough to understand adjustment-related issues among recipients of a transplant or their donors. Moreover, studies which examined the long-term implications of liver transplantation and donation have assessed recipients and donors at different times after surgery [19, 84].

Evidence also suggests that high levels of psychological problems such as anxiety and depres-sion negatively influence quality of life directly or as a mediator among recipients of a liver transplant and their donors. One explanation for this evidence is that high levels of these problems impair quality of life directly or as a mediator by, for example, maintaining the sick role [60]. Another explanation is that anxiety and depression may reduce compliance with treatment, and this in turn reduces quality of life [61].

Despite numerous studies on the extent of psychological problems and quality of life, attempts to predict these outcomes have fallen short. There is little evidence to conclude from quantitative studies that particular factors predict outcome. Therefore, more research is needed. The construct of beliefs could guide future attempts to explain these outcomes. A review on adjustment in end-stage renal failure (ESRF) [118] shows that although the variance explained in outcomes by beliefs is small, beliefs have been more consistent in predicting these outcomes than other variables such as social support. One exception for these small effects is the beliefs postulated by the self-regulatory model of illness [119, 120] which is developed on the basis of interviews with patients suffering from different types of chronic physical illnesses. This model includes beliefs about identity, cause, consequences, timeline and cure or controllability of a particular chronic physical illness. Future research may examine the ways in which these beliefs predict these outcomes.

An alternative approach to better understand these outcomes is to be guided by qualitative studies. In terms of beliefs, only one qualitative study [113] examined donors' beliefs about ESLF, transplantation and organ donation surgery. More qualitative research is needed, in particular about recipients' beliefs about ESLF and transplantation.

Overall, qualitative findings suggest that candidates or recipients of a liver transplant and their donors experience ESLF and/or transplantation surgery or organ donation surgery and the process of organ donation in ways that are not identified by quantitative research. God's will, blaming oneself, blaming physicians as causes for recipients' ESLFl, doing the right thing, being healed as reasons for being a donor, the views that others are frightened of getting infected by ESLF and insensitive, experience of positive emotions, ways of improving, worsening aspects of character and close relationships are among findings which extend quantitative findings. These findings can be used not only to develop ESLF-specific quality of life or emotional well-being questionnaires but also patient- or donor-derived interventions to improve poor outcomes.

Conflict of interest

There is no conflict of interest.

Author details

Margörit Rita Krespi

Address all correspondence to: margorit.boothby@khas.edu.tr

Kadir Has University, Istanbul, Turkey

References

[1] Falvo DR. Medical and Psychosocial Aspects of Chronic Illness and Disability. Jones and Bartlett Publishers, Inc., Burlington; 2018

[2] Radley A. Making Sense of Illness: The Social Psychology of Health and Disease. London: Sage Publications Ltd.; 1994

[3] Songer TJ. The economics of diabetes care. In: Alberti KGM, DeFronzo RA, Keen H, Zimmet P, editors. International Textbook of Diabetes Mellitus. Vol. 2. Chichester: John Wiley & Sons; 1992. pp. 1643-1673

[4] Bryan S, Ratcliffe J, Neuberger J, Burroughs A, Gunson B, Buxton M. Health-related quality of life following liver transplantation. Qualitative Life Research. 1998;**7**:115-120

[5] Charlton M, Kasparova P, Weston S, et al. Frequency of nonalcoholic steatohepatitis as a cause of advanced liver disease. Liver Transplantation. 2001;**7**:608-614

[6] Keeffe EB. Liver transplantation: Current status and novel approaches to liver replacement. Gastroenterology. 2001;**120**:749-762

[7] Sagmeister M, Mullhaupt B, Kadry Z, Kullak-Ublick GA, Clavien PA, Renner EL. Cost-effectiveness of cadaveric and living-donor liver transplantation. Transplantation. 2002;**73**:616-622

[8] Huang CH, Hu RH, Shih FJ, Chen HM. Motivations and decision-making dilemmas of overseas liver transplantation: Taiwan recipients' perspectives. Transplantation Proceedings. 2011;**43**:1754-1756

[9] Lo CM. Complications and long-term outcome of living liver donors: A survey of 1508 cases in five Asian centers. Transplantation. 2003;**75**:12-15

[10] Huang J. Ethical and legislative perspectives on liver transplantation in the People's Republic of China. Liver Transplantation. 2007;**13**:193-196

[11] Marcos A, Ham JM, Fisher RA, Olzinski AT, Posner MP. Single-center analysis of the first 40 adult-to-adult living donor liver transplants using the right lobe. Liver Transplantation. 2000;**6**:296

[12] Renz JF, Roberts JP. Long-term complications of living donor liver transplantation. Liver Transplantation. 2000;**6**:73-76

[13] Adam R, Cailliez V, Majno P, Karam V, McMaster P, Caine RY, et al. Normalised intrinsic mortality risk in liver transplantation: European liver transplant registry study. Lancet. 2000;**356**:621-627

[14] Adcock L, Macleod C, Dubay D, Greig PD, Cattral MS, McGilvray I. Adult living liver donors have excellent long-term medical outcomes: The University of Toronto liver transplant experience. American Journal of Transplantation. 2010;**10**:364-371

[15] Chen P-X, Yan L-N. Health-related quality of life in living liver donors after transplantation. Hepatobiliary Pancreatic Disease International. 2011;**10**(4):356-361

[16] Ran S, Wen TF, Yan LN, Li B, Zengi Y, Chen ZY. Risks faced by donors of right lobe for living donor liver transplantation. Hepotabiliary Pancreatic Disease International. 2009;**8**:581-585

[17] Seek AL, Sullivan MA, Pomfret EA. Transplantation of the right hepatic lobe. New England Journal of Medicine. 2002;**347**:615-618

[18] Erim Y, Malagó M, Valentin-Gamazo C, Senf W, Broelsch CE. Guidelines for the psychosomatic evaluation of living liver donors: Analysis of donor exclusion. Transplantation Proceedings. 2003;**35**(3):909-910

[19] Pascher A, Sauer IM, Walter M, et al. Donor evaluation, donor risks, donor outcome and donor quality of life in adult-to-adult living donor liver transplantation. Liver Transplantation. 2002;**8**:829

[20] Shrestha R. Psychosocial assessment of adult living liver donors. Liver Transplantation. 2003;**9**:8

[21] Brown RS. Live donors in liver transplantation. Gastroenterology. 2008;**134**(6):1802-1813

[22] Trotter JF, Wachs M, Trouillot T, Steinberg T, Bak T, Everson GT, Kam I. Evaluation of 100 patients for living donor liver transplantation. Liver Transplantation. 2000;**6**:290-295

[23] Grover S, Sarkar S. Liver transplant: Psychiatric and psychosocial aspects. Journal of Clinical and Experimental Hepatology. 2012;**2**(4):382-392

[24] Gish RG, Lee AH, Keeffe EB, Rome H, Concepcion W, Esquivel CO. Liver transplantation for patients with alcoholism and end-stage liver disease. American Journal of Gastroenterology. 1993;**88**:1337-1342

[25] Lopez-Navas A, Ríos A, Riquelme A, et al. Psychological characteristics of patients on the liver transplantation waiting list with depressive symptoms. Transplantation Proceedings. 2011;**43**:158-160

[26] Pelgur H, Atak N, Kose K. Anxiety and depression levels of patients undergoing liver transplantation and their need for training. Transplantation Proceedings. 2009;**41**: 1743-1748

[27] Singh N, Gayowski T, Wagener MM, Marino IR. Depression in patients with cirrhosis: Impact on outcome. Digestive Diseases Sciences. 1997;**42**:1421-1427

[28] Surman OS, Purtilo R. Reevaluation of organ transplantation criteria: Allocation of scarce resources to borderline candidates. Psychosomatics. 1992;**33**(2):202-212

[29] Telles-Correia D, Barbosa A, Mega I, Direitinho M, Morbey A, Monteiro E. Psychiatric differences between liver transplant candidates with familial amyloid polyneuropathy and those with alcoholic liver disease. Progress in Transplantation. 2008;**18**:134-139

[30] Telles-Correia D, Barbosa A, Mega I, Monteiro E. Importance of depression and active coping in liver transplant candidates' quality of life. Progress in Transplantation. 2009;**19**: 85-89

[31] Trzepacz PT, Maue FR, Coffman G, Van Thiel DH. Neuropsychiatric assessment of liver transplantation candidates: Delirium and other psychiatric disorders. International Journal of Psychiatry and Medicine. 1986;**16**:101-111

[32] Trzepacz PT, Brenner R, Van Thiel DH. A psychiatric study of 247 liver transplantation candidates. Psychosomatics. 1989;**30**:147-153 (32)

[33] DiMartini A, Twillman R. Organ transplantation and paranoid schizophrenia. Psychosomatics. 1994;**35**:159-161

[34] Yates W, LaBreque D, Pfab D. Personality disorder as a contradiction for liver transplantation. Psychosomatics. 1998;**39**:501-511

[35] Chiu N-M, Chen C-L, Cheng ATA. Psychiatric consultation for post-liver-transplantation patients. Psychiatry and Clinical Neuroscience. 2009;**63**:471-477

[36] Fukunishi I, Sugawara Y, Takayama T, Makuuchi M, Kawarasaki H, Surman OS. Psychiatric disorders before and after living-related transplantation. Psychosomatics. 2001;**42**:337-343

[37] Fukunishi I, Sugawara Y, Takayama T, Makuuchi M, Kawarasaki H, Surman OS. Association between pretransplant psychological assessments and posttransplant psychiatric disorders in living-related transplantation. Psychosomatics. 2002;**43**(1):49-54

[38] Rothenhausler H-B, Ehrentraut S, Kapfhammer H-P, et al. Psychiatric and psychosocial outcome of orthotopic liver transplantation. Psychotherapy and Psychosomatics. 2002;**71**:285-297

[39] Commander M, Neuberger J, Dean C. Psychiatric and social consequences of liver transplantation. British Journal of Psychiatry. 1992;**166**:521-524

[40] Collis I et al. Psychiatric and social consequences of liver transplantation. British Journal of Psychiatry. 1995;**166**:521-524

[41] Russell RT, Feurer ID, Wisawatapnimit P, Salomon RM, Pinson CW. The effects of physical quality of life, time, and gender on change in symptoms of anxiety and depression after liver transplantation. Journal of Gastrointestinal Surgery. 2008;**12**:138-144

[42] Menegaux F, Keeffe EB, Andrews BT, et al. Neurological complications of liver transplantation in adult versus pediatric patients. Transplantation. 1994;**58**:447-450

[43] Moore KA, Burrows GD, Hardy KJ. Anxiety in chronic liver disease: Changes post transplantation. Stress in Medicine. 1997;**13**:49-57

[44] Santos Junior R, Miyazaki MCOS, Domingos NAM, Valério NI, Silva RF, Silva RCMA. Patients undergoing liver transplantation: Psychosocial characteristics, depressive symptoms, and quality of life. Transplantation Proceedings. 2008;**40**:802-804

[45] Perez-San-Gregorio MA, Martin-Rodríguez A, Asián-Chavez E, Gallego-Corpa A, Pérez-Bernal J. Psychological adaptation of liver transplant recipients. Transplantation Proceedings. 2005;**37**:1502-1504

[46] Bravata DM, Olkin I, Barnato AE, Keeffe EB, Owens DK. Health-related quality of life after liver transplantation: A metaanalysis. Liver Transplantation Surgery. 1999;**5**:318-331

[47] Hunt S, McEwen J, McKenna S. Perceived health: Age and sex comparisons in a community. Journal of Epidemiology and Community Health. 1984;**38**:156-160

[48] Hunt SM, McEwen J, McKenna SP. Measuring health status: A new tool for clinicians and epidemiologists. Journal of Royal College of General Practice. 1985;**35**:185-188

[49] Estraviz B, Quintana JM, Valdivieso A, et al. Factors influencing change in health-related quality of life after liver transplantation. Clinical Transplantation. 2007;**21**:481

[50] Sainz-Barriga M, Baccarani U, Scudeller L, et al. Quality of life assessment before and after liver transplant. Transplantation Proceedings. 2005;**37**:2601

[51] Tome S, Wells JT, Said A, Lucey MR. Quality of life after liver transplantation: A systematic review. Journal of Hepatology. 2008;**48**:567-577

[52] Younossi ZM, McCormick M, Price LL, et al. Impact of liver transplantation on health-related quality of life. Liver Transplantation. 2000;**6**:779

[53] Tarter RE, Erb S, Biuller PA, Switala J, Van Thiel DH. The quality of life following liver transplantation: A preliminary report. Gastroenterology of Clinics North America. 1998; **17**(1):207-217

[54] Belle SH, Porayko MK, Hoofnagle JH, Lake JR, Zetterman RK. Changes in quality of life after liver transplantation among adults. Liver Transplantation Surgery. 1997;**3**:93-104

[55] Moore KA, Jones RM, Burrows GD. Quality of life and cognitive function of liver transplant patients: A prospective study. Liver Transplantation. 2000;**6**:633-642

[56] Ratcliffe J, Longworth L, Young T, Bryan S, Burroughs A, Buxton M. Cost-effectiveness of liver transplantation team assessing health-related quality of life pre and post-liver transplantation: A prospective multicenter study. Liver Transplantation. 2002;**8**:263-270

[57] Lewis MB, Howdle PD. Cognitive dysfunction and health-related quality of life in long-term liver transplant survivors. Liver Transplantation. 2003;**9**:1145-1148

[58] Pereira SP, Howard LM, Muiesan P, Rela M, Heaton N, Williams R. Quality of life after liver transplantation for alcoholic liver disease. Liver Transplantation. 2000;**6**:762-768

[59] O'Carroll RE, Couston M, Cossar J, Masterton G, Hayes PC. Psychological outcome and quality of life following liver transplantation: A prospective, national, single-center study. Liver Transplantation. 2003;**9**(7):712-720

[60] Nickel R, Wunsch A, Egle UT, Lohse AW, Otto G. The relevance of anxiety, depression, and coping in patients after liver transplantation. Liver Transplantation. 2002;**8**(1):63-71

[61] Bunzel B, Laederach-Hofmann K. Solid organ transplantation: Are there predictors for posttransplant. Transplantation. 2000;**70**:711-716

[62] Wainwright SP. Transcending chronic liver disease: A qualitative study. Journal of Clinical Nursing. 1997;**6**(1):49-53

[63] Robertson G. Individuals' perception of their quality of life following a liver transplant: An exploratory study. Journal of Advanced Nursing. 1999;**30**(2):497-505

[64] Bjork IT, Naden D. Patients' experiences of waiting for a liver transplantation. Nursing Inquiry. 2008;**15**:289e98

[65] Brown J, Sorrell JH, McClaren J, et al. Waiting for a liver transplant. Qualitative Health Research. 2006;**16**:119e36

[66] Chou CY, Chen YC, Chen CL, et al. Family experience of waiting for living donor liver transplantation: From parental donor perspective. Journal of Clinical Nursing. 2009;**18**:1684e92

[67] McGregor LM, Swanson V, Hayes PC, et al. Considering adult living donor liver transplantation: A qualitative study of patients and their potential donors. Psychology and Health. 2008;**25**:75166

[68] Sargent S, Wainwright SP. A qualitative study exploring patients perceived quality of life following an emergency liver transplant for acute liver failure. International Critical Care Nursing. 2007;**23**:272-280

[69] Weng LC, Huang HL, Wang YW, et al. Primary caregiver stress in caring for a living-related liver transplantation recipient during the postoperative stage. Journal of Advanced Nursing. 2011;**67**:1749e57

[70] Tankurt A, Krespi Boothby MR, Acarlı K, Kalayoğlu M, Kanmaz T, Yankol Y. Liver transplantation: Recipients' evaluation of life from the perspective of living donors. Transplantation Proceedings. 2016;**48**:107-110

[71] Simmons RG, Klein SD, Simmons RL. Gift of Life: The Social and Psychological Impact of Organ Transplantation. Brunswick, NJ: Transaction Books; 1987

[72] Erim Y, Beckmann M, Valentin-Gamazo C, et al. Selection of donors for adult living-donor liver donation: Results of the assessment of the first 205 donor candidates. Psychosomatics. 2008;**49**(2):143-151

[73] Jendrisak MD, Hong B, Shenoy S, et al. Altruistic living donors: Evaluation for nondirected kidney or liver donation. American Journal of Transplantation. 2006;**6**(1):115-120

[74] Valentin-Gamazo C, Malago M, Karliova M, et al. Experience after the evaluation of 700 potential donors for living donor liver transplantation in a single center. Liver Transplantation. 2004;**10**(9):1087-1096

[75] DiMartini A, Cruz RJ Jr, Dew MA, et al. Motives and decision making of potential living liver donors: Comparisons between gender, relationships and ambivalence. American Journal of Transplantation. 2012;**12**(1):136-151

[76] Hayashi A, Noma S, Uehara M, et al. Relevant factors to psychological status of donors before living-related liver transplantation. Transplantation. 2007;**84**(10):1255-1261

[77] Kusakabe T, Irie S, Ito N, Kazuma K. Feelings of living donors about adult-to-adult living donor liver transplantation. Gastroenterology Nursing. 2008;**31**(4):263-272

[78] Lee SH, Jeong JS, Ha HS, et al. Decision-related factors and attitudes toward donation in living related liver transplantation: Ten-year experience. Transplantation Proceedings. 2005;**37**(2):1081-1084

[79] Simpson A, Kendrick J, Verbesey JE, et al. Ambivalence in living liver donors. Liver Transplantation. 2011;**17**(10):1226-1233

[80] Gordon EJ, Daud A, Caicedo J C, Cameron KA, Jay C; Fryer J, Beauvais N, Skaro A, Baker T. Informed consent and decision-making about adult-to-adult living donor liver transplantation: A systematic review of empirical research. Transplantation. 2011; **92**(12):1285-1296

[81] Karliova M, Malago M, Valentin-Gamazo C, et al. Living- related liver transplantation from the view of the donor: A 1-year followup survey. Transplantation. 2002;**73**:1799-1804

[82] Reichman TW, Fox A, Adcock L, et al. Anonymous living liver donation: Donor profiles and outcomes. American Journal of Transplantation. 2010;**10**(9):2099-2104

[83] Sevmis S, Diken T, Boyvat F, et al. Right hepatic lobe donation: Impact on donor quality of life. Transplantation Proceedings. 2007;**39**:826

[84] Trotter JF, Talamantes M, McClure M, et al. Right hepatic lobe donation for living donor liver transplantation: Impact on donor quality of life. Liver Transplantation. 2001;**7**(6):485-493

[85] Beavers KL, Sandler RS, Fair JH, et al. The living donor experience: Donor health assessment and outcomes after living donor liver transplantation. Liver Transplantation. 2001; **7**:943

[86] DuBay DA, Holtzman S, Adcock L, et al. Adult right-lobe living liver donors: Quality of life, attitudes and predictors of donor outcomes. American Journal of Transplantation. 2009;**9**(5):1169-1178

[87] Verbesey JE, Simpson MA, Pomposelli JJ, et al. Living donor adult liver transplantation: A longitudinal study of the donor's quality of life. American Journal of Transplantation. 2005;**5**(11):2770-2777

[88] Chan SC, Liu CL, Lo CM, Lam BK, Lee EW, Fan ST. Donor quality of life before and after adult-to-adult right liver live donor liver transplantation. Liver Transplantation. 2006;**12**(10):1529-1536

[89] DuBay DA, Holtzman S, Adcock L, et al. Cosmesis and body image after adult right lobe living liver donation. Transplantation. 2010;**89**(10):1270-1275

[90] Erim Y, Beckmann M, Valentin-Gamazo C, et al. Quality of life and psychiatric complications after adult living donor liver transplantation. Liver Transplantation. 2006; **12**(12):1782-1790

[91] Trotter JF, Hill-Callahan MM, et al. Severe psychiatric problems in right hepatic lobe donors for living donor liver transplantation. Transplantation. 2007;**83**(11):1506-1508

[92] Walter M, Bronner E, Steinmuller T, Klapp BF, Danzer G. Psychosocial data of potential living donors before living donor liver transplantation. Clinical Transplantation. 2002;**16**(1):55-59

[93] Basaran O, Karakayali H, Emiroğlu R, Tezel E, Moray G, Haberal M. Donor safety and quality of life after left hepatic lobe donation in living-donor liver transplantation. Transplantation Proceedings. 2003;**35**:2768-2769

[94] Feltrin A, Pegoraro R, Rago C, et al. Experience of donation and quality of life in living kidney and liver donors. Transplantation International. 2008;**21**(5):466-472

[95] Walter M, Bronner E, Pascher A, et al. Psychosocial outcome of living donors after living donor liver transplantation: A pilot study. Clinical Transplantation. 2002;**16**(5):339-344

[96] Hsu HT, Hwang SL, Lee PH, Chen SC. Impact of liver donation on quality of life and physical and psychological distress. Transplantation Proceedings. 2006;**38**(7):2102-2105

[97] Walter M, Dammann G, Papachristou C, Pascher A, Neuhaus P, Danzer G, Klapp BF. Quality of life of living donors before and after living donor liver transplantation. Transplantation Proceedings. 2003;**35**(8):2961-2963

[98] Erim Y, Beckmann M, Kroencke S, et al. Sense of coherence and social support predict living liver donors' emotional stress prior to living-donor liver transplantation. Clinical Transplantation. 2008;**22**(3):273-280

[99] Schultz KH, Kroencke S, Beckmann M, et al. Mental and physical quality of life in actual living liver donors versus potential living liver donors: A prospective, controlled, multicenter study. Liver Transplantation. 2009;**15**(12):1676-1687

[100] Erim Y, Beckmann M, Kroencke S, et al. Psychological strain in urgent indications for living donor liver transplantation. Liver Transplantation. 2007;**13**:886

[101] Kim-Schluger L, Florman SS, Schiano T, et al. Quality of life after lobectomy for adult liver transplantation. Transplantation. 2002;**73**(10):1593-1597

[102] Kousoulas L, Emmanouilidis N, Klempnauer J, Lehner F. Living-donor liver transplantation: Impact on donor's health-related quality of life. Transplantation Proceedings. 2011;**43**:3584-3587

[103] Parikh ND, Ladner D, Abecassis M, Butt Z. Quality of life for donors after living donor liver transplantation: A review of the literature. Liver Transplantation. 2010; **16**(12):1352-1358

[104] Sterneck MR, Fischer L, Nischwitz U, et al. Selection of the living liver donor. Transplantation. 1995;**60**(7):667-671

[105] Azoulay D, Bhangui P, Andreani P, et al. Short and longterm donor morbidity in right lobe living donor liver transplantation: 91 consecutive cases in a European Center. American Journal of Transplantation. 2011;**11**(1):101-110

[106] De Bona M, Ponton P, Ermani M. The impact of liver disease and medical complications on quality of life and psychological distress before and after liver transplantation. Journal of Hepatology. 2000;**33**:609-615

[107] Diaz GC, Renz JF, Mudge C, et al. Donor health assessment after living-donor liver transplantation. Annals of Surgery. 2002;**236**(1):120-126

[108] Crowley-Matoka M, Siegler M, Cronin DC. Long-term quality of life issues among adult-to-pediatric living liver donors: A qualitative exploration. American Journal of Transplantation. 2004;**4**:744-750

[109] Walter M, Papachristou C, Danzer G, et al. Willingness to donate: An interview study before liver transplantation. Journal of Medical Ethics. 2004;**30**:544-550

[110] Fujita M, Akabayashi A, Taylor Slingsby B, Kosugi S, Fujimoto Y, Tanaka K. A model of donors' decision-making in adult-to-adult living donor liver transplantation in Japan: Having no choice. Liver Transplantation. 2006;**12**:768-774

[111] Fujita M, Slingsby BT, Akabayashi A. Three pattern of voluntary consent in the case of adult-to adult living related liver transplantation in Japan. Transplant Proceedings. 2004;**36**:1425e8

[112] Papachristou C, Walter M, Dietrich K, Danzer G, Klupp J, Klapp BF, Frommer J. Motivation for living-donor liver transplantation from the donor's perspective: An in-depth qualitative research study. Transplantation. 2004;**78**:1506-1514

[113] Krespi MR, Tankurt A· Acarlı K, Kanmaz T, Yankol Y, Kalayoğlu M. Beliefs of living donors about recipients' end-stage liver failure and surgery for organ donation. Transplantation Proceedings. 2017;**49**:1369-1375

[114] Papachristou C, Walter M, Frommer J, Klapp BF. Decision-making and risk-assessment in living liver donation: How informed is the informed consent of donors? A qualitative study. Psychosomatics. 2010;**51**(4):312-319

[115] Walter M, Papachristou C, Pascher A, Danzer G, Neuhaus P, Klapp BF, Frommer J. Impaired psychosocial outcome of donors after living donor liver transplantation: A qualitative case study. Clinical Transplantation. 2006;**20**:410-415

[116] Krespi MR, Tankurt A, Acarlı K, Yankol Y, Munci K, Kanmaz T. Post-donation evaluation of life of donors of liver transplantation. Cogent Psychology. 2016;**3**:1262724

[117] Papachristou C, Walter M, Schmid G, Frommer J, Klapp BF. Living donor liver transplantation and its effect on the donor–recipient relationship: A qualitative interview study with donors. Clinical Transplantation. 2009;**23**:382-391

[118] Krespi Boothby MR. Shift in paradigm: Understanding of dialysis patients. Anatolian Journal of Psychiatry. 2017;**18**:292-299

[119] Leventhal H, Zimmerman R, Gutmann M. Compliance: A self regulation perspective. Handbook of Behavioral Medicine. 1984. pp. 369-436

[120] Meyer D, Leventhal H, Gutmann M. Common-sense models of illness: The example of hypertension. Health Psychology. 1985;**4**:115-135

12

Evaluation and Surgical Management of Hepatocellular Carcinoma

Adrian Bartoș, Cristian Cioltean, Caius Breazu and
Dana Bartoș

Abstract

Hepatocellular carcinoma (HCC) is the most frequent primary malignant tumor of the liver, being the sixth most common cancer in the world and the third cause of cancer mortality. Most of the patients with HCC have an established background of cirrhosis and chronic liver disease. Magnetic resonance imaging (MRI) is the best technique for evaluation of the liver nodules in patients with cirrhosis, especially when a HCC is suspected. HCC staging is mandatory to select the appropriate primary and adjuvant therapy and to evaluate the prognosis. Hepatic resection is the treatment of choice in non-cirrhotic patients who have been diagnosed with HCC. In this chapter we underline the main diagnostic methods used for HCC staging, together with the treatment possibilities, highlighting the importance of surgical management, conventional or minimally invasive.

Keywords: hepatocellular carcinoma, hepatic resections, laparoscopy, ablative therapy

1. Introduction: generalities

Hepatocellular carcinoma (HCC) is the most frequent primary malignant tumor of the liver, which is arising from hepatocytes, the liver's parenchymal cells. Most of the patients with HCC have an established background of cirrhosis and chronic liver disease due to hepatitis B virus or hepatitis C virus. HCC is the sixth most common cancer in the world and the third cause of cancer mortality [1].

2. Diagnosis

Clinical features of HCC may include pain in the upper right quadrant and weight loss. Most of the patients diagnosed with HCC are patients known with liver cirrhosis. Despite this fact, there is a rare complication such as rupture of a liver tumor with intra-abdominal bleeding, which will need immediate surgical care [2]. These patients will present with acute abdominal pain, peritoneal irritation and hypotension. Other patients present with nonspecific signs such as fever, jaundice, ascites, anorexia or encephalopathy [3].

Clinical examination can reveal an abdominal mass in the upper right quadrant or hepatomegaly. Obstructive jaundice can indicate tumor extension into the extrahepatic biliary structures [4].

HCC can metastasize to any organ, the most frequent being metastasis to bone, lung or other abdominal viscera; so, patients can present with various clinical signs and symptoms related to the affected organs. Watery diarrhea is more common in patients with cirrhosis and HCC because of the increased production of intestinal secretory substances such as gastrin and vasoactive intestinal peptide (VIP) [5, 6].

Alpha-1 fetoprotein is the most commonly used marker for HCC. Patients with AFP > 400 ng/ml tend to have a greater size, bilobar involvement, portal vein thrombosis and decreased survival [7]. If the tumor producing AFP is left untreated, the AFP value will increase over the time, so this marker can be used for detecting tumor progression. APF may be increased in a variety of other malignancies and in patients with chronic liver disease without HCC, particularly in hepatitis C [8]. The sensitivity, specificity and positive predictive value of AFP range from 39 to 64%, 76 to 91% and 9 to 32% [8]. Patients with values of AFP greater than 1000 ng/ml have a higher incidence of vascular invasion (61%) compared with patients with values of AFP <1000 ng/ml [9].

Other clinical biomarkers used for the diagnosis of HCC are: microRNAs [10], des-gamma-carboxyprothrombin (DCP) [11], glypican-3 (GPC3) [12], proteomic profiling [13], and alpha-L-fucosidase [14].

Imaging has an important role in the diagnosis of HCC. Even if over the past decades the imaging technology has improved and the hepatic lesions are better characterized, detection of the small tumors continues to be difficult especially in patients with liver cirrhosis whose parenchymal architecture is abnormal. The most common imaging techniques used for evaluation of the liver parenchyma are as follows: ultrasound scanning (US), CT scan, MRI, and angiography.

Ultrasound scanning is the most used technique, and it is performed as a routine test for screening focal hepatic lesions. Ultrasound imaging has now been replaced in diagnosis by CT scan and MRI. Contrast-enhanced ultrasound (CEUS) uses contrast agents such as intra-arterial dioxide carbon and helium. Also, application of color Doppler sonography can be useful in the assessment of intrahepatic vascular flow and the Doppler of the portal vein can differentiate bland thrombus from tumor invasion.

Contrast-enhanced ultrasonography (CEUS) can offer information about the nature of the liver tumor which cannot be obtained with conventional ultrasonography. CEUS is safe, and it is usually performed after detection of a focal lesion on standard US. The characterization of the hepatic lesion depends on all phases of contrast enhancement.

Most of the HCC are characterized by arterial phase enhancement and wash-out of the contrast during the late phase. According to some studies, more the differentiated a lesion is, the more gradually it is to washout [15, 16].

CEUS is an alternative for CT and MRI especially when there are contraindications for these investigations and it offers equivalent accuracy to CT and MRI if there is an experienced and skilled operator [17, 18].

CT scan is an important investigation for the characterization of the HCC. It includes 4 phases: pre-contrast, hepatic arterial phase, portal venous and delayed phases.

HCC must be differentiated from regeneration nodules, hemangioma, focal fat, dysplastic nodules and peliosis [19].

Factors such as injection of the contrast, tumor size and vascularity can affect the diagnostic accuracy of the HCC. In small tumors (less than 2 cm), the efficacy of CT is diminished due to the hypo-vascularization of small-sized tumors. The sensitivity of four phase CT in detecting HCC was up to 100% for tumors larger than 2 cm, 93% for tumors size between 1 and 2 cm and 60% for tumors less than 1 cm [20–22].

Multidetector helical CT (MDCT) is a new technique. which allows collection of early (18–28 s after administration of the contrast agent) and late or early parenchymal (35–45 s) arterial phase images. This new technique has improved the sensitivity and positive predictive values [23, 24]. Vascular tumors appear hypodense compared with liver parenchyma during the equilibrium phase (3–5 min after the administration of the contrast agent) and this technique is compared with MRI for early detection of small HCC (<1 cm) [24, 25].

Magnetic resonance imaging (MRI) is the best technique for evaluation of the liver nodules in patients with cirrhosis. HCC aspect varies on MRI because of the following factors: hemorrhage, degree of fibrosis and necrosis and histologic pattern. MRI is more accurate than CT or ultrasonography in detecting and characterization of HCC even for patients with liver cirrhosis. HCC appears hyper-intense on T2-weighted images while in T1-weighted images it may appear hypointense, isointense or hyperintense.

The sensitivity of MRI depends on tumor size, and it is about 95% in tumors larger than 2 cm and reduced to 30% for tumors, which are less than 2 cm in size [26].

Even if the MRI is the best investigation to characterize a liver nodule and to put the diagnosis of HCC, often the nodules might not be distinguished so a histological examination or advance imaging modalities will be necessary.

Angiography can be used to define hepatic anatomy before surgical resection.

Liver biopsy is performed with fine needle aspiration biopsy (FNAB) under ultrasonography or CT guidance and is considered the best method for a sure diagnosis of HCC. The sensitivity and specificity are about 96 and 95%, respectively, superior to any other test [27]. Sometimes, because the HCC lesions cannot be accurately located by radiographic methods, it is necessary to perform open surgical biopsy. The most important complications are the risk of tumor spreading along the needle tract, estimated at up 3%, important bleeding or infectious complications [7] [28–30]. Contraindications for liver biopsy are platelet count <50,000 per mm^3 or the international normalizing ratio (INR) > 2 [7].

3. Diagnostic guidelines

According to European Association for the Study of the Liver (EASL):

- HCC lesions of greater than 2 cm in diameter can be diagnosed non-invasively in patients with cirrhosis based on radiographic criteria;

- Nodules with arterial hypervascularization in two imaging modalities or in only single imaging modality associated with values of AFP > 400 ng/ml in the cirrhotic liver is considered HCC [31];

- Evaluation of the liver nodules should be performed by US, CT and MRI; liver biopsy is not mandatory [32];

- EASL recommend repeated US every 3 months for lesions which are smaller than 1 cm, until it grows [31];

- Nodules between 1 and 2 cm in size are more likely to be HCC and confirmation by liver biopsy is recommended [33].

According to American Association for the Study of Liver Disease (AASLD):

- AFP > 200 ng/ml should lead to diagnostic suspicion of HCC and requires more investigation;

- Nodules <1 cm should be repeatedly imaged for up to 2 years;

- Nodules between 1 and 2 cm should be investigated with two techniques: CEUS, CT scan, MRI. If there is a hypervascularity with washout in the portal venous phase the lesion can be diagnosed as HCC [34];

- Nodules larger than 2 cm can be diagnosed as HCC with a use of only one imaging modality (arterial hypervascularity with wash-out in the early or delayed venous phase) [35];

- Liver biopsy is recommended if the vascular pattern is not characteristic for HCC on imaging modalities [34].

4. Stadialization

HCC staging is mandatory to select the appropriate primary and adjuvant therapy and to evaluate the prognosis. There are eight different staging systems available for the management of HCC but none of them are universally accepted. The currently available staging systems for

HCC include: pathologic tumor-node-metastasis (pTNM) [36], Okuda [37], Cancer of the Liver Italian Program (CLIP) [38] and Barcelona Clinic Liver Cancer (BCLC) [39].

BCLC staging system seems to be the best for selection of early-stage HCC that should benefit from orthotopic liver transplantation, hepatic resection or local ablation while the CLIP score may be more useful at stratifying patients who are not candidates for resection or transplantation.

5. Treatment

Nowadays, many of the patients with HCC are diagnosed at an early stage when there are no signs of an advanced cancer. In the past, most of the patients were diagnosed only when they became symptomatic and no treatment had a chance of being effective or to improve the survival rates. There are a number of treatments available which seems to improve the survival rates, but to achieve the best results a careful selection of the patients is needed. Liver transplantation is the best option treatment for the patients with solitary HCC in the setting of decompensated cirrhosis and for those with early multifocal disease (up to 3 lesions, none larger than 3 cm) [40, 41], while for the patients with solitary tumors in well-compensated cirrhosis the best treatment strategy is under debate [42]. Treatments which offer the best survival rate are surgical resection, liver transplantation, percutaneous ablation and transarterial chemoembolization [40, 43]. Systemic chemotherapy has been demonstrated that has no benefits on survival rates [44, 45], while agents like tamoxifen [43], anti-androgens [46] or octreotide [47] are completely ineffective.

Hepatic resection is the treatment of choice in non-cirrhotic patients who have been diagnosed with HCC (**Figure 1a** and **b**). Patients with cirrhosis have to be very well selected for surgical resection due to the high risk of postoperative liver failure which can lead to death after the surgery. Cirrhotic patients have a higher rate of decompensation if they are operated with right hepatectomy than if a left hepatectomy is performed; however, the 5-year survival rate after resection can exceed 50% [42, 48, 49]. Before the surgery there are some specific factors which need to be considered:

- Stage of the tumor;

- Size of the tumor;

- Presence/absence of a chronic liver disease and portal hypertension assessed clinically or by hepatic vein catheterization. If the upper endoscopy shows varices or diuretic treatment is necessary, the portal hypertension is severe and there is no need for catheterization of the hepatic veins;

- Quality and volume of the future functional liver remnant.

The most important causes of death after liver resections are postoperative hemorrhages, liver failure and sepsis, but all these complications have a lower incidence due to the improvements of the surgical techniques (Pringles maneuver), the development of ultrasonic dissectors and vascular staplers.

To perform a *right hepatic resection*, you have to mobilize completely the right lobe of the liver to have control on the right hepatic vein before the parenchymal transection. Sometimes the

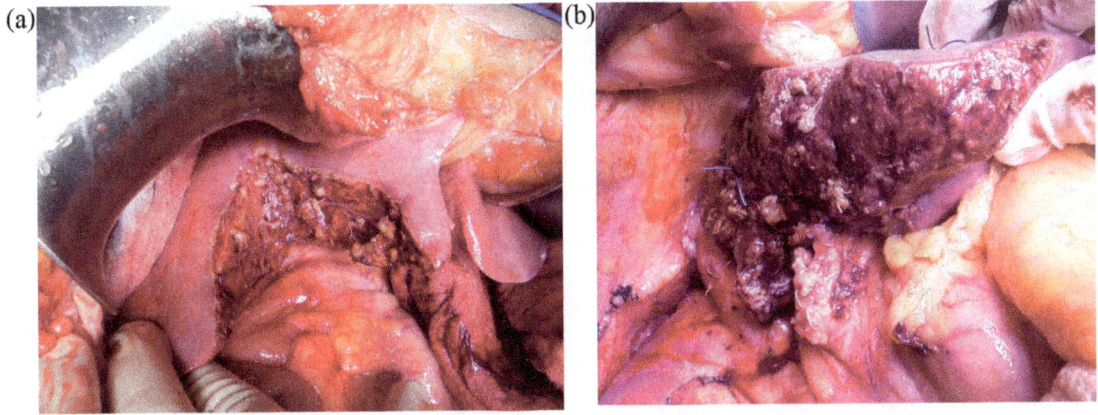

Figure 1. (a) Segment V resection. Intraoperative aspect after removal of the specimen (from the personal archive of the authors). (b) Right hepatectomy. Intraoperative aspect after removal of the specimen (from the personal archive of the authors).

size of the tumors does not permit to mobilize the right lobe of the liver and to expose the anterior surface of the inferior vena cava, so the surgeon has to perform an anterior approach. The anterior approach implies initial completion of parenchymal transection before mobilizing the right lobe of the liver and after hilar dissection is performed to control the right hepatic artery and portal vein. Intraoperative ultrasound is useful to mark on the Glisson capsule the plane of parenchymal transection. Transection is performed from the anterior surface of the liver down to right side of the liver hilum and down to the anterior surface of the inferior vena cava; then the right hepatic vein is isolated, clamped, divided and sutured. Only after the specimen is removed from the inferior vena cava, the right hepatic lobe is mobilized from the abdominal cavity by dividing the triangular ligament and other posterior attachments [50, 51].

Even if the anterior approach can be potentially dangerous because of the massive bleeding which can occur when deeper plane of the parenchyma is transected, it is an effective alternative when difficulty is encountered during liver mobilization using the conventional technique [52].

One of the most important factors which can lead to recurrence are microportal invasion and intrahepatic metastasis, these being associated with a poor prognosis. Anatomic resection implies the systematic removal of a hepatic segment or segments bearing the tumors (**Figure 2**). This technique has been shown to be effective in eradicating intrahepatic metastasis of HCC and it is associated with a prolonged survival. From the oncological perspective, anatomical resections which include satellite lesions are more efficient than limited resections without a surrounding margin [53].

Laparoscopic liver resection was initially used for non-anatomic liver resection for peripheral benign tumors (**Figure 3**), but nowadays, with the development of instrumentation and techniques, it has become a safe and feasible option for both benign and malignant liver lesions [54]. Regarding the advantages of laparoscopic liver resection, there are some advantages comparing with conventional liver resection such as reduced postoperative pain, less blood loss, less operative morbidity and a shorter length of hospitalization, while the long-term outcomes are similar especially for cirrhotic patients [55, 56].

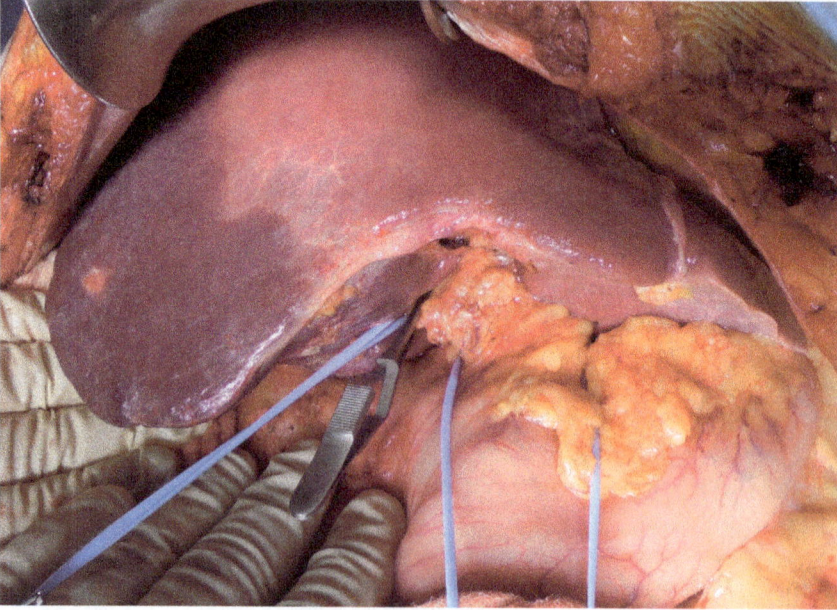

Figure 2. Anatomical resection of the VI–VII segments. Delimitation of the transection line after clamping the VI–VII pedicle (from the personal archive of the authors).

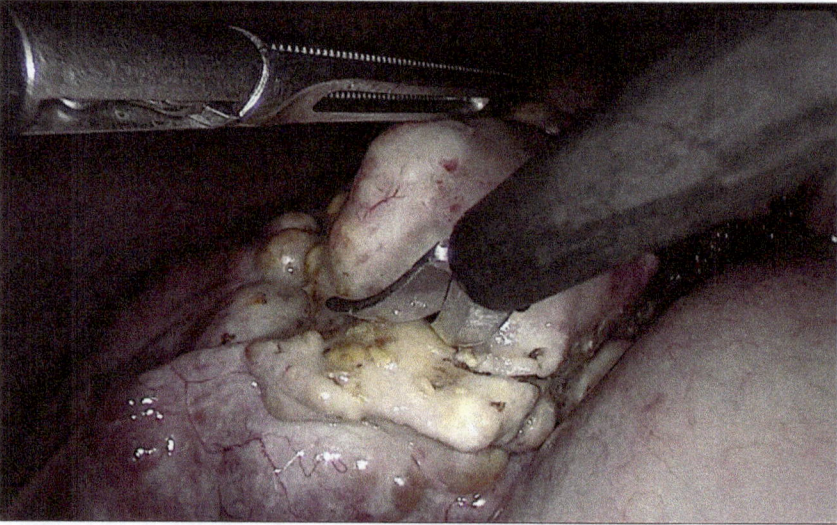

Figure 3. Laparoscopic liver resection of a HCC nodule (sg V) (from the personal archive of the authors).

Most of the patients with HCC are not suitable for the surgery due to the extent of the disease and because there is a high risk of liver failure. However, the patients with HCC who undergo surgery have a high risk of recurrence. The 5-year recurrence rate is about 77–100% and the median survival after the recurrence is between 7 and 28 months [57].

Predictors factors for the poor outcomes in HCC are the same for all therapeutic methods and they are: more than three tumors, tumor larger than 5 cm, portal vein invasion, intrahepatic metastases, absence of a tumor capsule, advanced TNM stage (III or IV), hepatitis C viral infection, and Child-Pugh class C [58, 59].

Liver resection may be used before the liver transplantation in three situations:

- Resection is used as primary treatment and liver transplantation will be an option for patients who develop liver failure or recurrence of the tumor;

- Resection is used as an initial treatment for patients who may undergo for liver transplantation according to detailed examination of the history pathological examination;

- Resection is used as pre-treatment for the patients which are already enlisted for liver transplantation.

Liver transplantation is the best treatment option for patients diagnosed with HCC and cirrhosis Child-Pugh B and C. The Milan criteria [60] are a generally accepted set of criteria used to assess suitability in patients for liver transplantation with cirrhosis and HCC. These criteria are:

- single tumor with diameter ≤ 5 cm, or up to 3 tumors each with diameter ≤ 3 cm;

- no extra-hepatic involvement;

- no major vessel involvement.

Living-donor liver transplantation is a liver transplantation option which has developed over the last years due to the limited availability of deceased-donor organs and can be offered for patients with HCC if the waiting time is long enough to allow tumor progression leading to exclusion from the waiting list [61]. This technique uses the right or left hemiliver from a healthy donor and should be performed by expert surgeons to ensure the lowest morbidity and best outcome. Complications may appear in 20–40% of the donors, while the mortality risk for the donor is still 0.3–0.5% [62].

One of the main problems after the liver transplantation for HCC is the risk for recurrence of the tumor which occurs in 8–20% of the patients. Usually, the recurrence appears in the first 2 years after liver transplantation and is associated with a median survival less 1 year [63].

For better results of the liver transplantation, there are some treatment options which can be performed before liver transplantation, such as liver resections or alcohol injection, radiofrequency ablation (RFA), transarterial chemoembolization (TACE), and transarterial radioembolization/selective internal radiotherapy (TARE/SIRT). The main purpose of this treatment strategy is to reduce the size and number of the tumors in patients who do not have the accepted criteria for liver transplantation [64]. Most of the above techniques have been used as locoregional therapy for HCC recurrence in patients with limited disease.

Ablative techniques are useful for patients, which are not suitable for resection or liver transplantation. Ablation can be done percutaneous, in open surgery or by laparoscopic approach and its purpose is to destruct the tumor cells by modifying the local temperature. The efficacy of the percutaneous ablation is evaluated after 1 month with a CT scan (absence of the contrast uptake within the tumor reflecting tumor necrosis, while the persistence of contrast uptake indicates treatment failure) [31]. Recurrence rate is higher after ablation and the recurrence will occur nearby of the treated nodule due to the presence of microscopic satellites. Ablation must be performed under ultrasound guidance (**Figure 4**). Ablation techniques use chemical substances (ethanol, acetic acid, boiling saline) or surgical devices which modify the temperature of the tissue (radiofrequency, microwave, laser and cryotherapy).

Ethanol injection is highly effective for small HCC and has a low rate of complications, while the necrosis rate is about 90–100% of the HCC smaller than 2 cm. If the tumor size is between 2 and 3 cm, the necrosis rate is reduced to 70 and 50%, respectively, for the tumor size between 3 and 5 cm [65, 66]. Patients with Child-Pugh A class and HCC with successful tumor necrosis can achieve a 50% survival at 5 years [67, 68].

Radiofrequency ablation (RFA) is an option of treatment which has better result than ethanol injection and requires fewer treatment sessions [69, 70]. This type of treatment requires an insertion of single or multiple cooled tip electrodes or single electrodes with j-hooked needles that deliver heat around a wide region inducing necrosis of the tumor. This treatment is more efficient than ethanol injection but has a higher cost and a higher rate of complications such as

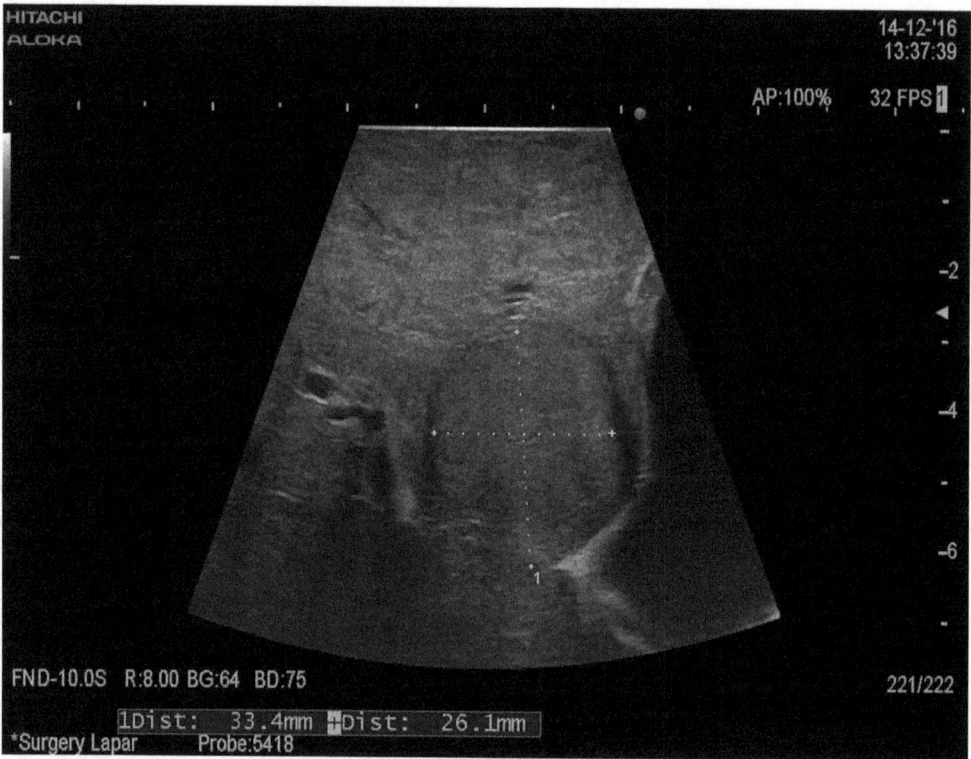

Figure 4. Intraoperative laparoscopic ultrasound of the liver showing a HCC nodule in segment V, next to the gallbladder (from the personal archive of the authors).

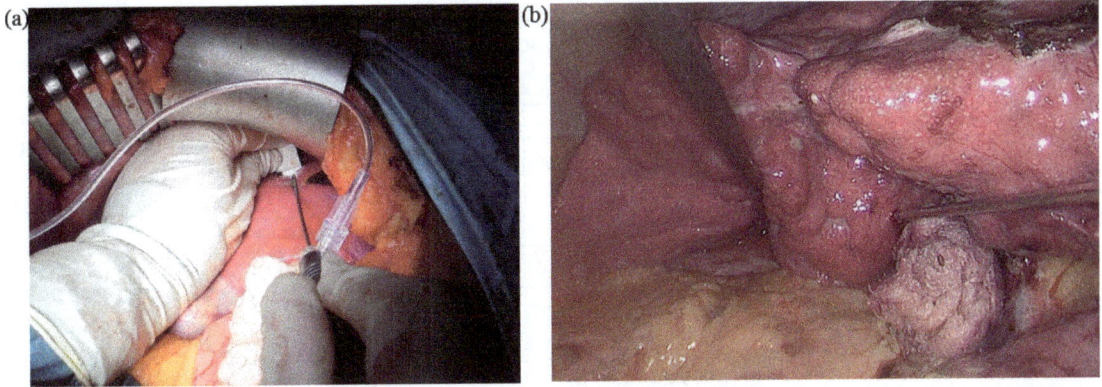

Figure 5. (a) US-guided intraoperative RFA of a liver tumor (from the personal archive of the authors). (b) Laparoscopic RFA of a HCC nodule. Intraoperative aspect (from the personal archive of the authors).

peritoneal bleeding or pleural effusion [69–72]. RFA can be performed by percutaneous under ultrasound guidance, open surgical approach or laparoscopic approach (**Figure 5a** and **b**). Some of the HCC cannot undergo for RFA due to their localization.

Transarterial embolization and chemoembolization are types of treatment which have developed over the last years because HCC exhibits intense neo-angiogenic activity and should be considered for patients who are not suitable for surgical resection or percutaneous ablation [61]. In patients with early-stage HCC, the blood supply comes from the portal vein and only when the tumor is larger it has an arterial blood supply from hepatic artery. This treatment purpose is to obstruct the hepatic artery to induce ischemia to the tumor. Hepatic artery obstruction is performed during an angiographic procedure and is known as transarterial embolization (TAE). If the transarterial embolization (TAE) is associated with the injection of chemotherapeutic agents in the hepatic artery, the procedure is known as transarterial chemoembolization (TACE). The procedure needs advanced catheterization of the hepatic artery and the specific lobar and segmental branches to be as selective as possible and to reduce the damages of the nontumoral liver parenchyma. Chemotherapic agents such as adriamycin or cisplatin must be injected prior to arterial obstruction [73]. Contraindication for TAE/TACE is the lack of portal blood flow due to portal vein thrombosis, portosystemic anastomoses or hepatofugal flow [61]. Also, patients which advanced staged disease (Child-Pugh B and C) should not be considered for this treatment due to the high risk of hepatic failure. Side effects of intraarterial injection of the chemotherapeutic agents are nausea, vomiting, alopecia and sometimes, renal failure. After the transarterial embolization, the so-called post-embolization syndrome can appear, which consists of fever, abdominal pain and ileus. Post-embolization syndrome is usually self-limited in less than 48 hours, but sometimes patients can develop hepatic abscess or cholecystitis. Regarding the response to this treatment there are no significant differences between TAE and TACE, the reported rate of objective response ranging from 16 to 60%, with a significant improvement in survival [43, 73].

Treatment algorithm is described in the next figure based on the Barcelona Clinic Liver Cancer (BCLC) staging classification [74]:

HCC

Stage 0
PST 0, Child-Pugh A

Stage A-C
PST 0–2, Child-Pugh A–B

Stage D
PST >2, Child-Pugh C

Very early stage (0)
Single <2 cm
carcinoma in situ

Early stage (A)
Single or 3 nodules
<3 cm, PST 0

Intermediate
stage (B)
Multinodular, PST 0

Advanced stage (C)
Portal invasion,
N1, M1, PST 1-2

PST
End stage (D)

Single

3 nodules
≤3 cm

Portal
pressure/
bilirubin → Increased → Associated
diseases

Normal   No   Yes

Resection

Liver transplantation
(CLT/LDLT)

PEI/RF

TACE

Sorafenib

Symptomatic
treatment (20%)
Survival <3 months

Curative treatments (30%)
5-yr survival: 40–70%

Randomized controlled trials (50%)
Median survival 11–20 months

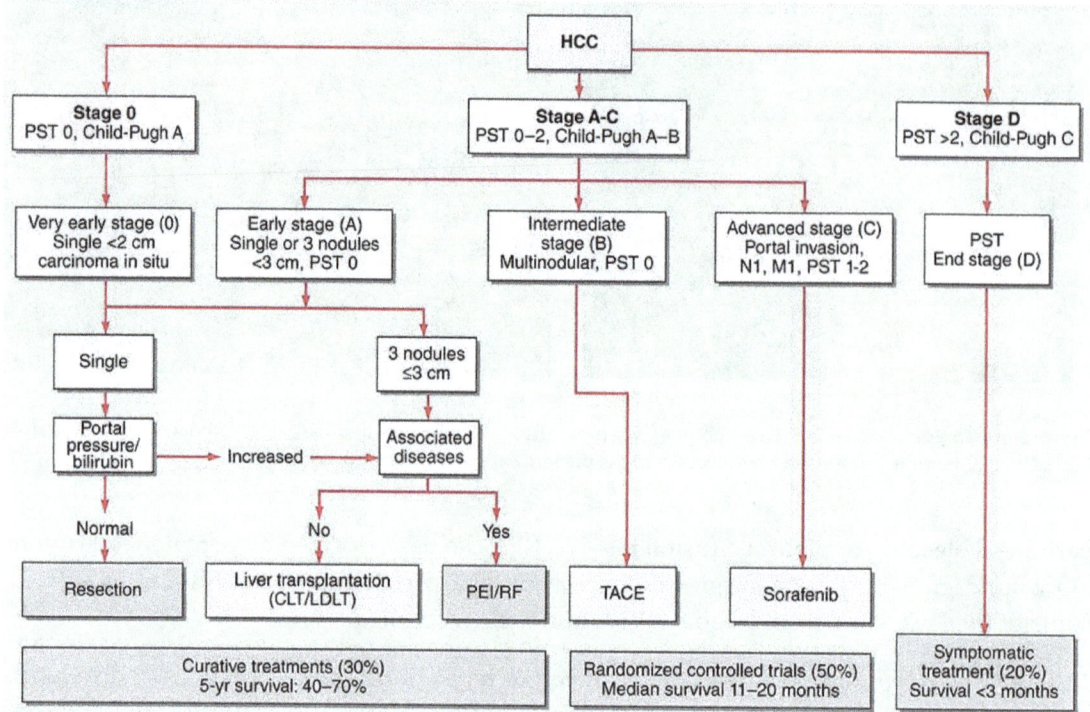

6. Perspectives

There are several areas where active research is needed, starting from molecular pathogenesis, to detection, diagnosis and treatment. Despite recent progress in the management of HCC, treatment of patients with portal vein thrombosis remains still a challenging area. Current clinical guidelines recommend Sorafenib only. However, besides Sorafenib, various therapies including surgery, TACE, external radiation therapy, hepatic artery infusion chemotherapy (HAIC) and radio-embolization may be considered in selected patients; the usefulness of combined treatment needs to be verified. Newer therapeutic options such as immunotherapeutic agent and oncolytic virus are under investigation [75].

7. Conclusions

Management of HCC continues to be improved due to development of newer therapies which are combined with liver resection and liver transplantation. These therapies become better tolerated and more precise even in patients with advanced liver disease. Better surveillance of cirrhotic patients allowed an early detection of HCC and permitted treatments to have a higher rate of cure. For the patients who present with HCC and moderate to severe liver insufficiency, liver transplant remains a critical method to eliminate the cancer and cure the underlying liver disease with a lower risk of recurrence than resection or ablation. The best results for liver resection are obtained in patients with small solitary tumors, but there is a high rate of disease recurrence due to cell dissemination prior to treatment. Improved survival for patients treated with Sorafenib for advanced disease increases enthusiasm for additional therapies for HCC.

Nowadays, the improvement of the surveillance will allow detection of the early stage of HCC when the loco-regional treatment is effective and transplantation is reserved only for selected cases. Alfa-fetoprotein and ultrasound scan should be used every 6 months for surveillance in high-risk individuals.

Acknowledgements

Adrian Bartoș is the coordinator of this chapter.

Author details

Adrian Bartoș[1]*, Cristian Cioltean[1], Caius Breazu[1] and Dana Bartoș[1,2]

*Address all correspondence to: bartos.adi@gmail.com

1 Regional Institute of Gastroenterology and Hepatology "Prof Dr. Octavian Fodor", Surgery Department, Cluj-Napoca, Romania

2 Anatomy and Embriology Department, UMF "Iuliu Hațieganu", Cluj-Napoca, Romania

References

[1] Ferlay J, Soerjomataram I, Dikshit R, Eser S, Mathers C, Rebelo M, et al. Cancer incidence and mortality worldwide: Sources, methods and major patterns in GLOBOCAN 2012. International Journal of Cancer. 2015;**136**(5):E359-E386

[2] Chen ZY, Qi QH, Dong ZL. Etiology and management of hemmorrhage in spontaneous liver rupture: A report of 70 cases. World Journal of Gastroenterology. 2002;**8**(6):1063-1066

[3] Trevisani F, D'Intino PE, Grazi GL, Caraceni P, Gasbarrini A, Colantoni A, et al. Clinical and pathologic features of hepatocellular carcinoma in young and older Italian patients. Cancer. 1996;**77**(11):2223-2232

[4] Murata K, Shiraki K, Kawakita T, Yamamoto N, Okano H, Sakai T, et al. Hepatocellular carcinoma presenting with obstructive jaundice: A clinicopathological study of eight cases. Hepato-Gastroenterology. 2003;**50**(54):2057-2060

[5] Bruix J, Castells A, Calvet X, Feu F, Bru C, Sole M, et al. Diarrhea as a presenting symptom of hepatocellular carcinoma. Digestive Diseases and Sciences. 1990;**35**(6):681-685

[6] Steiner E, Velt P, Gutierrez O, Schwartz S, Chey W. Hepatocellular carcinoma presenting with intractable diarrhea. A radiologic-pathologic correlation. Archives of Surgery. 1986;**121**(7):849-851

[7] Bialecki ES, Di Bisceglie AM. Diagnosis of hepatocellular carcinoma. HPB: The Official Journal of the International Hepato Pancreato Biliary Association. 2005;7(1):26-34

[8] Collier J, Sherman M. Screening for hepatocellular carcinoma. Hepatology. 1998;27(1): 273-278

[9] Sakata J, Shirai Y, Wakai T, Kaneko K, Nagahashi M, Hatakeyama K. Preoperative predictors of vascular invasion in hepatocellular carcinoma. European Journal of Surgical Oncology. 2008;34(8):900-905

[10] Chen X, Ba Y, Ma L, Cai X, Yin Y, Wang K, et al. Characterization of microRNAs in serum: A novel class of biomarkers for diagnosis of cancer and other diseases. Cell Research. 2008;18(10):997-1006

[11] Carr BI, Kanke F, Wise M, Satomura S. Clinical evaluation of lens culinaris agglutinin-reactive alpha-fetoprotein and des-gamma-carboxy prothrombin in histologically proven hepatocellular carcinoma in the United States. Digestive Diseases and Sciences. 2007;52(3):776-782

[12] Li B, Liu H, Shang HW, Li P, Li N, Ding HG. Diagnostic value of glypican-3 in alpha fetoprotein negative hepatocellular carcinoma patients. African Health Sciences. 2013;13(3):703-709

[13] Kimhofer T, Fye H, Taylor-Robinson S, Thursz M, Holmes E. Proteomic and metabonomic biomarkers for hepatocellular carcinoma: A comprehensive review. British Journal of Cancer. 2015;112(7):1141-1156

[14] Takahashi H, Saibara T, Iwamura S, Tomita A, Maeda T, Onishi S, et al. Serum alpha-L-fucosidase activity and tumor size in hepatocellular carcinoma. Hepatology. 1994;19(6): 1414-1417

[15] Claudon M, Cosgrove D, Albrecht T, Bolondi L, Bosio M, Calliada F, et al. Guidelines and good clinical practice recommendations for contrast enhanced ultrasound (CEUS)— Update 2008. Ultraschall in der Medizin. 2008;29(1):28-44

[16] Fan ZH, Chen MH, Dai Y, Wang YB, Yan K, Wu W, et al. Evaluation of primary malignancies of the liver using contrast-enhanced sonography: Correlation with pathology. AJR American Journal of Roentgenology. 2006;186(6):1512-1519

[17] Pompili M, Riccardi L, Semeraro S, Orefice R, Elia F, Barbaro B, et al. Contrast-enhanced ultrasound assessment of arterial vascularization of small nodules arising in the cirrhotic liver. Digestive and Liver Disease: Official Journal of the Italian Society of Gastroenterology and the Italian Association for the Study of the Liver. 2008;40(3):206-215

[18] Quaia E. Microbubble ultrasound contrast agents: An update. European Radiology. 2007;17(8):1995-2008

[19] Brancatelli G, Baron RL, Peterson MS, Marsh W, Helical CT. Screening for hepatocellular carcinoma in patients with cirrhosis: Frequency and causes of false-positive interpretation. AJR American Journal of Roentgenology. 2003;180(4):1007-1014

[20] Franca AV, Elias Junior J, Lima BL, Martinelli AL, Carrilho FJ. Diagnosis, staging and treatment of hepatocellular carcinoma. Brazilian Journal of Medical and Biological Research. 2004;37(11):1689-1705

[21] Ikeda K, Saitoh S, Koida I, Tsubota A, Arase Y, Chayama K, et al. Imaging diagnosis of small hepatocellular carcinoma. Hepatology. 1994;20(1 Pt 1):82-87

[22] Ohashi I, Hanafusa K, Yoshida T. Small hepatocellular carcinomas: Two-phase dynamic incremental CT in detection and evaluation. Radiology. 1993;189(3):851-855

[23] Murakami T, Kim T, Takahashi S, Nakamura H. Hepatocellular carcinoma: Multidetector row helical CT. Abdominal Imaging. 2002;27(2):139-146

[24] Saar B, Kellner-Weldon F. Radiological diagnosis of hepatocellular carcinoma. Liver International. 2008;28(2):189-199

[25] Mitsuzaki K, Yamashita Y, Ogata I, Nishiharu T, Urata J, Takahashi M. Multiple-phase helical CT of the liver for detecting small hepatomas in patients with liver cirrhosis: Contrast-injection protocol and optimal timing. AJR American Journal of Roentgenology. 1996;167(3):753-757

[26] Ebara M, Ohto M, Watanabe Y, Kimura K, Saisho H, Tsuchiya Y, et al. Diagnosis of small hepatocellular carcinoma: Correlation of MR imaging and tumor histologic studies. Radiology. 1986;159(2):371-377

[27] Borzio M, Borzio F, Macchi R, Croce AM, Bruno S, Ferrari A, et al. The evaluation of fine-needle procedures for the diagnosis of focal liver lesions in cirrhosis. Journal of Hepatology. 1994;20(1):117-121

[28] Bravo AA, Sheth SG, Chopra S. Liver biopsy. The New England Journal of Medicine. 2001;344(7):495-500

[29] Takamori R, Wong LL, Dang C, Wong L. Needle-tract implantation from hepatocellular cancer: Is needle biopsy of the liver always necessary? Liver Transplantation. 2000;6(1):67-72

[30] Chang S, Kim SH, Lim HK, Kim SH, Lee WJ, Choi D, et al. Needle tract implantation after percutaneous interventional procedures in hepatocellular carcinomas: Lessons learned from a 10-year experience. Korean Journal of Radiology. 2008;9(3):268-274

[31] Bruix J, Sherman M, Llovet JM, Beaugrand M, Lencioni R, Burroughs AK, et al. Clinical management of hepatocellular carcinoma. Conclusions of the Barcelona-2000 EASL conference. European Association for the Study of the Liver. Journal of Hepatology. 2001;35(3):421-430

[32] Talwalkar JA, Gores GJ. Diagnosis and staging of hepatocellular carcinoma. Gastroenterology. 2004;127(5, Suppl 1):S126-S132

[33] Bru C, Maroto A, Bruix J, Faus R, Bianchi L, Calvet X, et al. Diagnostic accuracy of fine-needle aspiration biopsy in patients with hepatocellular carcinoma. Digestive Diseases and Sciences. 1989;34(11):1765-1769

[34] Bruix J, Hessheimer AJ, Forner A, Boix L, Vilana R, Llovet JM. New aspects of diagnosis and therapy of hepatocellular carcinoma. Oncogene. 2006;**25**(27):3848-3856

[35] Bruix J, Sherman M. Practice Guidelines Committee AAftSoLD. Management of hepatocellular carcinoma. Hepatology. 2005;**42**(5):1208-1236

[36] Sobin LH, Fleming ID. TNM classification of malignant tumors, fifth edition (1997). Union Internationale Contre le Cancer and the American Joint Committee on Cancer. Cancer. 1997;**80**(9):1803-1804

[37] Okuda K, Ohtsuki T, Obata H, Tomimatsu M, Okazaki N, Hasegawa H, et al. Natural history of hepatocellular carcinoma and prognosis in relation to treatment. Study of 850 patients. Cancer. 1985;**56**(4):918-928

[38] Llovet JM, Bruix J. Prospective validation of the Cancer of the Liver Italian Program (CLIP) score: A new prognostic system for patients with cirrhosis and hepatocellular carcinoma. Hepatology. 2000;**32**(3):679-680

[39] Llovet JM, Bru C, Bruix J. Prognosis of hepatocellular carcinoma: The BCLC staging classification. Seminars in Liver Disease. 1999;**19**(3):329-338

[40] Llovet JM, Burroughs A, Bruix J. Hepatocellular carcinoma. Lancet. 2003;**362**(9399): 1907-1917

[41] Mazzaferro V, Regalia E, Doci R, Andreola S, Pulvirenti A, Bozzetti F, et al. Liver transplantation for the treatment of small hepatocellular carcinomas in patients with cirrhosis. The New England Journal of Medicine. 1996;**334**(11):693-699

[42] Llovet JM, Bruix J, Gores GJ. Surgical resection versus transplantation for early hepatocellular carcinoma: Clues for the best strategy. Hepatology. 2000;**31**(4):1019-1021

[43] Llovet JM, Bruix J. Systematic review of randomized trials for unresectable hepatocellular carcinoma: Chemoembolization improves survival. Hepatology. 2003;**37**(2):429-442

[44] Nerenstone SR, Ihde DC, Friedman MA. Clinical trials in primary hepatocellular carcinoma: Current status and future directions. Cancer Treatment Reviews. 1988;**15**(1):1-31

[45] Okada S, Okazaki N, Nose H, Yoshimori M, Aoki K. Prognostic factors in patients with hepatocellular carcinoma receiving systemic chemotherapy. Hepatology. 1992;**16**(1): 112-117

[46] Grimaldi C, Bleiberg H, Gay F, Messner M, Rougier P, Kok TC, et al. Evaluation of antiandrogen therapy in unresectable hepatocellular carcinoma: Results of a European Organization for Research and Treatment of cancer multicentric double-blind trial. Journal of Clinical Oncology: Official Journal of the American Society of Clinical Oncology. 1998;**16**(2):411-417

[47] Yuen MF, Poon RT, Lai CL, Fan ST, Lo CM, Wong KW, et al. A randomized placebo-controlled study of long-acting octreotide for the treatment of advanced hepatocellular carcinoma. Hepatology. 2002;**36**(3):687-691

[48] Arii S, Yamaoka Y, Futagawa S, Inoue K, Kobayashi K, Kojiro M, et al. Results of surgical and nonsurgical treatment for small-sized hepatocellular carcinomas: A retrospective and nationwide survey in Japan. The Liver Cancer Study Group of Japan. Hepatology. 2000;32(6):1224-1229

[49] Grazi GL, Ercolani G, Pierangeli F, Del Gaudio M, Cescon M, Cavallari A, et al. Improved results of liver resection for hepatocellular carcinoma on cirrhosis give the procedure added value. Annals of Surgery. 2001;234(1):71-78

[50] Lai EC, Fan ST, Lo CM, Chu KM, Liu CL. Anterior approach for difficult major right hepatectomy. World Journal of Surgery. 1996;20(3):314-317 discussion 8

[51] Liu CL, Fan ST, Lo CM, Tung-Ping Poon R, Wong J. Anterior approach for major right hepatic resection for large hepatocellular carcinoma. Annals of Surgery. 2000;232(1):25-31

[52] Ishizawa T, Kokudo N, Makuuchi M. Right hepatectomy for hepatocellular carcinoma: Is the anterior approach superior to the conventional approach? Annals of Surgery. 2008;247(2):390-391 author reply 1-2

[53] Nakashima Y, Nakashima O, Tanaka M, Okuda K, Nakashima M, Kojiro M. Portal vein invasion and intrahepatic micrometastasis in small hepatocellular carcinoma by gross type. Hepatology Research. 2003;26(2):142-147

[54] Nguyen KT, Gamblin TC, Geller DA. World review of laparoscopic liver resection-2,804 patients. Annals of Surgery. 2009;250(5):831-841

[55] Lee KF, Chong CN, Wong J, Cheung YS, Wong J, Lai P. Long-term results of laparoscopic hepatectomy versus open hepatectomy for hepatocellular carcinoma: A case-matched analysis. World Journal of Surgery. 2011;35(10):2268-2274

[56] Truant S, Bouras AF, Hebbar M, Boleslawski E, Fromont G, Dharancy S, et al. Laparoscopic resection vs. open liver resection for peripheral hepatocellular carcinoma in patients with chronic liver disease: A case-matched study. Surgical Endoscopy. 2011;25(11):3668-3677

[57] Takayama T, Sekine T, Makuuchi M, Yamasaki S, Kosuge T, Yamamoto J, et al. Adoptive immunotherapy to lower postsurgical recurrence rates of hepatocellular carcinoma: A randomised trial. Lancet. 2000;356(9232):802-807

[58] Sogawa H, Shrager B, Jibara G, Tabrizian P, Roayaie S, Schwartz M. Resection or transplant-listing for solitary hepatitis C-associated hepatocellular carcinoma: An intention-to-treat analysis. HPB: The Official Journal of the International Hepato Pancreato Biliary Association. 2013;15(2):134-141

[59] Poon RT, Fan ST, Lo CM, Ng IO, Liu CL, Lam CM, et al. Improving survival results after resection of hepatocellular carcinoma: A prospective study of 377 patients over 10 years. Annals of Surgery. 2001;234(1):63-70

[60] Mazzaferro V, Bhoori S, Sposito C, Bongini M, Langer M, Miceli R, et al. Milan criteria in liver transplantation for hepatocellular carcinoma: An evidence-based analysis of 15 years of experience. Liver Transplantation. 2011;17(Suppl 2):S44-S57

[61] Bruix J, Sherman M. American Association for the Study of Liver D. Management of hepatocellular carcinoma: An update. Hepatology. 2011;**53**(3):1020-1022

[62] Trotter JF, Wachs M, Everson GT, Kam I. Adult-to-adult transplantation of the right hepatic lobe from a living donor. The New England Journal of Medicine. 2002;**346**(14): 1074-1082

[63] Zimmerman MA, Ghobrial RM, Tong MJ, Hiatt JR, Cameron AM, Hong J, et al. Recurrence of hepatocellular carcinoma following liver transplantation: A review of preoperative and postoperative prognostic indicators. Archives of Surgery. 2008;**143**(2):182-188; discussion 8

[64] Ravaioli M, Grazi GL, Piscaglia F, Trevisani F, Cescon M, Ercolani G, et al. Liver transplantation for hepatocellular carcinoma: Results of down-staging in patients initially outside the Milan selection criteria. American Journal of Transplantation. 2008;**8**(12):2547-2557

[65] Livraghi T, Bolondi L, Lazzaroni S, Marin G, Morabito A, Rapaccini GL, et al. Percutaneous ethanol injection in the treatment of hepatocellular carcinoma in cirrhosis. A study on 207 patients. Cancer. 1992;**69**(4):925-929

[66] Vilana R, Bruix J, Bru C, Ayuso C, Sole M, Rodes J. Tumor size determines the efficacy of percutaneous ethanol injection for the treatment of small hepatocellular carcinoma. Hepatology. 1992;**16**(2):353-357

[67] Sala M, Llovet JM, Vilana R, Bianchi L, Sole M, Ayuso C, et al. Initial response to percutaneous ablation predicts survival in patients with hepatocellular carcinoma. Hepatology. 2004;**40**(6):1352-1360

[68] Livraghi T, Giorgio A, Marin G, Salmi A, de Sio I, Bolondi L, et al. Hepatocellular carcinoma and cirrhosis in 746 patients: Long-term results of percutaneous ethanol injection. Radiology. 1995;**197**(1):101-108

[69] Livraghi T, Goldberg SN, Lazzaroni S, Meloni F, Solbiati L, Gazelle GS. Small hepatocellular carcinoma: Treatment with radio-frequency ablation versus ethanol injection. Radiology. 1999;**210**(3):655-661

[70] Lencioni RA, Allgaier HP, Cioni D, Olschewski M, Deibert P, Crocetti L, et al. Small hepatocellular carcinoma in cirrhosis: Randomized comparison of radio-frequency thermal ablation versus percutaneous ethanol injection. Radiology. 2003;**228**(1):235-240

[71] Giorgio A, Tarantino L, de Stefano G, Coppola C, Ferraioli G. Complications after percutaneous saline-enhanced radiofrequency ablation of liver tumors: 3-year experience with 336 patients at a single center. AJR American Journal of Roentgenology. 2005;**184**(1): 207-211

[72] Tateishi R, Shiina S, Teratani T, Obi S, Sato S, Koike Y, et al. Percutaneous radiofrequency ablation for hepatocellular carcinoma. An analysis of 1000 cases. Cancer. 2005;**103**(6): 1201-1209

[73] Bruix J, Sala M, Llovet JM. Chemoembolization for hepatocellular carcinoma. Gastroenterology. 2004;**127**(5, Suppl 1):S179-S188

[74] Llovet JM, Fuster J, Bruix J. Barcelona-clinic liver cancer G. The Barcelona approach: Diagnosis, staging, and treatment of hepatocellular carcinoma. Liver Transplantation. 2004;**10**(2 Suppl 1):S115-S120

[75] Woo HY, Heo J. New perspectives on the management of hepatocellular carcinoma with portal vein thrombosis. Clinical and Molecular Hepatology. 2015;**21**(2):115-121

Permissions

The contributors of this book come from diverse backgrounds, making this book a truly international effort. This book will bring forth new frontiers with its revolutionizing research information and detailed analysis of the nascent developments around the world.

We would like to thank all the contributing authors for lending their expertise to make the book truly unique. They have played a crucial role in the development of this book. Without their invaluable contributions this book wouldn't have been possible. They have made vital efforts to compile up to date information on the varied aspects of this subject to make this book a valuable addition to the collection of many professionals and students.

This book was conceptualized with the vision of imparting up-to-date information and advanced data in this field. To ensure the same, a matchless editorial board was set up. Every individual on the board went through rigorous rounds of assessment to prove their worth. After which they invested a large part of their time researching and compiling the most relevant data for our readers.

The editorial board has been involved in producing this book since its inception. They have spent rigorous hours researching and exploring the diverse topics which have resulted in the successful publishing of this book. They have passed on their knowledge of decades through this book. To expedite this challenging task, the publisher supported the team at every step. A small team of assistant editors was also appointed to further simplify the editing procedure and attain best results for the readers.

Apart from the editorial board, the designing team has also invested a significant amount of their time in understanding the subject and creating the most relevant covers. They scrutinized every image to scout for the most suitable representation of the subject and create an appropriate cover for the book.

The publishing team has been an ardent support to the editorial, designing and production team. Their endless efforts to recruit the best for this project, has resulted in the accomplishment of this book. They are a veteran in the field of academics and their pool of knowledge is as vast as their experience in printing. Their expertise and guidance has proved useful at every step. Their uncompromising quality standards have made this book an exceptional effort. Their encouragement from time to time has been an inspiration for everyone.

The publisher and the editorial board hope that this book will prove to be a valuable piece of knowledge for researchers, students, practitioners and scholars across the globe.

List of Contributors

Luis Sendra, María José Herrero and Salvador F. Aliño Pellicer
Pharmacology Department, Medicine Faculty, University of Valencia, Valencia, Spain
Pharmacogenetics Unit, La Fe Health Research Institute, La Fe University and Polytechnic Hospital, Valencia, Spain

Luis Martí-Bonmatí
Radiology Department and Biomedical Imaging Research Group (GIBI230), La Fe University and Polytechnic Hospital, Valencia, Spain

Eva M. Montalvá and Rafael López-Andújar
Unit of Hepato-Biliary-Pancreatic Surgery and Transplantation, La Fe University and Polytechnic Hospital, Valencia, Spain

Matteo Frasson and Eduardo García-Granero
Department of General Surgery, Digestive Surgery Unit, La Fe University and Polytechnic Hospital, Valencia, Spain

Hiroya Shiomi and Ryoong-Jin Oh
Miyakojima IGRT Clinic, Osaka, Japan

Hiroshi Doi
Miyakojima IGRT Clinic, Osaka, Japan
Department of Radiation Oncology, Kindai University Faculty of Medicine, Osaka, Japan

Shahinul Alam, Golam Mustafa, Mahabubul Alam and Nooruddin Ahmad
Department of Hepatology, Bangabandhu Sheikh Mujib Medical University, Dhaka, Bangladesh

Thupten Kelsang Lama
Civil Service Hospital, Kathmandu, Nepal

Adrian Bartoş
Regional Institute of Gastroenterology and Hepatology, Surgery Department, Cluj-Napoca, Romania

Paula Iruzubieta, Marta González, Joaquín Cabezas, María Teresa Arias-Loste and Javier Crespo
Department of Gastroenterology and Hepatology, Marqués de Valdecilla University Hospital, Centro de Investigación Biomédica en Red de Enfermedades Hepáticas y Digestivas (CIBERehd), Infection, Immunity and Digestive Pathology Group, Research Institute Marqués de Valdecilla (IDIVAL), Santander, Spain

Hiroteru Kamimura, Tomoyuki Sugano, Ryoko Horigome, Naruhiro Kimura, Masaaki Takamura, Hirokazu Kawai, Satoshi Yamagiwa and Shuji Terai
Division of Gastroenterology and Hepatology, Niigata University Graduate School of Medical and Dental Sciences, Niigata, Japan

Kaori Minehira
Nestlé Institute of Health Sciences, Lausanne, Switzerland

Philippe Gual
Université Côte d'Azur, INSERM, U1065, C3M, Team 8, Chronic liver diseases associated with obesity and alcohol, Nice, France

Ali Ibrahim Yahya
Teaching Hospital, Zliten, Libya

Marco Antonio López Hernández
Internal Medicine Department, Tacuba General Hospital, Mexico City, Mexico

Monjur Ahmed
Thomas Jefferson University, Philadelphia, PA, USA

Caius Breazu
Regional Institute of Gastroenterology and Hepatology, ICU Department, Cluj-Napoca, Romania

Ioana Iancu
Regional Institute of Gastroenterology and Hepatology, Surgery Department, Cluj-Napoca, Romania
Anatomy and Embryology Department, UMF, Cluj-Napoca, Romania

Margörit Rita Krespi
Kadir Has University, Istanbul, Turkey

Adrian Bartoş, Cristian Cioltean and Caius Breazu
Regional Institute of Gastroenterology and Hepatology "Prof Dr. Octavian Fodor", Surgery Department, Cluj-Napoca, Romania

Dana Bartoş
Regional Institute of Gastroenterology and Hepatology, Surgery Department, Cluj-Napoca, Romania Anatomy and Embriology Department, UMF "Iuliu Haţieganu", Cluj-Napoca, Romania

Index

www.ingramcontent.com/pod-product-compliance
Lightning Source LLC
Chambersburg PA
CBHW061938190326

41458CB00009B/2765